Alcohol,
Immunity,
and
Cancer

Alcohol, Immunity, and Cancer

Edited by

Raz Yirmiya, Ph.D.
Assistant Professor
Department of Psychology
The Hebrew University of Jerusalem
Jerusalem, Israel

Anna N. Taylor, Ph.D.
Professor of Anatomy and Cell Biology
School of Medicine
University of California at Los Angeles
and
Chief of the Alcohol Research Laboratory
Brentwood Division
West Los Angeles Veterans Administration Medical Center
Los Angeles, California

CRC Press
Boca Raton   Ann Arbor   London   Tokyo

Library of Congress Cataloging-in-Publication Data

Alcohol, immunity, and cancer / edited Raz Yirmiya, Anna N. Taylor.
     p.   cm.
     Includes bibliographical references and index.
     ISBN 0-8493-5761-6
     1. Alcohol—Carcinogenicity.   2. Alcohol—Immunology.
   3. Immunosuppression.   4. Fetal alcohol syndrome—Pathophysiology.
   5. Fetal Alcohol Syndrome.
    [DNLM: 1. Alcohol, Ethyl—adverse effects.   2. Immunity, Cellular—
-drug effects.   3. Neoplasma—chemically induced.   QZ 202 A3545]
   RC268.7.A42A45   1992
   616.99'4071—dc20
   DNLM/DLC
   for Library of Congress   92-15535
                                                                  CIP

Direct all inquiries to CRC Press, Inc. 2000 Corporate Blvd., N.W., Boca Raton, Florida, 33431.

© 1993 by CRC Press, Inc.

International Standard Book Number 0-8493-5761-6

Library of Congress Card Number 92-15535

Printed in the United States of America 1 2 3 4 5 6 7 8 9 0

Printed on acid-free paper

We
Dedicate
This Book
To Our Mentors

PREFACE

Chronic alcoholism afflicts approximately 7% of the adult population in the U.S. and an even larger proportion in other countries. Most alcohol-dependent individuals experience negative psychosocial consequences, such as job or car accidents, marital problems, and problems with the law from this addiction. Devastating health problems are also associated with alcoholism, and include significant alterations in the immune and psychoneuroendocrine systems leading to increased morbidity and mortality from infections and cancer.

Clinically, an association between alcohol use and infections has been observed for centuries. Controlled clinical studies conducted over the last few decades confirmed these observations, indicating that alcoholism predisposes to bacterial and viral infections and increases their severity. These findings suggest that alcohol suppresses the host immune defense mechanisms. Recent experimental studies of the effects of alcohol on immunity indicate that alcohol alters (usually suppresses) most immune parameters examined to this date. The first part of the book provides data from studies of animals as well as from controlled studies of humans which review the effects of alcohol on several immune functions, including cellular immunity, natural killer cell (NK) activity, cytokine secretion, and tumor necrosis factor (TNF).

Alterations of immune function can result not only from alcohol consumption by the adult human or animal, but also from fetal alcohol exposure (FAE). Clinical observations in children indicate that FAE is associated with long-lasting immune deficits, which may be responsible for reduced resistance to infection and carcinogenesis. Similar findings have been demonstrated in animal models of FAE, which show alterations in the development of the immune system and the function of various immune parameters. The second part of this book reviews the consequences of FAE on immunity and on the interaction between the immune and nervous systems.

Considerable data suggest an association between alcohol consumption and increased cancer risk. The evidence for this association derives from epidemiological and clinical studies in humans and experimental studies in animals. The third part of this book provides comprehensive reviews of the effects of alcohol on human cancers and on experimental tumor models, particularly models of esophageal, hepatic, rectal, pancreatic, and metastatic breast cancers. Additionally, the mechanisms mediating alcohol's effects in these models are discussed, with particular emphasis on alcohol-induced immunosuppression as the mechanism underlying its effects on tumor development.

Collectively, the chapters in this book demonstrate that chronic exposure to alcohol, either in adulthood or *in utero*, can dramatically affect immune function and the incidence and progression of several types of cancer. Moreover, animal studies suggest that alcohol may affect immunity and neoplasia not only after chronic consumption, but also after acute exposure. If such findings are applicable to human alcohol consumption, the implications are far reaching, because alcohol is consumed on an occasional basis by large proportions of the population. Thus, even temporary alcohol-induced immune suppression may be responsible for less resistance to infectious diseases and possibly even to the progression of tumors.

Raz Yirmiya
Anna N. Tayor

THE EDITORS

Raz Yirmiya, Ph.D., is an Assistant Professor in the Department of Psychology at The Hebrew University of Jerusalem.

Dr. Yirmiya graduated in 1981 from the University of Haifa with a B.A. degree in psychology. He obtained his M.Sc. degree in physiology from the Technion–Israel Institute of Technology, in Haifa, in 1984, and received his Ph.D. in neuroscience from the University of California at Los Angeles (UCLA) in 1988. After completing two years of post-doctoral training in psychoneuroimmunology at UCLA, he was appointed Assistant Professor of Psychology at the Hebrew University of Jerusalem in 1990.

Dr. Yirmiya is a member of the International Brain Research Organization, the International Society for Neuroimmunomodulation, the Society for Neuroscience, and the Society for the Study of Ingestive Behavior.

He has been the recipient of the Rothschild Fellowship (1984 to 1985) and the Fulbright Scholarship (1984 to 1989).

Dr. Yirmiya has been the recipient of research grants from the UCLA Psychoneuroimmunology Task Force, the National Institute for Psychobiology in Israel, the Israel Cancer Association, the Israel Ministry of Science and Technology and the Israel Foundation Trustees. He has published more than 40 papers. His current research interests focus on the modulation of immunity and cancer by behavioral processes and psychoactive drugs, particularly opiates and alcohol.

Anna Newman Taylor, Ph.D., is a Professor of Anatomy and Cell Biology in the School of Medicine of the University of California at Los Angeles (UCLA), and Chief of the Alcohol Research Laboratory in the Brentwood Division of the West Los Angeles Veterans Administration (VA) Medical Center.

Dr. Taylor attended Radcliffe College and graduated with a B.A. degree from Mather College of Case-Western Reserve University, Cleveland, Ohio, in 1955. She obtained the Ph.D. degree in physiology from Case-Western Reserve University in 1961. After postdoctoral work in the Laboratory of Neurophysiology at the Hôpital Henri Rousselle, Paris, France, she was appointed Assistant Professor in the Departments of Anatomy and Psychiatry at Baylor University College of Medicine, Houston, Texas, in 1965. In 1967, she moved to UCLA where, in 1970, she became Associate Professor and in 1979, Professor. In 1979, she also was appointed to her current position at the VA.

Dr. Taylor is a member of the American Association for the Advancement of Science, the American Physiological Society, the Endocrine Society, the American Association of Anatomists, the Society for Neuroscience, the Research Society on Alcoholism, the International Society of Neuroendocrinology, the International Brain Research Organization, the International Society for Psychoneuroendocrinology, and the International Society for Biological Research on Alcoholism. She is a Fellow of the American Association for the Advancement of Science and has served on its Council.

Dr. Taylor has been the recipient of research grants from the National Institutes of Health, the National Science Foundation, the Alcohol, Drug Abuse and Mental Health Administration, and the Veterans Administration. She is the author of more than 80 papers. Her current research interests focus on the role of developmental insults, such as prenatal alcohol exposure, in the ontogeny of the central nervous system and consequent neuroendocrine, neuroimmunological, and neurobehavioral outcomes.

CONTRIBUTORS

Gregory Bagby, Ph.D.
Department of Physiology and
  Medicine
Louisiana State University Medical
  Center
New Orleans, Louisiana

Shamgar Ben-Eliyahu, Ph.D.
Department of Psychology
University of California at
  Los Angeles
Los Angeles, California

Sally E. Blank, Ph.D.
Department of Pharmaceutical
  Sciences
College of Pharmacy
Washington State University
Pullman, Washington

Mei-Ping Chang, Ph.D.
GRECC
Veterans Administration Medical
  Center
          and
Department of Medicine
University of California at
  Los Angeles
Los Angeles, California

Francesco Chiappelli, Ph.D.
Department of Anatomy and Cell
  Biology
School of Medicine
University of California at Los
  Angeles
Los Angeles, California

Sandra J. Ewald, Ph.D.
Department of Pathobiology
Auburn University
Auburn, Alabama

Zehava Gottesfeld, Ph.D.
Department of Neurobiology and
  Anatomy
The University of Texas Medical
  School at Houston
Houston, Texas

Charles J. Grossman, Ph.D.
Department of Veterans Affairs
Veterans Affairs Medical Center
Cincinnati, Ohio

Thomas R. Jerrells, Ph.D.
Department of Cellular Biology and
  Anatomy
Louisiana State University Medical
  Center
Shreveport, Louisiana

Carol Mason, M.D.
Department of Pulmonary/Critical
  Care Medicine
Louisiana State University Medical
  Center
New Orleans, Louisiana

Gary G. Meadows, Ph.D.
Department of Pharmaceutical
  Sciences
College of Pharmacy
Washington State University
Pullman, Washington

**Charles L. Mendenhall, M.D.,
  Ph.D.**
Department of Hepatic Research
Veterans Affairs Medical Center
Cincinnati, Ohio

Siraj I. Mufti, Ph.D.
Department of Pharmacology and
 Toxicology
College of Pharmacy
University of Arizona
Tucson, Arizona

Chester Nakamura, B.S.
Department of Pulmonary/Critical
 Care Medicine
Louisiana State University Medical
 Center
New Orleans, Louisiana

Steve Nelson, M.D.
Department of Pulmonary/Critical
 Care Medicine
Louisiana State University Medical
 Center
New Orleans, Louisiana

Dean C. Norman, M.D.
GRECC
Veterans Administration Medical
 Center
 and
Department of Medicine
University of California at
 Los Angeles
Los Angeles, California

Gary Roselle, M.D.
Department of Internal Medicine
University of Cincinnati Medical
 Center
 and
Medical Service
Veterans Affairs Medical Center
Cincinnati, Ohio

Helmut K. Seitz, M.D.
Department of Medicine
Salem Medical Center
University of Heidelberg
Heidelberg, Germany

Ulrich A. Simanowski, M.D.
Department of Medicine
Marienkrankenhaus Herne
Ruhr University Bochum
Herne, Germany

Akira Takada, M.D.
Department of Internal Medicine
Kanazawa Medical University
Uchinada, Ishikawa, Japan

Shujiro Takase, M.D.
Department of Internal Medicine
Kanazawa Medical University
Uchinada, Ishikawa, Japan

Anna N. Taylor, Ph.D.
Department of Anatomy and Cell
 Biology
School of Medicine
University of California at
 Los Angeles
 and
Brentwood Division
West Los Angeles Veterans
 Administration Medical Center
Los Angeles, California

Mikihiro Tsutsumi, M.D.
Department of Internal Medicine
Kanazawa Medical University
Uchinada, Ishikawa, Japan

Corjan J. T. Visser, M.Sc.
Department of Biological
 Toxicology
TNO-CIVO Toxicology and
 Nutrition Institute
Zeist, The Netherlands

Ronald R. Watson, Ph.D.
Department of Family and
  Community Medicine
  and
Alcohol Research Center
University of Arizona
Tucson, Arizona

Bernhard Watzl, Ph.D.
Institute of Nutrition
Tustus-Liebig University
Giessen, Germany

Carol Wong, D.D.S.
Department of Periodontics
School of Dentristry
University of Michigan
Ann Arbor, Michigan

Ruud A. Woutersen, Ph.D.
Department of Biological
  Toxicology
TNO-CIVO Toxicology and
  Nutrition Institute
Zeist, The Netherlands

Raz Yirmiya, Ph.D.
Department of Psychology
The Hebrew University of
  Jerusalem
Jerusalem, Israel

TABLE OF CONTENTS

PART III. ALCOHOL AND CANCER

PART I
Alcohol and Immunity

Chapter 1

EFFECTS OF ALCOHOL ON IMMUNITY AND CANCER

Gary Roselle, Charles L. Mendenhall, and Charles J. Grossman

"I intend to die in a tavern;
let the wine be placed near my dying mouth,
so that when the choirs of angels come, they may say,
'God be merciful to this drinker!'"
Walter Mapes (Circa 1140–1210)
DeNugis Curilium

TABLE OF CONTENTS

5761-6/93/$0.00 + $.50
© 1993 by CRC Press, Inc.

3

I. INTRODUCTION

The linkage between intemperate use of alcohol and human morbidity and mortality has been accepted by both the scientific community and the general population through the centuries. In more recent times, this linkage has been primarily defined by alcoholic liver disease, with the recognized sequelae of alcoholic hepatitis, alcoholic cirrhosis, and, finally, hepatic failure and death.

More recently, however, morbidity and abnormal pathologic sequelae associated with intemperate alcohol use has become more prominent. Although not universally accepted, an association between alcohol consumption and a variety of malignant tumors in several different organ systems has been proposed. For a number of tumor types, this linkage appears to be well-founded and has become accepted in the general scientific literature. Though currently suggested, universal acceptance of a relationship between alcohol and other tumor types will require further data in the published literature.

The association between alcohol consumption and defects in host immunologic response has been postulated for several years. Over the last decade, the concept of abnormal host response in alcoholics has become more accepted by the scientific community, and indeed appears to be real, both in the adult alcoholic and in the offspring of alcoholic mothers. The clinical relevance of these defects in host response continues to remain somewhat unclear.

While not directly within the purview of this chapter, the association between alcohol-related host response defects and infection in the alcoholic remains controversial,[21] with specific linkages between host immune defects in the alcoholic and infection still unproven. Perhaps then, the interrelationship of host immune response deficits in alcoholics and malignancy could be important in our understanding of the underlying pathophysiologic connection between excess ethanol consumption and cancer.

In this chapter we will provide an overview of alcohol-related tumors, with a specific effort made to clarify the evidence associating each tumor type with alcohol. In addition, we also will try to define the effects of ethanol consumption on host immune response. Finally, the general relationship between alcohol, host immunologic response, and cancer will be explored. Comments also will be made regarding any current theories about mechanistic links that may be postulated to explain the observed phenomena. Possible etiologic cofactors, including ethnicity and alcoholic beverage type, also will be considered. Other chapters within this book will deal in much greater detail with specific tumors and components of the immune response in relation to ethanol ingestion, both in animal models and humans.

It is important to remember that studies of alcohol use in both humans and animal models are often confounded by difficulties in control of a variety of variables. These include, but are not limited to, nutrition, vitamin deficiencies, source of alcohol used, genus and species of the animal models, the route of administration of either the carcinogen or alcohol, hormonal responses to the trauma of administration, and use of different outcome parameters. While these problems make the literature often difficult to interpret, they are frequently beyond the ability of the scientist to control. Therefore, one should not expect absolute answers to questions posed regarding alcohol, cancer, and host response. The data provided in this section should allow the reader to assess the current scientific evidence in the field, and perhaps plan future initiatives to answer some of the questions that will, by necessity, be left unresolved.

II. ALCOHOL AND CANCER

A. ALCOHOL AND UPPER GASTROINTESTINAL TRACT

In humans, many authors have shown an association between ethanol consumption and upper gastrointestinal tract tumors.[1,17,28,49,59,73,87,93,95,104,111,115] Merletti et al.[73] reported, in a population-based study in Italy, a correlation between the consumption of 120 or more grams of ethanol daily, and the incidence of oral and oropharyngeal tumors. Gingival cancer has also been linked with ethanol use, particularly in association with smokeless tobacco use. In New York, Graham et al.[28] found a link between ethanol consumption and esophageal cancer. In their study, beer was the only alcoholic beverage type to be consistently coupled with this tumor.

The linkage between category of alcoholic beverage and type of upper gastrointestinal cancer has also been reported by others.[18,110] In a study by Leclerc et al.[59] in France, mouth cancers were associated with wine consumption, pharyngeal and supraglottic tumors with spirits, and glottic cancer lesions with whiskey or fortified wine.

These relationships may be related to different carcinogenic substances in these alcoholic beverages. In certain brandies and some whiskey, specific carcinogens, particularly nitrosamines, contaminate up to 20 to 50% of samples.[29] As an example, in a study by Bull et al.[17] in Chile, red wines contained mutagenic substances at double the frequency of Chilean white wines. These carcinogens can mediate increased carcinogenic potential in association with ethanol, most notably seen in animal models of promotion of chemically induced malignant lesions.[28]

The relationship between ethanol and upper gastrointestinal tract cancer has been studied extensively in animal models.[6,30,39,55,76,107] While ethanol itself does not appear to be carcinogenic, even in this high-risk location, there does seem to be a distinct relationship between malignant tumors of the upper gastrointestinal tract and ethanol promotion of tumors induced by known carcinogens. Notably, although some data suggest that simultaneous administration of ethanol with a carcinogen may have a protective effect, clearly ethanol does promote tumors induced by a variety of carcinogens including, but not limited to, N-nitrosomethylbenzylamine,[76] and N-methyl-N'-nitro-N-nitrosoguanidine.[39,107] Furthermore, this effect appears to be influenced both by timing of ethanol administration in relation to the carcinogen and method of administration.

Ethanol consumption relates most clearly to promotion of upper gastrointestinal tract cancer in both human and animal models. Controversy still exists regarding the effect of ethanol consumption on the initiation of tumorigenesis, if given concomitantly with the carcinogen in an experimental model. This issue is perhaps of little clinical relevance in humans, since ethanol consumption would normally occur both with tumor initiation, as well as continue temporally through promotion of the malignant process.

B. ALCOHOL AND LIVER CANCER

Many animal models have been studied to establish and verify a relationship between ethanol and tumor initiation or promotion and specific hepatic carcinogens.[24,68,106,108,122] Using a variety of tumor initiators, including aflatoxin B_1,[108] diethylnitrosamine,[24,106] or N-nitrosopyrrolidine,[68] hepatic neoplastic foci were increased in animals treated with ethanol after exposure to the carcinogen. This occurred both in rats and golden hamsters using appropriate, similar experimental conditions.

All data are not consistent, however. In a paper by Yanagi et al.,[122] ethanol did not enhance hepatic carcinogenesis induced by 3'-methyl-4-dimethylaminoazobenzene, in the absence of liver injury. This study, done in Wistar rats, used a variety of concentrations of ethanol in drinking water, with the initiator placed in the rats' food over a four-week period. To differentiate initiation and promotion, the ethanol-laced drinking water was introduced after two weeks of carcinogen. Perhaps these disparate results concerning enhanced carcinogenesis can be explained by the method of carcinogen administration or timing of alcohol administration that may well influence amplification of tumor formation or growth.

In humans, the issue of enhancement of tumorigenesis in the liver is extraordinarily complex. Confounding variables, some of which relate to alcohol consumption, including infection with hepatitis B virus, liver fibrosis, geographical exposure to carcinogens, ethnicity, and diet, may all influence results of studies of the association of hepatic carcinoma and alcohol consumption.[9,11,16,32,40,52,80,81,84]

In investigations from a variety of countries, including Sweden, the United States, Uganda, and the Philippines, an increased risk of hepatocellular carcinoma was associated with alcohol consumption.[11] However, in the tropics, exposure to aflatoxin was implicated, while in the Far East and the United Kingdom, a relationship with hepatitis B virus has also been found, including inclusion of segments of the hepatitis virus genome in the hepatic tumor.[9,11,16,32,40,80,84] However, these correlates have raised questions. For example, in a paper by Horiike et al.,[38] the authors did not find a clear association between hepatitis B virus and hepatocellular carcinoma in Japan. The data from the paper by Walter et al.[114] raised similar questions by revealing no molecular evidence for the contribution of hepatitis B virus in the development of hepatocellular carcinoma in patients with alcoholic liver disease.

Nonomura et al.[80,81] found the incidence of hepatocellular carcinoma unrelated to total alcohol intake, but instead related to the development of macronodules and a decrease in liver weight. These data leave unclear the question whether alcohol itself acts as an enhancer of tumorigenesis in the liver or, rather, whether the liver injury itself is the culprit. Indeed, perhaps the primary entity responsible for the purported relationship between alcohol and liver cancer rests with the consequences of liver injury independent of etiology, whether induced by alcohol or viral infection.

In addition, regional differences in initiation or potentiation of liver tumors may vary depending on geographic locale. For instance, hepatitis B viral infection, carcinogen exposures, such as those related to aflatoxin, and perhaps other geoethnic characteristics may account for the observed disparity in epidemiologic human data. The number of confounding variables make clarification of the contribution of each to hepatocellular carcinoma a monumental task that is not easily accomplished.

C. ALCOHOL AND PANCREATIC CANCER

While early studies indicated an association between alcohol consumption and pancreatic cancer, more recent research fails to verify this linkage.[14,82,112,120] However, these were primarily case-control studies in which patients with pancreatic cancer were compared to patients without this tumor.

In a review of the subject of Velema et al.[112] in 1986, the authors felt that insufficient evidence was provided in the body of literature to link causally alcohol and pancreatic tumors. In a more recent paper Bouchardy et al.[14] reviewed studies of pancreatic cancer from Italy, France, and Switzerland. This allowed for consideration of data from almost 500 cancer patients with over 1700 controls. A variety of parameters were reviewed, including age, sex, smoking history, socioeconomic status, and source of alcohol consumed, including wine, beer, or spirits. The authors concluded after review of the data that there was no clear evidence of linkage between alcohol consumption and pancreatic cancer.

While these data are reassuring, the issue of alcohol and pancreatic cancer is still not settled, particularly when considering results of studies using animal models. Woutersen et al.[120] (see also Chapter 13, this volume) assessed both paraneoplastic foci and carcinoma in the pancreas of animals fed alcohol after a carcinogen exposure. Of special interest was the additional experimental condition in which the animals ate either a low-fat or a high-fat diet. Notably, rats fed a high-fat diet exhibited an increase in number and size of basophilic paraneoplastic foci. Furthermore, there appeared to be a greater overall incidence of carcinoma *in situ* in rats fed a high-fat diet. In hamsters, the effect of ethanol and high-fat diet was less pronounced, but there was a significant increase in number of early lesions in hamster pancreas induced by laboratory injection of a carcinogen. In an interesting Swedish study,[82] humans who had a high consumption frequency of fried or grilled meat had an increased risk of pancreatic cancer compared to controls. However, no consistent association was found with alcohol ingestion in the same study.

Therefore, it remains unclear whether alcohol does contribute to the incidence of pancreatic cancer, particularly in association with other co-factors such as dietary variables. While the general association may be somewhat weak based on current data, differences in alcohol consumption, dietary habits, and possibly geoethnic co-factors in various regions of the world, may impact the overall incidence of pancreatic tumors.

D. ALCOHOL AND COLON AND RECTAL CANCER

The relationship between alcohol consumption and colo-rectal cancer is far clearer than that relating pancreatic cancer and alcohol. Both animal model and human data confirm the relationship. However, certain specific carcinogens when given with ethanol yielded conflicting results with respect to colon cancer.

In studies by Hamilton et al.,[33-35] during the preinduction and induction phase of tumor produced by azoxymethane treatment, dietary ethanol inhibited tumorigenesis, despite high doses of the carcinogen. The authors speculate that this may be related to changes in carcinogen metabolism, but this postulate has not been confirmed. The same investigative group compared laboratory ethanol with beer as the laboratory carbohydrate source in an animal study, and found no difference between beer and laboratory ethanol in tumor protection beyond that already related to ethanol concentration.

In a paper and a letter to the editor by Sietz et al.[97,98] (see also Chapter 12 of this volume), it is indicated that ethanol consumption enhanced rectal carcinogenesis induced by acetoxymethylmethylnitrosamine in Sprague-Dawley rats. While the mechanism for this enhancement is not yet clear, the author speculates in a later letter to the editor that the effect on rectal carcinogenesis by ethanol may be mediated through the local action of ethanol or acetaldehyde on rectal mucosa. In contrast, McGarrity et al.[69] did not find an association between cancer and ethanol, using 1,2-dimethylhydrazine.

In humans, Klatsky[54] studied the incidence of cancers of the colon and rectum in over 100,000 men and women in California. A variety of parameters were reviewed to assess a possible positive association with these cancers. Controlling for age, sex, race, body-mass index, coffee use, total serum cholesterol, and education, alcohol showed a positive association with both colon and rectal cancer. This association was observed in both men and women, and the risk of cancer was not different among drinkers of wine, beer, or spirits. However, those who preferred beer had a slightly increased risk of rectal cancer, while those who preferred wine had a slightly increased risk of developing colon cancer.

In another large human study, Kabat et al.[50] reviewed over 200 patients with rectal cancer and over 500 controls for a possible association between beer consumption and rectal tumor. Beer consumption was found to be significantly associated with an increased risk of rectal cancer in males, but not females. However, when correction was made for potentially confounding variables, the relative risk was reduced slightly. Therefore, this study did not conclusively define a causal relationship between beer consumption and rectal carcinoma.

Kikendall et al.[53] reviewed the association between cigarettes and alcohol as risk factors for colonic adenomas. Both cigarette smoking and beer drinking showed independently statistically significant associations with colonic adenomas.

It thus would appear that the results generated from animal studies may be obscured by the use of different species of animals and different carcinogens. On the other hand, epidemiologic data using human subjects support the relationship between ethanol consumption and colo-rectal carcinoma.

E. ALCOHOL AND LUNG CANCER

The effect of alcohol and the carcinogen, *N*-nitrosodimethylamine (NDMA), was studied in male, strain A mice given ethanol simultaneously with chronic, oral NMDA.[7] The mice had a statistically significant enhancement of lung tumorigenesis. When the ethanol administration followed the carcinogen, there was no evidence for promotion of the tumors induced by NDMA. Therefore, the author speculates that the mechanism for this tumor enhancement may be related to alcohol-associated, competitive inhibition of NDMA metabolism in the liver, instead of promotion of tumorigenesis by direct effect of alcohol on tumor cells themselves. It should be noted, however, that confirmatory data linking lung cancer to alcohol consumption have not been convincingly presented.[12,56]

F. ALCOHOL AND BREAST CANCER

The relationship between alcohol consumption and breast cancer has been strikingly controversial.[2,36,37,62,71,85,101,102,121] In a recent review by Lowenfels,[62] published in 1989, the author evaluated published reports dating from 1974 through 1987, dealing with a linkage between alcohol consumption and breast cancer. This extensive review did not find persuasive, consistent evidence of a direct relationship between alcohol consumption and breast cancer, though some studies did reveal a strong relationship. However, in a paper by Hiatt[36] published in 1988, a cohort of 69,000 women was studied in Northern California from 1979 through 1984. In this rather large group, there was a significant association with breast cancer and heavy alcohol consumption among certain groups of women. The review did not find a linkage between source of alcohol consumed, such as wine, beer, or spirits, and the breast cancer.

Therefore, any substantiated linkage between alcohol consumption and breast cancer continues to be elusive. The disparity of the results among the studies may be related to the populations investigated. For example, in the study by Hiatt[36] the strongest associations were among white, postmenopausal women. Therefore, other co-factors may be conclusively participatory in breast cancer risk-enhancement associated with alcohol ingestion.

G. ALCOHOL AND URINARY TRACT TUMORS

Kunze et al.,[58] in Germany, sought a relationship between lower urinary tract tumor risk and alcohol consumption, using an appropriate control group matched for age and sex. After adjustment for smoking, multiple logistic regression analysis indicated that beer consumption was significantly associated with lower urinary tract tumors. While there was some tumor increase with consumption of spirits, this did not reach statistical significance. The authors speculate that this phenomenon may be related to nitrosamines that are widely found in beer, though the specific causal relationship among beer, nitrosamines, and lower urinary tract tumors in humans remains unproven.

III. ALCOHOL AND HOST RESPONSE

The effects of ethanol on host response are legion. Since, for the most part, they will be covered in detail in other sections of this text, only an overview will be given in this chapter. Ethanol appears to effect virtually all studied constituents of the immune system in both humans and animal models. Unfortunately, the extent and clinical significance of each of the individual alterations remains controversial.

A. ALCOHOL, LYMPHOCYTE SUBSETS, AND THYMOCYTES

Many authors have found alterations in lymphocyte subsets in patients with alcoholic liver disease. Most authors have found decreases in total T-lymphocytes or their percents in hospitalized patients with alcoholic liver disease, including both alcoholic hepatitis and alcoholic cirrhosis.[41,48,77,91] There has been some disparity in these results with respect to more defined lymphocyte subset abnormalities.[103] While some authors have found no general changes in either the absolute number of helper or suppressor/cytotoxic cells[41] or their ratio,[48] others have found decreases in CD4 and CD8 cells.[91] When found, these abnormalities may be in part reversible over varying periods of time after abstinence from ethanol ingestion.[91]

In addition to peripheral blood lymphocyte abnormalities, in animal models, alcohol also adversely effects thymic weight and cellularity.[66] and response of T cells to mitogenic stimulation.[19,31,41-46] In the rat, this was true of splenic cells as well.[43] Abnormalities of number and function of thymocytes in rats with fetal alcohol syndrome have also been shown.[5,26] In addition, abnormalities of expression of differentiation antigens occur.[20]

In both humans[8] and in rodent models[31] of alcohol treatment, the response of peripheral blood lymphocytes to mitogenic stimulation is generally decreased. The clinical significance of these consistent abnormalities is yet to be determined.

B. ALCOHOL AND B CELLS

Hypergammaglobulinemia is a well-recognized phenomenon in alcoholics with liver disease, especially cirrhosis.[83] The mechanism underlying this occurrence is still speculative, but may include increased exposure to gut flora, or increased responsiveness to a variety of immunogenic stimuli or tumor.[42] Though of probably equal importance, the effects of alcohol on B cell activity and production of immunoactive substances have been less well-studied compared with many other parameters of host response. While consumption of alcohol quantitatively impacted antibody production following immunization of alcoholic patients, the results of different studies demonstrated some interesting disparities. In patients receiving pneumococcal vaccine (polysaccharide), response to immunization has been respectable, with normal or greater than normal titers developed to the vaccine components. In patients immunized with hepatitis B vaccine (protein), antibody response to immunization is quantitatively decreased compared to controls.[72] Perhaps this is based on the requirement for T cell help for response to protein antigens. This is in contradistinction to the lack of such a requirement for response to polysaccharide antigens. Lastly, specific B cell metabolic abnormalities could explain these findings. However, Aldo-Benson[3-5] recently has reported data in the mouse model, revealing specific abnormalities of B cell proliferation in response to antigens. She did not find that alcohol inhibited membrane depolarization induced by antigen cross-linking immunoglobulin receptors, or inhibited activation of the phosphatidyl and acetyl pathways by receptor cross-linking. Obviously, more work is needed to define the interactions of B cells and T cells in alcoholics, and the specific effect of ethanol on B cell activity. This topic will receive more attention in other sections of this text.

C. ALCOHOL AND NATURAL KILLER CELL ACTIVITY

Meadows et al.[70] and others, have shown abnormalities of natural killer cell (NK) function related to ethanol. Specifically, Meadows[70] (see also Chapter 4 of this volume) has shown that ethanol impairs both baseline and interleukin 2 (IL-2)-stimulated splenic NK cell activity in rodents after one- and two-week test periods of ethanol ingestion. Linkage between the abnormalities in NK cell activity could not be made with any specific parameter, including average daily intake of alcohol, blood alcohol concentrations, or the number of alcohol derived calories each animal ingested. However, controversy remains concerning the real impact of alcohol consumption on NK cell activity, since occasional investigators have found an enhancement of NK cell activity using modest ethanol doses.[94] Of special note concerning malignancy is the observation that NK cell abnormalities may play a critical role in the control of distant tumor metastasis.

The low dose-enhancing effect of ethanol may be of importance, since similar results have occasionally been reported by other investigators using diverse parameters of cellular immunity. Dehne et al.[22] found a comparable effect in cutaneous hypersensitivity reactions (skin tests) in rats fed a low dose ethanol diet. In the higher dose ranges, a depression of the skin test response took place. The mechanism underlying these seemingly disparate dose-related results remains to be elucidated.

D. ALCOHOL AND MACROPHAGES

Watson et al.[117,118] have shown a decrease in percentage of peripheral blood and spleen cells expressing markers for macrophage cell type and their activation after treatment of rodents with alcohol. In a recent study by Morland and Morland,[74] short exposure of human monocytes to ethanol led to changes in a specific subpopulation of cells with the IgG FcR marker. The authors felt that this probably represented a decrease in functional receptors on the surface of the monocytes.

Of particular interest is the work by Wickramasinghe,[119] who identified specific ethanol metabolism in the macrophage. In this setting, mediation of ethanol metabolism is via the cytochrome P450 dependent mitochondrial ethanol-oxidizing system. Such an observation suggests that the products of ethanol metabolism may play a central role in defined macrophage functional abnormalities.

Bagasra et al.[10] found the ability of macrophages from alcohol-ingesting rats to phagocytize particles, using the C3b and Fc receptors significantly impaired. The ability of peritoneal macrophages from alcohol-treated animals to ingest nonopsonized *Candida albicans* and to reduce nitrablue tetrazolium (NBT) dye was also diminished. In this study, there were increases in receptor density for Fc and C3b on the cell surface in the alcohol rats compared to litter-mate controls. Therefore, clearly, ethanol can impact both number and function of macrophages, at least in animal models. It remains unclear whether the oxidative metabolites of ethanol that would be found in the macrophage microenvironment are of functional or clinical relevance in this setting.

E. ALCOHOL AND CYTOKINES

Recently, a variety of investigators has generated a large body of data on the impact of alcohol consumption on cytokine activity.[46,51,75,90] Early studies showed abnormalities in migration inhibitory-factor activity in the ferret and rat,[90] even after short-term ethanol ingestion. More recent investigations have concentrated on the interleukins and tumor necrosis factor, both better-defined systems in which to work. In a novel study by Kaplan,[51] ethanol suppressed the ability of preformed IL-2 to stimulate proliferation of T cells that had previously acquired IL-2 receptors. Neither production of IL-2 nor generation of IL-2 receptors was different in this study.

Jerrells et al.[46] have focused extensively on IL-2 in the rodent model, and found abnormalities associated with alcohol ingestion. These data and that of others will be discussed in detail in another chapter in this text and need not be considered here in detail.

F. ALCOHOL AND NEUTROPHILS

Extensive work has been accomplished in the area of neutrophils and alcohol,[63,66,79] particularly related to chemotaxis and adherence. Ethanol inhibits *in vitro* adherence of neutrophils to endothelial monolayers when stimulated by *N*-formyl-L-methionyl-L-leucyl-L-phenylalanine (fMLP). Ethanol, however, does not affect either resting adherence or resting surface expression of the adhesive glycoprotein, Mac-1. Up regulation of Mac-1 by fMLP, however, was inhibited in a dose-dependent manner by the addition of ethanol. A dose-dependent ethanol inhibition of primary and secondary granule release after cell activation was also reported.[66]

These findings by MacGregor et al.[63] have been confirmed to some extent in patients with alcoholic liver disease. Again, random motility of neutrophils was similar for alcoholic patients and controls. However, cells from cirrhotic patients exhibited reduced endotoxin activated chemotaxis.[64] The poor response appeared to be related to a serum inhibitor which also reduced the chemotactic activity of control serum. This constituent had no effect on chemotaxis induced by fMLP. In this study, however, delivery of polymorphonuclear leukocytes into skin chambers was similar in alcoholics and controls. The disparity in results between the ethanol inhibition of stimulated chemotaxis *in vitro* and the *in vivo* response in skin windows is not clear. This may be caused by the direct impact of ethanol in the media on neutrophil activity, instead of the expected effect of serum inhibitors found in some patient serum after long-term ethanol use.

G. ALCOHOL AND HISTOCOMPATIBILITY ANTIGEN EXPRESSION

Singer et al.[100] and Parent and co-workers[86] studied the expression of major histocompatibility antigens in some detail. They have consistently found an enhanced expression of cell surface class I major histocompatibility complex antigens in a variety of cell lines. In addition, the changes in cell surface antigen levels are reflected in increased intracellular protein synthesis and increased steady state messenger ribonucleic acid (mRNA) levels. It should also be noted that these effects are present when using *in vitro* ethanol concentrations that are physiologically attainable. In addition, data using cells obtained from human alcoholics support these findings.

These issues may be vital, since class I transplantation antigens are primary restriction elements for recognition of viral antigens in certain reactions, and may play a major role in tumor control and graft rejection.

H. ALCOHOL, CANCER, AND IMMUNITY, MECHANISTIC RELATIONSHIP

Several recent articles have described a cornucopia of conceivable mechanistic relationships between alcohol and cancer, and alcohol and host response.[13,15,23,27,57,60,61,65,78,88,89,92,96,105,110,113,116,123] While it is not at all clear that alcohol is a specific carcinogen, there is accumulating evidence that alcohol may contribute to either the initiation or potentiation of carcinogenesis linked to other compounds. This must be complex, and in all likelihood related to a variety of cellular systems. As a candidate, the microsomal cytochrome P 450 biotransformation system has been suggested as a possible intermediary in the co-carcinogenesis of many compounds. This would explain the putative co-carcinogenic effects of ethanol in anatomic areas distant from sites that may be in direct contact with alcohol per se, such as the mouth or pharynx.[61,96] The mechanism of this potentiation may be dependent on the stimulation of the microsomal system and increased metabolism of known carcinogens to their toxic metabolites. This may be particularly true for the polycyclic aromatic hydrocarbons and nitrosamines.[65,105]

Ethanol may also function directly at the DNA level, specifically generating chromosomal aberrations, perhaps via acetaldehyde, leading to tumor promotion. In addition, ethanol may inhibit the capacity of injured cells to repair DNA damage related to carcinogens.[61,67]

With respect to hepatocellular carcinoma, the alcoholic is at particular risk, probably involving several of the mechanisms noted previously. As an adjunct to these associations with carcinogenesis, hepatitis B virus also may be linked to hepatic cancer. In some cases, hepatitis B virus DNA sequences are integrated into the genome of the cancerous liver cells. While this may not be related directly to alcohol consumption, the incidence of hepatitis B virus infection is higher in patients with alcoholism than in nonalcohol controls. Furthermore, the extensive hepatocellular damage linked to underlying alcoholism, or viral liver disease, may be permissive for the development of hepatocellular carcinoma.[61]

There are also multiple direct effects of alcohol on the upper gastrointestinal tract. In addition to the cellular mechanisms noted above, alcohol may influence the presentation of carcinogens into at-risk alimentary tract cells based on changes in cell membranes with consequent alteration of penetration of carcinogens into the cell cytoplasm or organelles.[95,99]

The specific mechanistic linkage between immunomodulation and cancer in the alcoholic is more difficult to define. As noted in the sections above, and in other chapters of this text, it is clear that alcohol does modulate host response by a variety of mechanisms. Whether these alterations are important in tumor surveillance or have other physiologic significance in man is much less clear. Of particular note in the area of tumor cell destruction would be the changes in NK cell and macrophage function. Both of these cell types are important in removal of abnormal cells of every variety, and often have tumoricidal activity. The effect of ethanol on activity of cytokines, such as tumor necrosis factor (TNF), is probably of equal or greater importance, though more data are required before final conclusions can be drawn. Further work is required to clarify the impact of ethanol on polymorphonuclear leukocyte migration and/or killing that may be critical components of neoplastic housekeeping *in vivo*.

In conclusion, it is perfectly clear that alcohol consumption can be linked to a variety of neoplastic diseases in humans. The effect of alcohol on mucosal cells directly, the modulation of subcellular components related to carcinogen metabolism, the effect on subnuclear constituents such as DNA stability and repair, even at sites distant from the direct effects of alcohol, and the impact on immunoactive cells and cytokine production or activity, are excellent candidates that may be responsible for the enhancement of tumorigenesis in the alcoholic patient. It is likely that these components, functioning in concert, actively modulate the malignant process.

While intemperate alcohol use also negatively effects host immune function, it remains unclear whether direct linkage exists between host immune defects and cancer initiation or promotion. Only further work specifically related to this issue will allow solid confirmation of the role of alcohol and altered host response in human carcinogenesis.

REFERENCES

1. **Abdulgamidov, M. M., et al.,** Alcohol as an etiological factor in carcinogenesis, *ICRDB,* 1, 46, 1980.
2. Alcohol consumption and breast cancer, *Nutr. Rev.,* (editorial), 46, 9, 1988.
3. **Aldo-Benson, M., Scheiderer, L., and Dwulet, F. E.,** 2,4-Dinitrophenyl (DNP)-specific continuous B cell lines as a model system for studying B cell activation and tolerance, *Eur. J. Immunol.,* 16, 69, 1986.
4. **Aldo-Benson, M.,** Mechanisms of alcohol-induced suppression of B-cell response, *Alcohol. Clin. Exp. Res.,* 13, 469, 1989.
5. **Aldo-Benson, M.,** Investigations of intrinsic abnormalities in DNA-specific B lymphocytes from autoimmune mice, *J. Autoimmunity,* 2, 269, 1989.
6. **Alexandrov, V. A., Novikov, A. I., Zabezhinsky, M. A., et al.,** The stimulating effect of acetic acid, alcohol and thermal burn injury on esophagus and forestomach carcinogenesis induced by *N*-nitrososarcosin ethyl ester in rats, *Cancer Lett.,* 47, 179, 1989.
7. **Anderson, L. M.,** Increased numbers of *N*-nitrosodimethylamine-initiated lung tumors in mice by chronic co-administration of ethanol, *Carcinogenesis,* 9, 1717, 1988.
8. **Area, B. R., De La Barrera, S., Del Carmen Sasiain, M., et al.,** Cell-mediated immunity in alcoholic liver cirrhosis, *Medicina,* 47, 27, 1987.

9. **Austin, H., Delzell, E., Grufferman, S., et al.,** A case-control study of hepatocellular carcinoma and the hepatitis B virus, cigarette smoking, and alcohol consumption, *Cancer Res.,* 46, 962, 1986.
10. **Bagasra, O., Howeedy, A., Kajdacsy-Ball, A., et al.,** Macrophage function in chronic experimental alcoholism. I. Modulation of surface receptors and phagocytosis, *Immunology,* 65(3), 405, 1988.
11. **Bassendine, M. F.,** Alcohol-a major risk factor for hepatocellular carcinoma? *J. Hepatol.,* 2, 513, 1986.
12. **Batkin, S. and Tabrah, F. L.,** Ethanol vapor modulation of Lewis lung carcinoma, a murine pulmonary tumour, *Cancer Res. Clin. Oncol.,* 116, 187, 1990.
13. **Bora, P. S., Spilburg, C. A., and Lange, L. G.,** Metabolism of ethanol and carcinogens by glutathione transferases, *Proc. Natl. Acad. Sci. U.S.A.,* 86, 4470, 1989.
14. **Bouchardy, C., Clavel, F., LaVecchia, C., et al.,** Alcohol beer and cancer of the pancreas, *Int. J. Cancer,* 45, 842, 1990.
15. **Boyland, E.,** Water could reduce the hazard of cancer from spirits, *Br. J. of Ind. Med.,* 46, 423, 1989.
16. **Brechot, C.,** Hepatitis B virus in alcoholic liver disease with hepatocellular carcinoma, *Hepatology,* 9, 514, 1989.
17. **Bull, P., Yanez, L., and Nervi, F.,** Mutagenic substances in red and white wine in Chile, a high risk area for gastric cancer, *Mutation Res.,* 187, 113, 1987.
18. **Carstensen, J. M., Bygren, L. O., and Hatschek, T.,** Cancer incidence among Swedish brewery workers, *J. Cancer,* 45, 393, 1990.
19. **Chang, M. P., Norman, D. C., and Makinodan, T.,** Immunotoxicity of alcohol in young and old mice. I. *In vitro* suppressive effects of ethanol on the activities of T and B immune cells of aging mice, *Alcohol. Clin. Exp. Res.,* 14, 210, 1990.
20. **Datta, R., Sherman, M. L., and Kufe, D. W.,** Regulation of proto-oncogene and tumor necrosis factor gene expression by ethanol in HL-60 myeloid leukemia cells, *Blood,* 76, 298, 1990.
21. **Davis, C. C., Mellencamp, M. A., and Preheim, L. C.,** A model of pneumococcal pneumonia in chronically intoxicated rats, *J. Infect. Dis.,* 63, 799, 1991.
22. **Dehne, N. E., Mendenhall, C. L., Roselle, G. A., et al.,** Cell-mediated immune responses associated with short term alcohol intake: time course and dose dependency, *Alcohol. Clin. Exp. Res.,* 13, 201, 1989.
23. **Driver, H. E. and Swann, P. F.,** Alcohol and human cancer, *Anticancer Res.,* 7, 309, 1987.
24. **Driver, H. E. and McLean, A. E. M.,** Dose-response relationships for initiation of rat liver tumors by diethylnitrosamine and promotion by phenobarbitone or alcohol, *Food Chem. Toxicol.,* 24, 241, 1986.
25. **Ewald, S. J. and Walden, S. M.,** Flow cytometric and histological analysis of mouse thymus in fetal alcohol syndrome, *J. Leukocyte Biol.,* 44, 434, 1988.
26. **Ewald, S.,** T lymphocyte populations in fetal alcohol syndrome, *Alcohol. Clin. Exp. Res.,* 13, 485, 1989.
27. **Garro, A. J. and Lieber, C. S.,** Alcohol and cancer, *Annu. Rev. Pharmacol. Toxicol.,* 30, 219, 1990.
28. **Graham, S., Marshall, J., Haughey, B., et al.,** Nutritional epidemiology of cancer of the esophagus, *Am. J. Epidemiol.,* 3, 454, 1990.
29. **Griciute, L., Castegnaro, M., and Bereziat, J. C.,** Influence of ethyl alcohol on carcinogenesis induced by volatile *N*-nitrosamines detected in alcoholic beverages, *IARC Sci. Publ.,* 84, 264, 1987.
30. **Griciute, L., Castegnaro, M., Bereziat, J. C., et al.,** Influence of ethyl alcohol on the carcinogenic activity of *N*-nitrosonornicotine, *Cancer Lett.,* 31, 267, 1986.
31. **Grossman, C. J., Mendenhall, C. L., and Roselle, G. A.,** Alcohol and immune regulation. I. *In vivo* effects of ethanol on concanavalin A sensitive thymic lymphocyte function, *Int. J. Immunopharmacol.,* 10, 187, 1988.

32. **Hadengue, A., N'Dri, N., and Benhamou, J.-P.,** Relative risk of hepatocellular carcinoma in HBsAg positive vs. alcoholic cirrhosis. A cross-sectional study, *Liver,* 10, 147, 1990.

33. **Hamilton, S. R., Hyland, J., McAvinchey, D., et al.,** Effects of chronic dietary beer and ethanol consumption on experimental colonic carcinogenesis by azoxymethane in rats, *Cancer Res.,* 47, 1551, 1987.

34. **Hamilton, S. R., Sohn, O. S., and Fiala, E. S.,** Effects of timing and quantity of chronic dietary ethanol consumption on azoxymethane-induced colonic carcinogenesis and azoxymethane metabolism in Fisher 344 rats, *Cancer Res.,* 47, 4305, 1987.

35. **Hamilton, S. R., Sohn, O. S., and Fiala, E. S.,** Inhibition by dietary ethanol of experimental colonic carcinogenesis induced by high-dose azoxymethane in 344 rats, *Cancer Res.,* 48, 3313, 1988.

36. **Hiatt, R. A., Klatsky, A. L., and Armstrong, M. A.,** Alcohol consumption and the risk of breast cancer in a prepaid health plan, *Cancer Res.,* 48, 2284, 1988.

37. **Hiatt, R. A.,** Alcohol consumption and breast cancer, *Med. Oncol. Tumor Pharmacother.,* 7, 143, 1990.

38. **Horiike, N., Michitaka, K., Onji, M., et al.,** HBV-DNA hybridization in hepatocellular carcinoma associated with alcohol in Japan, *J. Med. Virol.,* 28, 189, 1989.

39. **Iishi, H., Tatsuta, M., Baba, M., et al.,** Promotion by ethanol of gastric carcinogenesis induced by *N*-methyl-*N'*-nitro-*N*-nitrosoguanidine in Wistar rats, *Br. J. Cancer,* 59, 719, 1989.

40. **Imai, T., Carrillo, V. M., Yokoi, H., et al.,** Clinicopathological studies and operative results of hepatocellular carcinoma with liver cirrhosis, comparing HB-associated cirrhosis to alcoholic and post-transfusion cirrhosis, *Gastroenterol. Jpn.,* 25, 54, 1990.

41. **Ishimaru, H. and Matsuda, T.,** T cell subsets (Tc, Th, Ts, Tsi) and IL2 receptor-bearing cells in peripheral blood of patients in the acute phase of alcoholic hepatitis, *Alcohol and Alcoholism,* 25, 353, 1990.

42. **Ito, M., Hsu, C.-T., Shikuwa, S., et al.,** Multiple myeloma in alcoholic liver cirrhosis, *Tohoku J. Exp. Med.,* 157, 39, 1989.

43. **Jerrells, T. R., Marietta, C. A., Bone, G., et al.,** Ethanol-associated immunosuppression, *Adv. Biochem. Psychopharmacol.,* 44, 173, 1988.

44. **Jerrells, R., Perritt, D., Marietta, C., et al.,** Mechanisms of suppression of cellular immunity induced by ethanol, *Alcohol. Clin. Exp. Res.,* 13, 490, 1989.

45. **Jerrells, T. R., Smith, W., and Eckardt, M. J.,** Murine model of ethanol-induced immunosuppression, *Alcohol. Clin. Exp. Res.,* 14, 546, 1990.

46. **Jerrells, T. R., Marietta, C. A., Eckardt, M. J., et al.,** Effects of ethanol administration on parameters of immunocompetency in rats, *J. Leukocyte Biol.,* 39, 499, 1986.

47. **Jerrells, T. R., Perritt, D., Eckardt, M. J., et al.,** Alterations in interleukin-2 utilization by T-cells from rats treated with an ethanol-containing diet, *Alcohol. Clin. Exp. Res.,* 14, 245, 1990.

48. **Jovanovic, R., Worner, T., Lieber, C. S., et al.,** Lymphocyte subpopulations in patients with alcoholic liver disease, *Dig. Dis. Sci.,* 31, 125, 1986.

49. **Kabat, G. C. and Wynder, E. L.,** Type of alcoholic beverage and oral cancer, *Int. J. Cancer,* 43, 190, 1989.

50. **Kabat, G. C., Howson, C. P., and Wynder, E. L.,** Beer consumption and rectal cancer, *Int. J. Epidemiol.,* 15, 494, 1986.

51. **Kaplan, D. R.,** A novel mechanism of immunosuppression mediated by ethanol, *Cell. Immunol.,* 102, 1, 1986.

52. **Karhunen, P. J., Penttila, A., Liesto, K., et al.,** Occurrence of benign hepatocellular tumors in alcoholic men, *Acta Pathol. Microbiol. Immunol. Scand. Sect. A,* 94, 141, 1986.

53. **Kikendall, J. W., Bowen, P. E., Burgess, M. B., et al.,** Cigarettes and alcohol as independent risk factors for colonic adenomas, *Gastroenterology,* 97, 660, 1989.

54. **Klatsky, A. L., Armstrong, M. A., Friedman, G. D., et al.,** The relation of alcoholic beverage use to colon and rectal cancer, *Am. J. Epidemiol.,* 128, 1007, 1988.
55. **Konishi, N., Kitahori, Y., Shimoyama, T., et al.,** Effects of sodium chloride and alcohol on experimental esophageal carcinogenesis induced by *N*-nitrosopiperidine in rats, *Jpn. J. Cancer Res.,* 77, 446, 1986.
56. **Kristiansen, E., Clemmensen, S., and Meyer, O.,** Chronic ethanol intake and reduction of lung tumours from urethane in Strain A mice, *Food Chem. Toxicol.,* 28, 35, 1990.
57. **Kune, G. A. and Kune, S.,** The nutritional causes of colorectal cancer: an introduction to the Melbourne Study, *Nutr. Cancer,* 9, 1, 1987.
58. **Kunze, E., Claude, J., and Frentzel-Beyme, R.,** Association of cancer of the lower urinary tract with consumption of alcoholic beverages. A case-control study, *Carcinogenesis,* 7, 163, 1986.
59. **Leclerc, A., Brugere, J., Luce, D., et al.,** Type of alcoholic beverage and cancer of the upper respiratory and digestive tract, *Eur. J. Cancer Clin. Oncol.,* 5, 529, 1987.
60. **Lieber, C. S.,** Interaction of ethanol with drugs, hepatotoxic agents, carcinogens and vitamins, *Alcohol and Alcoholism,* 25, 157, 1990.
61. **Lieber, C. S., Garro, A., Leo, M. A., et al.,** Alcohol and cancer, *Hepatology,* 6, 1005, 1986.
62. **Lowenfels, A. B. and Zevola, S. A.,** Alcohol and breast cancer: an overview, *Alcohol.: Clin. Exp. Res.,* 13, 109, 1989.
63. **MacGregor, R. R., Safford, M., and Shalit, M.,** Effect of ethanol on functions required for the delivery of neutrophils to sites of inflammation, *J. Infect. Dis.,* 157, 682, 1988.
64. **MacGregor, R. R.,** *In Vivo* neutrophil delivery in men with alcoholic cirrhosis is normal despite depressed *in vitro* chemotaxis, *Alcohol.: Clin. Exp. Res.,* 14, 195, 1990.
65. **Maduagwu, E. N. and Uhegbu, F. O.,** *N*-nitrosamines and Nigerian habitual drinks and cancer, *Carcinogenesis,* 7, 149, 1986.
66. **Marietta, C. A., Jerrells, T. R., Meagher, R. C., et al.,** Effects of long-term ethanol inhalation on the immune and hematopoietic systems of the rat, *Alcohol.: Clin. Exp. Res.,* 12, 211, 1988.
67. **Matsushima, Y,.** Chromosomal aberrations in the lymphocytes of alcoholics and former alcoholics, *Neuropsychobiology,* 17, 24, 1987.
68. **McCoy, G. D., Hecht, S. S., and Furuya, K.,** The effect of chronic ethanol consumption on the tumorigenicity of *N*-nitrosopyrrolidine in male Syrian Golden Hamsters, *Cancer Lett.,* 33, 151, 1986.
69. **McGarrith, T. J., Peiffer, L. P., Colony, P. C., et al.,** The effects of chronic ethanol administration on polyamine content during dimethylhydrazine-induced colorectal carcinogenesis in the rat, *Carcinogenesis,* 9, 2093, 1988.
70. **Meadows, G. G., Bank, S. E., and Duncan, D. D.,** Influence of ethanol consumption on natural killer cell activity in mice, *Alcohol.: Clin. Exp. Res.,* 13, 476, 1989.
71. **Meara, J., et al.,** Alcohol, cigarette smoking and breast cancer, *Br. J. Cancer,* 60, 70, 1990.
72. **Mendenhall, C., Roselle, G. A., Lybecker, L., et al.,** Hepatitis B vaccination, response of alcoholic with and without liver injury, *Dig. Dis. Sci.,* 33, 263, 1988.
73. **Merletti, F., Boffetta, P., Ciccone, G., et al.,** Role of tobacco and alcoholic beverages in the etiology of cancer of the oral cavity/oropharynx in Torino, Italy, *Cancer Res.,* 49, 4919, 1989.
74. **Morland, B. and Morland, H.,** The interaction of ethanol with human monocyte IgG-Fc receptors, characterized by monoclonal antibodies raised against two distinct receptor subpopulations, *Scand. J. Immunol.,* 25(5), 573, 1989.
75. **Mozes, G., Beak, G., Lang, I., et al.,** Studies on the monocyte interleukin-1 and tumor necrosis factor-alpha production in patients with alcohol liver cirrhosis, *Acta Medica Hung.,* 46, 253, 1989.

76. **Mufti, S. I., Becker, G., and Sipes, I. G.**, Effect of chronic dietary ethanol consumption on the initiation and promotion of chemically-induced esophageal carcinogenesis in experimental rats, *Carcinogenesis,* 10, 303, 1989.
77. **Mufti, S. I., Prabhala, R., Moriguchi, S., et al.**, Functional and numerical alterations induced by ethanol in the cellular immune system, *Immunopharmacology,* 15, 85, 1988.
78. **Mufti, S. I., Darban, H. R., and Watson, R. R.**, Alcohol, cancer, and immunomodulation, *Crit. Rev. Oncol. Hematol.,* 9, 243, 1989.
79. **Nilsson, E., Lindstrom, P., Patarroyo, M., et al.**, Ethanol impairs certain aspects of neutrophil adhesion *in vitro:* comparisons with inhibition of expression of the CD18 antigen, *J. Infect. Dis.,* 163, 591, 1991.
80. **Nonomura, A., Hayashi, M., Takayanagi, N., et al.**, Correlation of morphologic subtypes of liver cirrhosis with excess alcohol intake, HBV infection, age at death, and hepatocellular carcinoma. A study on 234 autopsy cases in Japan. *Acta Pathol. Jpn.,* 36(5), 631, 1986.
81. **Nonomura, A., Hayashi, M., Watanabe, K., et al.**, Studies on the pathogenesis of hepatocellular carcinoma in HBV-negative alcoholic cirrhotics, *Acta Pathol. Jpn.,* 36, 1297, 1986.
82. **Norell, S. E., Ahlbom, A., and Erwald, R.**, Diet and pancreatic cancer: A case control study, *Am. J. Epidemiol.,* 124, 894, .
83. **Nouri-Aria, K. T., Alexander, G. J. M., Portmann, J. E., et al.**, T and B cell function in alcoholic liver disease, *J. Hepatol.,* 2, 195, 1986.
84. **Olm, M., Gonzalez, F. J., Fuster, J., et al.**, Primary liver and esophageal neoplasms in an alcoholic patient, *Am. J. Gastroenterol.,* 85, 108, 1990.
85. **Parazzini, F., et al.**, Methylxanthine, alcohol-free diet and fibrocystic breast disease: a factorial clinical trial, *Surgery,* 90, 576, 1986.
86. **Parent, L. J., Ehrlich, R., Matis, L., et al.**, Ethanol: an enhancer of major histocompatibility complex antigen expression, *FJ Res. Commun.,* 1, 469, 1987.
87. **Prior, P.**, Long-term cancer risk in alcoholism, *Alcohol and Alcoholism,* 23, 163, 1988.
88. **Radike, M. J., Stemmer, K. L., and Bingham, E.**, Effect of ethanol on vinyl chloride carcinogenesis, *Environ. Health Perspect.,* 41, 59, 1981.
89. **Rogers, A. E. and Conner, M. W.**, Alcohol and cancer, *Adv. Exp. Med. Biol.,* 206, 473, 1986.
90. **Roselle, G. A., Mendenhall, C. L., and Grossman, C. J.**, Ethanol and soluble mediators of host response, *Alcohol.: Clin. Exp. Res.,* 13, 494, 1989.
91. **Roselle, G., Mendenhall, C. L., Grossman, C. J., et al.**, Lymphocyte subset alterations in patients with alcoholic hepatitis, *J. Clin. Lab. Immunol.,* 26, 169, 1988.
92. **Rothman, K. J., Cann, C. I., and Fried, M. P.**, Carcinogenicity of dark liquor, *Am. J. Public Health,* 79, 1516, 1989.
93. **Sankaranarayanan, R., Duffy, S. W., and Padmakumary, G.**, Tobacco chewing, alcohol and nasal snuff in cancer of the gingiva in Kerala, India, *Br. J. Cancer,* 60, 638, 1989.
94. **Saxena, Q., Saxena, R., and Adler, W.**, Regulation of natural killer activity *in vivo,* Part IV, *Ind. J. Exp. Biol.,* 19, 1001, 1981.
95. **Seitz, H. K. and Simanowski, U. A.**, Ethanol and carcinogenesis of the alimentary tract, *Alcohol.: Clin. Exp. Res.,* 6 (Suppl.), 335, 1986.
96. **Seitz, H. K. and Simanowski, U. A.**, Alcohol and carcinogenesis, *Annu. Rev. Nutr.,* 8, 99, 1988.
97. **Seitz, H. K., Simanowski, U. A., Garzon, F. T., et al.**, Possible role of acetaldehyde in ethanol-related rectal cocarcinogenesis in the rat, *Gastroenterology,* 98, 406, 1990.
98. **Seitz, H. K., Simanowski, U. A., Garzon, F. T., et al.**, Alcohol and cancer letter, *Hepatology,* 7, 616, 1987.

99. **Silberman, S., McGarvey, T. W., Comrie, E., et al.,** The influence of ethanol on cell membrane fluidity, migration, and invasion of murine melanoma cells, *Exp. Cell. Res.,* 189, 64, 1990.

100. **Singer, D. S., Parent, L. J., and Kolber, M. A.,** Ethanol: an enhancer of transplantation antigen expression, *Alcohol.: Clin. Exp. Res.,* 13, 480, 1989.

101. **Skegg, D. C. G.,** Alcohol, coffee, fat, and breast cancer, *Br. Med. J.,* 295, 1011, 1987.

102. **Smith, D. I.,** Relationship between alcohol consumption and breast cancer morbidity rates in Western Australia, *Drug Alcohol Dependence,* 24, 61, 1989.

103. **Spinozzi, F., Rambotti, P., Gerli, R., et al.,** Immunoregulatory T cells in alcoholic liver disease: phenotypical dissection of circulating LEU3$^+$/T4$^+$ inducer T-lymphocytes, *J. Clin. Lab. Immunol.,* 23, 161, 1987.

104. **Stefani, E. D., Correa, P., Oreggia, F., et al.,** Black tobacco, wine and mate in oropharyngeal cancer. A case-control study from Uruguay, *Rev. Epidemiol. et Sante Publ.,* 36, 389, 1988.

105. **Swann, P. F., Graves, R. J., and Mace, R.,** ICPMEC working paper No. 15/6. Effect of ethanol on nitrosamine metabolism and distribution. Implications for the role of nitrosamines in human cancer and for the influence of alcohol consumption on cancer incidence, *Mutation Res.,* 186, 261, 1987.

106. **Takada, A., Nei, J., Takase S., et al.,** Effects of ethanol on experimental hepatocarcinogenesis, *Hepatology,* 6, 65, 1986.

107. **Takahashi, M., Hasegawa, R., Furukawa, F., et al.,** Effects of ethanol, potassium metabisulfite, formaldehyde and hydrogen peroxide on gastric carcinogenesis in rats after initiation with N-methyl-N'-nitro-N-nitrosoguanidine, *Jpn. J. Cancer Res.,* 77, 118, 1986.

108. **Tanaka, T., Nishikawa, A., Iwata, H., et al.,** Enhancing effect of ethanol on aflatoxin B$_1$-induced hepatocarcinogenesis in male ACI/N rats, *Jpn. J. Cancer Res.,* 80, 526, 1989.

109. **Tuyns, A. J.,** Beer consumption and rectal cancer, *Rev. Epidemiol. et Sante Publ.,* 36, 144, 1988.

110. **Tuyns, A. J.,** Cancer risks derived from alcohol, *Med. Oncol. and Tumor Pharmacother.,* 4, 241, 1987.

111. **Vecchia, C. L. A., Decarli, A., Mezzanotte, G., et al.,** Mortality from alcohol related disease in Italy, *J. Epidemiol. Community Health,* 40, 257, 1986.

112. **Velema, J. P., Walker, A. M., and Gold, E. B.,** Alcohol and pancreatic cancer, *Epidemiol. Rev.,* 8, 28, 1986.

113. **Walia, A. S. and Lamon, E. W.,** Ethanol inhibition of cell-mediated lysis of antibody-sensitized target cells at a calcium-dependent step (42975), *Proc. Soc. Exp. Biol. Med.,* 192, 177, 1989.

114. **Walter, E., Blum, H. E., Meier, P., et al.,** Hepatocellular carcinoma in alcoholic liver disease: no evidence for a pathogenetic role of hepatitis B virus infection, *Hepatology,* 8, 745, 1988.

115. **Wasunna, A. E. O.,** Carcinoma of the oesophagus: alcohol, tobacco and vitamins, *East African Med. J.,* 63, 569, 1986.

116. **Watson, R. R.,** Ethanol immunomodulation and cancer, *Prog. in Food and Nutr. Sci.,* 12, 189, 1988.

117. **Watson, R. R., Prabhala, R. H., Abril, E., et al.,** Changes in lymphocyte subsets and macrophage functions from high, short-term dietary ethanol in C57/BL6 mice, *Life Sci.,* 43, 865, 1988.

118. **Watson, R. R., Prabhala, R. H., Darban, H. R., et al.,** Changes in lymphocyte and macrophage subsets due to morphine and ethanol treatment during a retrovirus infection causing murine aids, *Life Sci.,* 43, 5, 1988.

119. **Wickramasinghe, S. N.,** Observations on the biochemical basis of ethanol metabolism by human macrophages, *Alcohol and Alcoholism,* 21, 57, 1986.

120. **Woutersen, R. A., van Garderen-Hoetmer, A., Bax, J., et al.,** Modulation of putative preneoplastic foci in exocrine pancreas of rats and hampsters. I. Interaction of dietary fat and ethanol, *Carcinogenesis,* 7, 1587, 1986.

121. **Wynder, E. L.,** American health foundation workshop on alcohol and breast cancer, *Prev. Med.,* 17, 667, 1988.

122. **Yanagi, S., Yamashita, M., Hiasa, Y., et al.,** Effects of ethanol on hepatocarcinogenesis initiated in rats with 3′-methyl-4-dimethylaminoazobenzene in the absence of liver injuries, *Int. J. Cancer,* 44, 681, 1989.

123. **Ziegler, R. G.,** Alcohol-nutrient interactions in cancer etiology, *Cancer,* 58, 1942, 1986.

Chapter 2

EFFECTS OF ETHANOL ON CELLULAR IMMUNITY AND ANTIMICROBIAL IMMUNE RESPONSES

Thomas R. Jerrells

TABLE OF CONTENTS

I. BACKGROUND

Many study findings have suggested that ethanol (ETOH) abuse results in changes in the immune system. Susceptibility to infectious diseases such as tuberculosis, opportunistic infections, tumors, and autoimmune diseases are believed to be sequelae of these changes.[1,2]

Published experimental data have helped to define the effects of ETOH on the immune system. It has been shown that ingestion of ETOH by human beings under experimental conditions, or administration of ETOH to experimental animals, results in a number of changes in the immune system. These changes include a loss of circulating lymphoid cells[1,3] and a loss of cells from the peripheral lymphoid organs, most notably the spleen and thymus.[3-8] Incidentally, it has also been shown that ETOH depletes bone marrow stem cells of the erythroid series and inhibits the function of these cells.[7] It is not clear whether ETOH has an effect on the granulocyte-monocyte precursor cells in the bone marrow. Available evidence, however, would lead one to believe that this cell lineage is not greatly affected.

Perhaps of more importance are the study findings that have established that ETOH affects lymphocyte function. Briefly, it has been shown that the proliferation of lymphocytes in both human beings and animals is diminished by *in vivo* exposure to ETOH.[3,7-10] Interestingly, the exposure of isolated lymphocytes to ETOH in culture has generally been shown to have no effect, or to be slightly stimulatory at low levels.[37]

The ability of an animal to generate a primary immune response in terms of antibody production to a foreign antigen has also been shown to be compromised by ETOH ingestion.[8,11,12] As will be described later, this defect seems to be selective for only certain antigens — in particular, those antigens under the control of helper T cells. Preliminary study findings from this laboratory have shown that the *in vitro* secondary response to a recall antigen (keyhole limpet hemocyanin), as measured by lymphocyte proliferation, is also diminished in immune animals administered ETOH.[13]

Although it is beyond the scope of this chapter, it has been shown that a number of nonspecific host defense mechanisms are affected by ETOH. These include changes in granulocyte function and mobility[1,4,5] and alterations in function of mononuclear phagocytes — most importantly, the phagocytic cells of the liver.[14] Recently, it has been reported that the production of the macrophage product tumor necrosis factor is diminished in animals treated acutely with ETOH.[15]

On the basis of existing information, it can be concluded that ETOH abuse has a profound negative effect on the immune system. It can be speculated that this negative effect of ETOH would lead to an increased incidence of infections and tumors. Very little information is available concerning the effect of ETOH on the development of autoimmune disease. Some workers believe that ETOH-associated liver disease is due to autoimmune reactivity.

The fact that lymphocytes from persons with liver disease respond to proteins derived from liver cells supports this contention. This intriguing area of research requires further study.

The purpose of this chapter is to describe recent studies that have provided insight into the mechanisms of the ETOH-associated alterations in lymphocyte functions. The emphasis will be on work performed in this laboratory. Where appropriate, however, other data will be described.

II. ANIMAL MODELS

The work done in this laboratory has used three animal models of ETOH administration or ingestion. The original studies were performed with the use of a rat model system developed by Majchrowicz.[16] In this model, ETOH is given for a relatively short period of time (4 to 5 days), but in relatively large amounts (8 to 11 g/kg body weight/day) by intubation. Treatment of rats by this protocol involves administering ETOH in fractional doses throughout the day to maintain intoxication. We described a profound effect of ETOH on the immune system using this model system,[8] including loss of thymocytes and spleen cells, and a functional loss of lymphocyte proliferative responses to T and B cell mitogens. We also demonstrated that the antibody production to T cell-dependent antigens, as measured by an antibody-producing cell assay[17] was markedly diminished by ETOH administration.

The administration of ETOH by the above method would have a major effect on the gastrointestinal tract, and perhaps alter the immune status of the animal. To overcome this problem we have studied the effects of ETOH using a model system in which ETOH is given to animals by inhalation.[7] The results of this study were essentially the same as those in our original study, except that the proliferation response to mitogens by peripheral blood mononuclear cells was not altered by ETOH. This system differs from the other system in that the blood ETOH levels remain constant and do not drop during periods when ETOH is not given in diet. This very likely results in a lack of withdrawal and the associated stress response. Two points are worthy of mention regarding this model. First, it can be surmised from these data that ETOH-associated immunosuppression is relatively independent of withdrawal stress, although this was not formally addressed in this study. Second, alterations in the immune system related to ETOH administration are independent of the effects of ETOH on the gastrointestinal system.

We have recently used a mouse-model system in which ETOH is given to the animals in Lieber-DeCarli diet, Bioserv, French, NJ, and the experiments are controlled by feeding another group of animals an isocaloric diet without ETOH in a paired-feeding design. This model system has shown immune system abnormalities similar to those described above.[18] This model system has the advantage of allowing exposure of animals to ETOH for various times, and perhaps of examining the effects of chronic ETOH ingestion on the immune system. Also, much is known about the murine immune system, and a large number of reagents are available for use. Additionally, inbred strains of animals are available, which differ in susceptibility to natural infectious agents and tumors, and perhaps in their response to ETOH.

III. EFFECTS OF ETOH ON LYMPHOCYTE SUBPOPULATIONS

As discussed earlier, one of the effects of ETOH is depletion of the thymus and spleen of mononuclear cells. The cell loss from the thymus in terms of cell numbers suggests that immature cells might be lost from this organ. To define the lymphocyte subpopulations that were lost from each organ, we performed flow cytometric analyses of cells from each tissue with the use of available monoclonal antibodies for specific populations of lymphocytes. We found that ETOH ingestion using the paired feeding design described above resulted in a loss of predominantly immature thymocytes ($CD4^+/CD8^+$ and PNA^+) from the thymus.[36] With the use of immunohistochemical techniques, this finding was confirmed with thin sections of the thymus. Changes in the mature T cell population in the thymus ($CD4^+/CD8^-$ or $CD4^-/CD8^+$) were evident only after prolonged exposure to ETOH, and both populations were proportionately lost from the thymus.

Surprisingly, the cells lost from the spleen in greatest numbers were cells with the characteristics of B cells (surface Ig^+). T cells were lost as well, but not in as great numbers as B cells, and no differences were noted in the class of T cells lost ($CD4^+$ or $CD8^+$). These observations were also confirmed by immunohistochemistry studies. Although B cells were lost in greatest numbers, the intrinsic function of these cells was not affected (see later section).

IV. EFFECTS OF CORTICOSTEROIDS

Because of the similarity between the effects of ETOH on the thymus and published data on the effects of corticosteroids, especially the loss of immature thymocytes, we investigated the role of corticosteroids in the observed phenomena associated with ETOH administration to experimental animals. Initial experiments used rats in whom adrenal glands had been removed surgically.[19] It was first noted that the animals who were adrenalectomized (ADX) did not tolerate ETOH as well as sham-ADX rats, and it was necessary to reduce the amount of ETOH in the diet given to each group. Nevertheless, the reduced ETOH diet was associated with a loss of cells from the thymus, and a defect in lymphocyte function, as measured by proliferation and the production of T cell-dependent antibody responses similar to those described in the earlier studies.[7,8] The administration of ETOH to ADX animals still produced a loss of spleen cells essentially of the same magnitude as that

TABLE 1
Effect of Adrenalectomy on the ETOH-Induced Loss of Spleen Cells and Thymus Cells[a]

	Control diet	ETOH diet
Spleen	$11 \pm 0.7 \times 10^{7b}$	$7.2 \pm 0.6 \times 10^7$
Thymus	$5.2 \pm 0.9 \times 10^7$	$2.6 \pm 0.4 \times 107$

[a] Adrenalectomized C57Bl/6 mice were fed either control diet, or a diet containing 5% (v/v) ETOH for eight days.

[b] Total cells/organ $\pm$ standard error of the mean. Each data point is the mean of five mice fed control diet and ten mice fed ETOH-containing diet.

observed in the control animals. The loss of thymocytes was partially reduced by adrenalectomy, but ETOH still induced approximately 50% loss of thymocytes. It has been shown in preliminary experiments with the use of flow cytometry, that the same cell populations are lost, regardless of whether the animal had adrenal glands, but adrenalectomy reduced the magnitude of the cells lost. Interestingly, adrenalectomy did not affect the suppression of antibody responses to the T-dependent antigen sheep erythrocytes, and ETOH did not affect the immune response to the T-independent antigen trinitrophenyl (TNP)-ficoll. The effect of adrenalectomy on the response to TNP-ficoll was to elevate further the number of antibody-producing cells. Proliferation of mature circulating lymphocytes in response to mitogens was essentially restored to normal levels by adrenalectomy. This finding suggested a role for corticosteroids in this effect. Whether the appropriate cell types (i.e., helper T cells) are responding to stimulation in ADX animals remains to be seen. The normal response of the cells to proliferative stimuli and the lack of T-dependent antibody response remains a paradox. It is possible, however, that, as mentioned above, the inappropriate cell type is proliferating, or the appropriate cytokines for B cell activation and differentiation are not being produced. These questions are currently being addressed.

The above studies were performed by using the model system of Majchrowicz[16] in which animals are intubated with large amounts of ETOH for short periods of time. Thus, the high levels of ETOH may have induced an artifact. To avoid high levels of ETOH, we studied C57Bl/6 mice that had been ADX and fed a liquid diet containing ETOH or an isocaloric control diet (Lieber-DeCarli diet, Bioserv, French, NJ). As before, the amount of ETOH in the diet was reduced to 5% v/v. Again, animals who were unable to produce adrenocorticosteroids showed a loss of spleen and thymus cells (Table 1). The loss of thymocytes was less than that seen in animals fed ETOH who retained their adrenal glands, but significantly ($p \leq 0.05$, Student's t test) greater than the cell loss from mice fed control diet.

The T-dependent antibody response to sheep erythrocytes was also depressed in these animals, regardless of whether they were ADX (Table 2).

TABLE 2
Effect of Adrenalectomy on the ETOH-Associated Suppression of Antibody Production to Sheep Erythrocytes[a]

Control diet	ETOH diet
$1.4 \pm 0.2 \times 10^{5b}$	$0.6 \pm 0.06 \times 10^5$

[a] See legend for Table 1.
[b] Mean IgM plaque-forming cell response/spleen $\pm$ standard error of the mean. Each data point is the mean response of five mice fed control diet and ten mice fed ETOH-containing diet.

We have not adequately studied the effects of adrenalectomy on lymphocyte proliferation in this model system, and cannot draw any conclusions regarding the effects of steroids on this parameter. We have shown, however, that ETOH ingestion in this system results in diminished lymphocyte proliferation to mitogens and alloantigens similar to that noted in our earlier studies.

V. MECHANISMS OF DECREASED LYMPHOCYTE PROLIFERATION

One of the most important aspects of T cell responses is the production of interleukin-2 (IL-2) and the expression of receptors for IL-2.[20,21] Because it was possible that the observed decrease in proliferation in ETOH-treated animals was due to alterations in IL-2 production or utilization, we measured the ability of the T cell to produce IL-2 in response to stimulation, and the ability of IL-2 receptor-bearing cells to respond to IL-2.[22] We found that ETOH did not affect the ability of the T cell to produce IL-2, and, if anything, IL-2 production was slightly greater in cells from ETOH-treated animals. It was found, however, that blast cells expressing IL-2 receptors did not proliferate in response to added recombinant IL-2, as would be expected. This was not due to the ability of the isolated T cell blasts to bind IL-2 but, in preliminary studies, perhaps due to internalize the bound IL-2. It is also possible that the defect is in the transduction of the IL-2 signal to the nucleus once the receptor-ligand complex is internalized. Studies are underway to address these two possibilities.

VI. EFFECTS OF ETOH ON PRIMARY ANTIBODY RESPONSES

We and others[8,11] have shown that ETOH affects the primary antibody response to sheep erythrocytes. This antibody response is dependent on functional helper T cells. It is interesting to note that the antibody response to TNP-ficoll, a T cell-independent antigen, is relatively unaffected by ETOH.[11,19]

We have confirmed the finding that the T cell-independent B cell response is relatively intact, with the use of a clonal precursor analysis approach to determine the frequency of lipopolysaccharide-responsive B cells in the spleens of ETOH-treated mice.[38] Recently, we have expanded this finding to the T-independent microbial antigen phosphorylcholine. These data support the tentative conclusion that ETOH is primarily affecting T cell-dependent immune functions.

VII. EFFECTS OF FETAL ALCOHOL EXPOSURE ON THE IMMUNE SYSTEM

In several laboratories, investigators are currently working to define the effects of *in utero* exposure to ETOH on the developing immune system. We and other workers propose that exposure to ETOH results in subtle changes in the immune system that result in impairments of the adult individual. Study results showing increased infections and changes in lymphocyte responses of children with fetal alcohol syndrome support this idea.[23,24]

Work by Ewald and co-workers[25,26] has shown that exposure of fetal mice to ETOH in the mothers' diet results in changes in the thymus lymphocyte populations. The extent or consequences of these changes has not been established.

It has also been shown that rats exposed to ETOH show an impairment in mature lymphocyte proliferation to IL-2 after stimulation with concanavalin A (ConA) stimulation.[27] My laboratory has established a collaboration with Dr. JoAnn Weinberg at the University of British Columbia to test the immune system of rats exposed to ETOH *in utero* using her protocols.[28] We have found and reported[29,30] that adult animals exposed to ETOH *in utero* have an impairment in their response to ConA, and an inability of blast cells recovered from stimulated cultures to respond to stimulation with IL-2. It is interesting to note that not all of the animals tested demonstrated an inability, and when the data were examined closely it was found that only the male animals showed the impairment. Furthermore, not all male animals were deficient in their proliferative response to ConA, but blast cells from all male animals responded poorly to IL-2. This surprising result is being studied further in my laboratory now. Gender differences also exist in the response to stress of fetal alcohol-exposed rats. Female animals are more responsive to stress than male animals.[31] Again, it is not clear how stress influences the observations we have made concerning the effects of fetal alcohol on the immune system.

VIII. EFFECTS OF ETHANOL ON *IN VIVO* RESPONSE

The majority of studies performed in this laboratory and other laboratories have documented the effect of ETOH on cellular immune mechanisms with the use of *in vitro* parameters of immunocompetence. To determine if the changes in T cell function described above exist *in vivo* and reflect relevant changes in the immune system, we studied the effect of ETOH on the development of immunity to the facultative intracellular bacterium *Listeria monocytogenes,* and responsiveness of splenic T cells to stimulation with anti-CD3 monoclonal antibody injected intravenously.

We used *Listeria monocytogenes* because of the well-documented role of cell-mediated immunity in clearance of this organism from the livers of infected mice.[32,33] Animals were fed an ETOH-containing or control diet for five days, at which time animals from each group were injected intravenously (i.v.) with 5×10^4 bacteria (1/2 lethal dose [LD][50]), and continued on the appropriate diet until studied. After two and five days of infection, serum enzyme levels, bacterial colony counts in the liver and spleen, and liver histologic studies were obtained.

The results of these studies dramatically show that ETOH has a profound effect on T cell function *in vivo*.[39]

Briefly, it was found that the numbers of bacteria in the livers and spleens of ETOH-treated animals were 100 to 1000 times higher than the numbers from the same organs obtained from control-diet treated animals. This was most obvious five days after infection. The numbers of bacteria were only slightly higher in ETOH-treated mice two days after infection. It was found that ETOH-treatment did not significantly alter the ability of the reticuloendothelial system to clear and nonspecifically kill most of the bacterial inoculum, as is characteristic of this system. These data suggest that initial bacterial replication was similar in both groups of mice, but ETOH treatment resulted in an inability to control bacterial growth.

When the livers were examined with histologic techniques, very interesting observations were made. Early in the infection (two days), both groups of mice showed numerous, large lesions in the liver, with morphology characteristic of abscesses. Numerous granulocytes and hepatocyte necrosis were evident. It has been suggested that ETOH inhibits chemotaxis of granulocytes to areas of inflammation, and at least in this murine model, of liver inflammation; this is apparently not a universal finding, as the lesions in the ETOH-treated animals contained similar numbers or slightly more granulocytes. Later in the infection (five days), the diet-treated mice had small, compact areas of inflammation, consisting of predominantly mononuclear cells with characteristic morphologic features of granulomas. The ETOH-treated animals, in contrast, showed large lesions containing mixed inflammatory cell infiltrates and numerous bacteria. Marked hepatocyte necrosis was still evident. Many of the lesions contained numerous lymphocytes and macrophages. These observations were confirmed by the finding of significantly higher bacterial counts in the livers of ETOH-treated mice (counts were found to be 10 to 100 times greater), and the enzymes aspartate aminotransferase (AST) and alanine aminotransferase (ALT) were also significantly higher in ETOH-treated, infected mice. These data support our hypothesis that ETOH inhibits the T cell-dependent clearance of bacteria from the liver and spleen.

In a second series of experiments, mice were immunized with a sublethal dose of *Listeria*. After one week to establish immunity, the immunized animals were placed on ETOH or control diet and, after five days of feeding, challenged with a lethal dose (10 LD_{50}) *Listeria* as before. As expected, the mice given the control diet readily cleared the bacterial inoculum as determined by bacterial colony counts, and this was associated with the formation of typical granulomas in the liver. As before, animals fed the ETOH diet were unable to resist the challenge, as determined with histological techniques, colony counts, and serum enzymes as described above. The histological examinations revealed large liver lesions in the ETOH-treated mice, with large areas of hepatocyte necrosis. Interestingly, the lesions in the livers of ETOH-treated mice contained predominantly mononuclear cells, and preliminary studies show that large numbers of T cells (Thy 1.2^+) and macrophages (Mac-1^+) were present in the liver lesions. These findings are consistent with our *in vitro* data[18] showing that T cell function is impaired by ETOH in this experimental animal model. It is also clear from our data that ETOH doesn't affect the ability of cells to migrate to sites of infection. However, it is likely that ETOH affects the T cell and/or macrophage response. Further work is in progress to address this possibility. From the data discussed above, we conclude that ETOH has a profound effect on the ability of animals to produce a primary immune response to *Listeria* and express a preexisting antilisterial immunity.

The effect of ETOH on *in vivo* T cell function has also been assessed in this laboratory by measuring T cell stimulation after injection of a monoclonal antibody (clone 145-2C11) with specificity for the CD3 molecule. This antibody has been shown to stimulate T cells *in vitro* and *in vivo*,[34,35] and this stimulation is analogous to the stimulation of the cell following recognition of an antigen-major histocompatibility protein complex by the T cell receptor. Preliminary studies were performed to determine the effect of ETOH on the *in vivo* responses of T cells to anti-CD3. Mice that were fed either control diet or ETOH diet for eight days were injected with 4μ of anti-CD3 monoclonal antibody and, at various times after *in vivo* stimulation ranging from 10 min to 18 h, ribonucleic acid (RNA) was extracted from spleen cells obtained from animals from each group. The expression of messenger RNA (mRNA) for the cytokine IL-2 and for the proto-oncogene C-rel was determined by slot-blot hybridization of cellular RNA with specific riboprobes prepared from IL-2, C-rel, and β-actin DNA.

It was found (Figure 1) that anti-CD3 monoclonal antibody stimulated the production of mRNA for IL-2 and C-rel in animals fed the control diet at the appropriate times after *in vivo* stimulation, essentially as shown by others.[34] In our experiments, this stimulation peaked between 2 and 4 h after injection of antibody. Interestingly, feeding ETOH to animals did not affect the production of IL-2 RNA at this early time point. This is in agreement with our previous study findings that showed that ETOH treatment of rats did not alter the ability of T cells to produce IL-2 *in vitro*.[22]

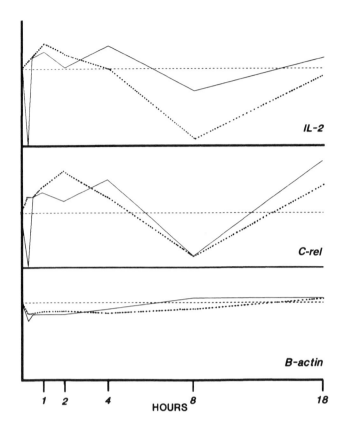

FIGURE 1. Relative expression of mRNA specific for IL-2, the proto-oncogene C-rel, and β-actin. The level of expression was quantified by densitometry of slot blots, and expressed relative to the level of message detected with the use of RNA obtained from spleens of animals that were not stimulated (- - -). Each point was obtained from three to five mice fed on ethanol-containing diet (· · ·) or control diet (——) for eight days. Each animal was injected by intravenous route with 4 μg of anti-CD3 antibody and spleen RNA obtained at the indicated times after injection. (From Jerrells, T. et al., *Alcohol*, 9, 1, 1992. With permission.)

We noted a later (18 h) peak of C-rel RNA in control animals that may be the result of T and/or B cell proliferation in response to the early production of T cell cytokines. Of interest was the finding that second peak of C-rel RNA production was markedly lower in ETOH-treated animals. It is possible that this is due to an inability of T cells or B cells to utilize cytokines essentially analogous to our *in vitro* findings. This intriguing possibility is under investigation at this time.

Our *in vivo* studies of T cell function in ETOH-treated animals have shown similar kinds of changes in T cell-dependent immune functions as did earlier studies performed with the use of *in vitro* parameters of immunity. The current approach should establish the range of effects ETOH has on T cell-dependent host defense mechanisms.

IX. SUMMARY

A number of study findings have shown that ETOH has a profound effect on the immune system. The work from my laboratory has established in animal models that the effect of ETOH is complex. It is well-established that ingestion of ETOH-containing diets results in a loss of lymphoid cells from the peripheral blood, spleen, and thymus. Some of the cell loss from the thymus is the result of corticosteroid release as a result of the withdrawal from ETOH, but the loss from the spleen and some of the thymocyte loss is independent of corticosteroids, as demonstrated by studies using ADX mice and rats.

We have also established that ETOH ingestion is associated with a loss of lymphocyte function, especially T cell-dependent immune responses. One aspect of the T cell defect is an inability to use IL-2, an important growth factor for T cells. Similar changes in lymphocyte function have been demonstrated in animals exposed to ETOH only *in utero*.

The inability of a person to respond immunologically in an appropriate fashion to foreign antigens has a profound effect on the survival of the person. It would be predicted that ETOH-associated immunosuppression would result in increased incidences of infections. From the data generated from my laboratory, it could also be predicted that these infections would be primarily opportunistic infections that are associated with defects in T cell function. The available literature would support these predictions. It is also likely that changes in T cell function would alter immunosurveillance mechanisms, with the end result being an increased incidence of tumors. Again, the available literature would support this prediction. Currently, we are attempting to establish a link between ETOH-induced immunosuppression and the predicted changes in the host with the use of *in vivo* parameters of T cell function.

ACKNOWLEDGMENTS

This work was supported in part by Grant AA-07731. The technical assistance of Rana Domiati-Saad and Eileen Clark is greatly appreciated.

REFERENCES

1. **MacGregor, R. R.,** Alcohol and immune defense, *JAMA,* 256, 1474, 1986.
2. **Eckardt, M. J., Hartford, T. C., Kaelber, C. T., et al.** Health hazards associated with alcohol consumption, *JAMA,* 246, 648, 1981.
3. **Tennenbaum, J. I., Ruppert, R. D., Pierre, R. St. Pierre, et al.,** The effect of chronic alcohol consumption on the immune responsiveness of rats, *J. Allergy,* 44, 272, 1969.
4. **Brayton, R. G., Stokes, P. E., Schwartz, M. S., et al.,** Effects of alcohol and various diseases on leukocyte mobilization, phagocytosis, and intracellular killing, *N. Engl. J. Med.,* 282, 123, 1970.

5. **Spagnuolo, R. J. and MacGregor, R. R.**, Acute ethanol effect on chemotaxis and other components of host defense, *J. Lab. Clin. Med.,* 86, 24, 1975.
6. **Slone, F. L., Smith, W. L., Jr., and VanThiel, D. H.**, The effects of alcohol and partial portal ligation on the immune system of the rat, *Gastroenterology,* 72, 1133, 1977.
7. **Marietta, C. A., Jerrells, T. R., Meagher, R. C., et al.**, Effects of long-term ethanol inhalation on the immune and hematopoietic systems of the rat, *Alcohol.: Clin. Exp. Res.,* 12, 211, 1988.
8. **Jerrells, T. R., Marietta, C. A., Eckardt, M. J., et al.**, Effects of ethanol administration on parameters of immunocompetency in rats, *J. Leukocyte Biol.,* 39, 499, 1986.
9. **Mutchnick, M. G. and Horchance, H. L.**, Impaired lymphocyte proliferation response to mitogen in alcoholic patients. Absence of a relation to liver disease activity, *Alcohol.: Clin. Exp. Res.,* 12, 155, 1988.
10. **Roselle, G. A. and Mendenhall, C. L.**, Ethanol-induced alterations in lymphocyte function in the guinea pig, *Alcohol.: Clin. Exp. Res.,* 8, 62, 1984.
11. **Bagasara, O., Howeedy, A., Dorio, R., et al.**, Functional analysis of T cell subsets in chronic experimental alcoholism, *Immunology,* 61, 63, 1987.
12. **Jerrells, T. R., Marietta, C. A., Bone, G., et al.**, Ethanol-associated immunosuppression, in *Psychological, Neuropsychiatric, and Substance Abuse Aspects of AIDS,* Bridge, T. P., Ed., Raven Press, New York, 1988, 173.
13. **Jerrells, T. R., Peritt, D., Marietta, C., et al.**, Mechanisms of suppression of cellular immunity induced by ethanol, *Alcohol.: Clin. Exp. Res.,* 13, 490, 1989.
14. **Galante, D., Adreana, A., Perna, P., et al.**, Decreased phagocytic and bactericidal activity of the hepatic reticuloendothelial system during chronic ethanol treatment and its restoration by levamisole, *J. Reticuloendothel. Soc.,* 32, 179, 1982.
15. **Nelson, S., Bagby, G. J., and Summer, W. R.**, Alcohol-induced suppression of tumor necrosis factor — A potential risk factor for secondary infection in the acquired immunodeficiency syndrome, in *Alcohol, Immunomodulation, and AIDS,* Seminara, D., Watson, R. R., and Pawlowski, A., Eds., Alan R. Liss, New York, 1990, 211.
16. **Majchrowicz, E.**, Induction of physical dependence upon ethanol and the associated behavioral changes in rats, *Psychopharmacologia,* 43, 245, 1975.
17. **Cunningham, A. M. and Szenberg, A.**, Further improvements in the plaque technique for antibody-forming cells, *Immunology,* 14, 599, 1968.
18. **Jerrells, T. R., Smith, W., and Eckardt, M. J.**, Murine model of ethanol-induced immunosuppression, *Alcohol.: Clin. Exp. Res.,* 14, 546, 1990.
19. **Jerrells, T. R., Marietta, C. A., Weight, F. F., and Eckardt, M. J.**, Effect of adrenalectomy on ethanol-associated immunosuppression, *Int. J. Immunopharmacol.,* 12, 435, 1990.
20. **Smith, K. A.**, Interleukin-2: inception, impact, and implications, *Science,* 242, 1169, 1988.
21. **Robb, R. J. and Greene, W. C.**, Internalization of interleukin-2 is mediated by the beta chain of the high-affinity interleukin-2 receptor, *J. Exp. Med.,* 165, 1201, 1987.
22. **Jerrells, T. R., Perritt, D., Eckardt, M. J., and Marietta, C. A.**, Alterations in interleukin-2 utilization by T cells from rats treated with an ethanol-containing diet, *Alcohol.: Clin. Exp. Res.,* 14, 245, 1990.
23. **Johnson, S., Knight, R., Marmer, D. J., et al.**, Immune deficiency in fetal alcohol syndrome, *Pediatr. Res.,* 15, 908, 1981.
24. **Monjan, A. A. and Mandell, W.**, Fetal alcohol and immunity: depression of mitogen-induced lymphocyte blastogenesis, *Neurobehav. Toxicol.,* 2, 213, 1980.
25. **Ewald, S. J. and Frost, W. W.**, Effect of prenatal exposure to ethanol on development of the thymus, *Thymus,* 9, 211, 1987.
26. **Ewald, S. J. and Walden, S. M.**, Flow cytometric and histologic analysis of mouse thymus in fetal alcohol syndrome, *J. Leukocyte Biol.,* 44, 434, 1988.

27. **Norman, D. C., Chang, M.-P., Castle, S. C., et al.,** Diminished proliferative response of Con A-blast cells to interleukin 2 in rats exposed to ethanol in utero, *Alcohol.: Clin. Exp. Res.,* 13, 69, 1989.
28. **Weinberg, J.,** Effects of ethanol and maternal nutritional status on fetal development, *Alcohol.: Clin. Exp. Res.,* 9, 49, 1985.
29. **Jerrells, T. R. and Weinberg, J.,** Suppression of immune responsiveness following prenatal ethanol exposure, *Alcohol.: Clin. Exp. Res.,* 13, 320, 1989.
30. **Weinberg, J. and Jerrells, T. R.,** Suppression of immune responsiveness: sex differences in prenatal ethanol effects, *Alcohol.: Clin. Exp. Res.,* 15, 525, 1991.
31. **Weinberg, J. and Gallo, P. V.,** Prenatal ethanol exposure: pituitary-adrenal activity in pregnant dams and offspring, *Neurobehav. Toxicol. Teratol.,* 4, 515, 1982.
32. **Sasaki, T., Mieno, M., Udono, H., Yamaguchi, K., Usui, T., Hara, K., Shiku, H., and Nakayama, E.,** Roles of CD4 + and CD8 + cells and the effect of administration of recombinant murine interferon γ in listerial infection, *J. Exp. Med.,* 171, 1141, 1990.
33. **Naher, H., Sperling, U., Takacs, L., and Hahn, H.,** Dynamics of T cells of L3T4 and Lyt 2 phenotype within granulomas in murine listeriosis, *Clin. Exp. Immunol.,* 60, 559, 198.
34. **Scott, D. E., Gause, W. C., Finkelman, F. D., and Steinberg, A. D.,** Anti-CD3 antibody induces rapid expression of cytokine genes *in vivo, J. Immunol.,* 145, 2183, 1990.
35. **Flamand, V., Abramowicz, D., Goldman, M., Biernaux, C., Huez, G., Urbain, J., Moser, M., and Leo, O.,** Anti-CD3 antibodies induce T cells from unprimed animals to secrete IL-4 both *in vitro* and *in vivo, J. Immunol.,* 144, 2875, 1990.
36. **Saad, A. J. and Jerrells, T. R.,** Ethanol-induced changes in the spleen and thymus: a flow cytometric and immunohistochemical study, *Alcohol.: Clin. Exp. Res.,* 15, 796, 1991.
37. **Jerrells, T. R.,** unpublished observations.
38. **Palafox, A. and Jerrells, T. R.,** unpublished observations.
39. **Saad, A. J. and Jerrells, T. R.,** Ethanol ingestion increases susceptibility of mice to *Listeria monocytes, Alcohol.: Clin. Exp. Res.,* in press.

Chapter 3

EFFECTS OF ALCOHOL ON T CELL IMMUNITY IN AGING MICE

Mei-Ping Chang and Dean C. Norman

TABLE OF CONTENTS

I. INTRODUCTION

Alcoholism remains a significant problem in the elderly population, and is a major factor contributing to a significant number of nursing home, psychiatric, and medical admissions in the elderly population. Ethanol exposure could compound the complexity of aging processes and enhance susceptibility of the elderly to certain infectious diseases and cancer. The question of whether the target cells affected most by aging are also the target for the effect of ethanol remains to be resolved. Our current knowledge of immunosenescence indicates that T cells appear to be the immune cells most vulnerable to the effects of aging.[1] An impairment of the proliferative response of T cells to antigen/mitogen stimulation appears to result from a decrease in production of lymphokines[2,13] and from altered biochemical and metabolic events, which precede the DNA replicative phase.[14-16] A great deal of evidence has shown that ethanol suppresses T cell proliferation and B cell antibody response to T cell-dependent antigenic sitmulation in normal young humans and experimental animals.[17,30] However, there is only a meager amount of information on the effect of ethanol on the activities of T and B cells obtained from aged humans and rodents.[31-34]

This chapter will present a brief overview of the age-related changes in T cell-mediated immunity and suppressive effects of ethanol on the activities of T cell functions in aged mice. An interpretative discussion on a mechanism of ethanol-mediated immunosuppression will then follow.

II. THE CELLULAR BASIS OF IMMUNOSENESCENCE

A. EFFECT OF AGE ON T CELLS AND THEIR GROWTH FACTOR (INTERLEUKIN-2)

Immune responses involve the coordinated efforts of three cell types: B cells, T cells, and macrophages, including a variety of macrophage-related cell types such as Langerhans cells and dendritic cells.

Changes in age-related immunologic activity could be due to an alteration in number or function of one or more of these interacting cells. The proliferative response of both T and B cells declines with age, but the decline in T cell response is greater than the decline in B cell response.[1] Many groups have found little or no change with age in subsets of T cell distribution.[6,35-39] On the other hand, studies also show an effect of age on the shift of T cell subsets, with some indicating a shift toward a decrease in CD4 cells,[40-42] and others toward increased proportions of CD8 cells.[43-45] However, the consensus is that changes in the relative proportions of T and B lymphocytes or in distribution of T cells between the CD4 and CD8 subsets are unlikely to explain age-related declines in immune function.

It has been shown that functionally meaningful cell subsets could exist within the aged individual.[36,38,39,46] Grossman et al.,[36] for example, while failing to find any age-dependent change in the relative proportions of CD3, CD4, or CD8 positive cells in human blood, did find an increase in a cell type expressing low levels of CD8 antigen and a decrease in a group of bright CD8[+] cells. Sidman et al.[39] found no change in the average density of CD4 or CD8 antigen on mouse T cells, but did note a loss with age in the average density of immunoglobulin IgM on B cells, and an increase in the density of H-2 histocompatibility antigens. The latter change was shown to be functionally significant, for the old cells with the higher H-2 antigen density became better able to respond to stimuli. Rabinowe et al.[38] have reported an age-related increase in the fraction of human peripheral blood T cells bearing the 3G5 glycolipid, from about 20 to 30% in young adults to over 50% in the elderly. Recently, Ernst et al.[46] have also demonstrated an alteration with age in mouse T cells expressing Pg-1 antigen, a marker for "memory" T cells. It has been well established that aging leads to a substantial decline in most T cell functions measured in both *in vitro* cell cultures[47-53] and *in vivo* systems.[49,54-56] The question remaining to be solved is what the nature of this functional deficit is in biochemical aspects.

It is known that upon activation by mitogenic (or antigenic) stimuli, T cells secrete a number of antigen-nonspecific growth and maturation factors known as lymphokines. Among these factors, interleukin 2 (IL-2), produced largely by the CD4 helper subset, seems to be required for T cell growth and differentiation, and plays a role in B cell growth, as well. Many groups have reported that T cells from old experimental animals or humans secrete less amounts of IL-2.[2-7,57-60] Evidence has also shown that the addition of IL-2 to *in vitro* cultures[6,61] or the injection of IL-2 into intact animals[62] can restore normal competence of T cells from old individuals. In many instances, however, addition of exogenous IL-2 leads only to a partial restoration of function in immune cells from old animals.[35,58,63,66] Furthermore, the number of T cells able to express IL-2 receptors (IL-2R) has also been shown to decline with age in humans and mice.[65,67] Recently Ernst et al.[46] have shown a decline in the number of murine T cells that can express IL-2R within both the CD4 and CD8 subsets. In addition, evidence has also shown that high-affinity IL-2R expression after exposure of human T cells to antigen or mitogen was diminished in the aged.[65,68] Findings generated by limiting dilution analysis have also shown that the number of antigen (or mitogen)-activated T cells, able to respond to saturating doses of IL-2, was diminished with age.[64,66] Thus, it has become clear that aging not only impairs production of IL-2 and expression of IL-2R, but also diminishes responsiveness to IL-2.

Why are T cells the most vulnerable to the effect of aging, and how are T cell functions diminished in aging? Before answering these questions, one could first ask whether age-related alterations affect all T cells equally and, if not, at what stage(s) of T cell activation impairment occurs? The findings generated by cytokinetic analyses have suggested that the number of T cells that can leave the G_0 resting phase and enter the mitotic cycle are decreased in aged individuals.[69-76] However, the results of Negoro et al.[65] on memory T cell responses to a tuberculin active protein (TAP) are an exception to this generalization. A decrease with age in the proportion of T cells that can respond to a stimulus was also confirmed by the limiting dilution analysis method.[64,66,74] In addition, it has been reported that aging leads to a decline in the number of activated T cells that are able to express IL-2R,[67] IL-2 messenger ribonucleic acid (mRNA),[13] and c-myc mRNA.[85] Taken together, these results thus suggest that aging leads to an accumulation of T cells that fail to enter the mitotic cycle when exposed to stimuli.

It is less clear, however, to what extent those T cells that do leave G_0 are functionally impaired at later points in the activation process. The findings of the limiting dilution studies on the frequency of IL-2 producing cells,[64] and clonal size of cytotoxic or proliferative T cells[66,74,75] suggest that there is little age-dependent decline in those T cells that can produce a detectable response. The data, however, based on cytokinetic analysis are more equivocal. For instance, while some groups report no change of normal cell kinetic parameters in old T cells that manage to enter G_1,[69,73,74] most report age-related impairment in cell cycle transition,[72] average length of cycle,[76] or numbers of cycles successfully negotiated.[36,65,75,76]

B. EFFECT OF AGE ON THE BIOCHEMICAL AND MOLECULAR EVENTS INVOLVED IN T CELL ACTIVATION

It is well established that the decreased T cell proliferation in aging individuals results from impaired production of lymphokines,[2-12] expression of IL-2 mRNA,[13] and IL-2R.[57,59,65,68] What could go wrong with earlier events in those old T cells that fail to respond to stimuli? The mitogen-induced rise in cytoplasmic Ca^{2+} is thought to be a key factor in triggering subsequent steps in the activation cascade. It is also known that an increase in cytoplasmic free calcium ion concentration occurring within the first few minutes is required for T cell activation upon stimulation with an activating mitogen (or antigen).

Evidence has shown age-related deficits in the generation of this Ca^{2+} signal in ConA-stimulated murine T cells.[14-16] What accounts for the defect in Ca^{2+} signal generation? It has been suggested that the decline with age in Ca^{2+} signal generation might be attributable to the decline in production of inositol triphosphate (IP_3) from its membrane phospholipid precursors.[77] Lerner et al.,[78] however, failed to detect any age-associated decline in production of either IP_3 or its immediate product, IP_4 in Concanavalin A (ConA)-stimulated mouse T cells. Furthermore, evidence has shown that an increased influx of Ca^{2+} from the extracellular medium within the first one minute of ConA addition, is also impaired in T cells from old mice.[79] The diminished calcium influx may reflect age-dependent alterations in G protein-mediated activation of phospholipase C. It has been shown that age-associated deficits in intracellular Ca^{2+} concentration can also be produced by treatment with ionomycin, a stimulus independent of transmembrane signal transduction.[77,79,80] This observation, thus, suggests that alterations in the calcium pump of the plasma membrane of T cells could result in sudden changes in intracellular Ca^{2+} levels.

The findings in human T cells may be somewhat different. Lustyik and O'Leary[37] were unable to detect any age-related change in the level of phytohaemagglutinin (PHA lectin mitogen) induced intracellular Ca^{2+} concentrations. Grossman et al.,[36] however, were able to demonstrate an age-associated decline in the level of intracellular Ca^{2+} concentrations in $CD4^+$ cells stimulated by anti-CD3 antibodies or PHA. However, the alterations in Ca^{2+} concentrations are unlikely to account for an age-associated decline in T cell proliferation because $CD8^+$ cells are affected more severely than $CD4^+$ cells.

The pathways by which changes in the level of intracellular cytoplasmic Ca^{2+} and activation of protein kinases eventually lead to new gene expression, DNA synthesis, and mitosis are still not clear. The mRNA expression coded for a nuclear, DNA-binding protein is thought to be critical in the activation of resting T cells. Augmented transcription of the c-myc proto-oncogene whose mRNA coded for this protein is detectable within an hour after mitogen stimulation. Buckler et al.[81] have shown an age-dependent decline in c-myc mRNA expression in ConA-stimulated mouse splenic cells. The impaired mRNA expression could not result from age-related alterations, either in mRNA stability or in rates of transcription. These data, however, would suggest the possibility of age-dependent changes in intranuclear stabilization and processing of the primary c-myc transcripts. Gamble[82] obtained similar results using PHA-stimulated human peripheral blood T cells, and suggested that the deficits in the expression of PHA-stimulated c-myc mRNA were due in part to a decline in the rate of transcription. Therefore, extension of these early findings to other genes or activators involved in T cell activation may provide better understanding as to how alcohol affects expression of genes that regulate normal T cell functions of aging individuals.

III. IMMUNOSUPPRESSIVE EFFECTS OF ALCOHOL IN AGING ANIMALS

Attempts have been made to assess the effect of ethanol on the immune responses of the fetal alcohol-exposed offspring,[83-87] and both chronic and acute alcohol exposure of humans[17-19,21,26-29,88] and experimental animals.[20,22-25,30-34] Evidence that ethanol suppresses T cell proliferation and B cell antibody response to T cell-dependent antigen in normal young individual humans[17-19,21] and rats[24,25] has been shown. Recently, it has also been shown that the ability of macrophages from alcoholic rats to phagocytize through C3b and Fc receptors was significantly impaired, although the macrophages from alcoholic rats have higher surface density of both C3b and Fc receptors.[89] However, there is a paucity of studies examining the effect of alcohol on the immune response of old individuals.

Chang et al.,[31] using a mouse model, demonstrated for the first time that alcohol suppresses the immune response of T and B cells from young and old mice. Roselle et al.,[33] using a rat model (Sprague-Dawley rat), demonstrated that splenic cells from rats fed an alcohol-containing liquid diet, diminished with age in their ability to proliferate in response to plant lectin. Norman et al.[91] also used the same strain of rats to demonstrate that both mitogen- and recombinant IL-2 (rIL-2) induced proliferative responses of T cells from these rats exposed to ethanol *in utero* were diminished with age. However, neither of these studies examined the mechanism of action of alcohol on the immune function of aging individuals at the cellular and molecular level.

In order to understand the immunosuppressive effect of alcohol on T cell immunosenescence, we used a mouse model. The reasons for selecting mice rather than human subjects for our studies are

1. The animals are amenable to self-administration of large amounts of alcohol.
2. Individual variation in alcohol preference within the same strain is relatively small.
3. The amount of alcohol consumed can be easily measured, as can the level of blood alcohol concentration, which is readily measurable in the serum.
4. Calorically controlled diets for the ethanol-containing diets are commercially available.

In addition, other advantages of the mouse T cell model are

1. Age-related alterations in T cells and T cell-mediated immune responses in mice are comparable to those in humans.
2. Stages of T cell proliferation that are vulnerable to modulation have been identified.[90]

Attempts were made in our laboratory to resolve the question of whether the altered immune response of aged mice results from a direct alcohol effect on the immune cells or from a consequence of these alcohol-associated conditions. We therefore undertook the task of resolving this issue by comparing the effect of alcohol on:

1. The primary antibody response to T cell-dependent antigen, sheep red blood cells (SRBC)
2. The proliferative capacity of T cells prepared from the spleens of alcohol-fed mice and from spleens of mice exposed *in vitro* to alcohol

For the *in vitro* alcohol exposure study,[31,32] splenic cells from young (3 to 5 months) and old (26 to 32 months) BALB/c mice were cultured in the absence or presence of various doses of alcohol, to determine their ability to produce IL-2 and proliferate in response to mitogenic stimulation. Then, splenic T blast cells from young and old mice, generated by ConA-activation, were assessed for their IL-2-dependent proliferative capacity in the presence of various doses of alcohol. Finally, splenic cells of young and old mice were assessed for their ability to generate plaque-forming cells (PFC) in response to sheep red blood cells (RBC) in the presence of various doses of alcohol. The results revealed that alcohol has a much greater suppressive effect on old that young splenic T cells (10 to 15 times), as judged by their ability to proliferate in response to mitogenic stimulation. The possibility exists that the reduced mitogenic response of splenic T cells of young and old mice exposed to alcohol *in vitro* is due to a cytolytic effect of alcohol. This notion was tested by culturing splenic cells in the absence or presence of alcohol (50, 150, and 200 mM) for different lengths of time, and by determining the number of viable cells. Our results showed no significant loss of viable cells in cultures with alcohol. Therefore, a reduction in the number of viable splenic T cells is not a likely cause for alcohol-mediated suppression of ConA-induced proliferation of splenic T cells of both young and old mice.

Previously, we found that ConA-stimulated T blast cells from young rats exposed to alcohol *in utero* have significantly diminished proliferative responses to both crude and recombinant IL-2.[83,87] It was therefore of interest to test whether the proliferative ability of ConA-activated T blast cells of young and old mice in response to exogenous IL-2 is also affected by alcohol exposure *in vitro*. The results showed that:

1. The IL-2-dependent proliferative response of ConA-activated T blast cells of old mice to exogenous IL-2 stimulated in the absence of alcohol was greatly reduced as compared to that of young mice.
2. The IL-2-dependent proliferative response of the T blast cells of both young and old mice was significantly suppressed by alcohol, and the suppression was dose-dependent.

However, the magnitude of suppression in old cells was only twofold greater than that of young cells. Furthermore, alcohol had only a minimal suppressive effect on IL-2 production by T cells of both young and old mice, even at the concentration of 100 mM. These findings would suggest that the alcohol-mediated suppression of T cell proliferation of both young and old mice is more likely due to an impairment of metabolic event(s) associated with or subsequent to the interaction of IL-2 and IL-2R leading to cellular replication. Splenic cells of young and old mice were also assessed *in vitro* for the ability to generate plaque-forming cells in response to the T cell-dependent antigen, sheep RBC, in the presence or absence of varying doses of alcohol. The results showed that the primary antisheep RBC antibody responses of young and old spleen cells were also significantly suppressed by alcohol, but the magnitude of suppression was comparable.

For the *in vivo* alcohol exposure study,[34] the effect of extended ethanol consumption by young and old BALB/c mice on the proliferative response to ConA and T cell-dependent antibody response of their spleen cells to sheep RBC stimulation was also determined. Both young and old mice were divided into three weight-matched groups and fed a different diet:

1. One group was fed *ad libitum* a high protein liquid diet (Bio-Serv Co., Frenchtown, NJ) that contained 5% w/v alcohol (100%). This diet is referred to as alcohol diet.
2. As nutritional control, a second group of mice was fed *ad libitum* with the same volume of liquid diet that was consumed by its weight-matched alcohol fed mice, except that an isocaloric amount of maltose-dextrin replaced ethanol. This diet is referred to as maltose diet.
3. The third group of mice was fed *ad libitum* a standard normal solid diet of murine chow. This diet is referred to as mouse chow diet. The reason that mouse chow diet instead of a high protein liquid diet was used for this study to feed the third group of mice is because we observed no significant difference in the mitogenic responses of splenic cells from mice fed with solid or liquid diet.

Mice used in this study were housed individually under constant environmental conditions (lights on at 0600 h, off at 1800 h; $22 \pm 1°C$) and maintained on these diets for the duration of 21 to 28 d. Ethanol consumption averaged 13.5 ± 1.8 ml/d for young mice, and 10.8 ± 3.7 ml/d for aged mice. At the time of sacrifice, tailtip blood samples were collected, and blood levels were determined spectrophotometrically with an alcohol dehydrogenase kit (Sigma Chemical Co., St. Louis, MO). Blood ethanol concentrations were 131 ± 48.8 mg/100 ml for young mice, and $134 \pm 38.9/100$ ml for old mice. When the immunological studies were performed, the average of body weight was not significantly different for all three weight-matched groups of young and old mice.

Splenic cells of young (3 months) and old (25 months) BALB/c mice, fed with one of three different diets (5% alcohol, maltose-substitute and standard mouse chow), were first cultured with ConA to assess T cell proliferation and production of IL-2. Then, ConA-activated T blast cells from young and old mice were assessed for their proliferative-responding capacity to exogenous human recombinant IL-2 and crude rat IL-2 supernatant. Finally, splenic cells of young and old mice were assessed for their ability to generate plaque-forming cells in response to sheep RBC. The results of this study revealed that both T cell mitogenesis and IL-2-dependent proliferation of T blast cells from young and old ethanol diet-fed mice were remarkably diminished as compared to that of young and old maltose-substituted diet (isocaloric control) fed mice, respectively. The ability of T cells from both young and old alcohol diet-fed mice to produce IL-2, however, was not affected. Therefore, the impaired T cell proliferation appears to result from a decrease in the responsiveness to IL-2, but not production of IL-2. Finally, the ability of young and old alcohol diet-fed mice to mount a primary antibody response to sheep RBC was also significantly reduced. These results taken together demonstrate for the first time that both the T cell proliferative activity and the T cell-dependent antibody response of young and old alcohol diet-fed mice are impaired. However, with respect to age, a differential effect of immunosuppression of alcohol was not noted.

Since our findings on the effects of *in vitro* and *in vivo* alcohol exposure on T cell proliferation were comparable, these results would suggest that alcohol has a direct impact on the immune response of young and old mice.

IV. MECHANISM OF ALCOHOL-MEDIATED SUPPRESSION OF T CELL PROLIFERATION

Findings of previous studies from this laboratory and others have established that alcohol ingestion by human beings or chronic consumption of alcohol by experimental animals results in diminished immune responses in general. However, most of these studies have been of a phenomenological nature, and did not examine the mechanism underlying the specific abnormality. The major effort in our laboratory is to study the mechanisms by which alcohol down-regulates T cell-mediated immune responses. By focusing on a young mouse model of excessive alcohol consumption, we have also shown that both ConA- and PHA-induced T cell mitogenesis and IL-2-dependent proliferation of T blast cells from alcohol diet-fed mice were remarkably diminished as compared to that of maltose-substituted diet (isocaloric control). These diminished proliferative responses of alcohol diet-fed mice were due not to a decreased number of splenic cells, nor to a loss of viable cells caused by a toxic effect of alcohol.[91] Although the ratio of ConA-induced $CD4^+CD8^+$ cells from alcohol-fed mice was altered, we could not rule out a possibility that an increase in the number of $CD8^+$ cells was attributable to a diminished ability of splenic cells from alcohol diet-fed mice to proliferate upon stimulation with lectins or a combination of phorbol-12-myristate-13 acetate (PMA) and ionomycin.[91] We also confirmed the findings that the impaired T cell proliferation induced by alcohol was due to a decrease in the responsiveness to, but not production of, IL-2, or expression of IL-2R.[19,32,34,92] Furthermore, using $^{125}[I]IL$-2 binding assay, we also showed that the Kd values and the number of low and high affinity IL-2R binding sites on the T cells from alcohol diet-fed mice is comparable to that of paired- and normal diet-fed mice.[104] Our observation that ethanol exposure *in vivo* suppressed T cell proliferation, but did not inhibit production of IL-2 and the expression of both low and high affinity IL-2R, suggests that the alcohol-mediated suppression of T cell proliferation is due to perturbation (or interference) in the events following the IL-2-IL-2R interaction.

It is well known that PMA can act as an analog of diacylglycerol to activate protein kinase C (PKC) translocation,[93] and ionomycin can substitute for the effect of inositol triphosphate, which causes release of Ca^{2+} from intracellular stores.[94,95] It is also known that neither PMA nor ionomycin alone is mitogenic for murine splenic cells. However, a combination of these two agents can synergistically induce murine splenic cells to proliferate, bypassing the requirement for an antigen or mitogen ligand-receptor interaction induced signal at the onset of T cell activation.[93] Thus, if the proliferative response of T cells triggered by a combination of PMA and ionomycin is not affected by alcohol, it would suggest that suppression of T cell proliferation by alcohol may be at the level of mitogenic receptor-mediated events. However, if the magnitude of suppression in the proliferative responses is similar to that of T cells stimulated by plant lectins, it would indicate that suppression of T cell proliferation by alcohol may be at the level of IL-2R mediated-transmembrane signal transduction. Therefore, our findings that the magnitude of alcohol-mediated suppression of T cell proliferation induced by a combination of PMA and ionomycin is comparable to that induced by lectin mitogens[91] (i.e., 51.3 ± 13.9% vs. 57.7 ± 8.6%), strongly suggest that alcohol suppresses the proliferative response of T cells by affecting the IL-2R-mediated (rather than mitogen receptor-mediated) process which leads to DNA synthesis and cell division via a common cellular pathway or similar events of T cell proliferation (Figure 1).

There are two major signal transduction pathways believed to be involved in cell proliferation. Both pathways share some similar biochemical components, and both involve activation of distinct protein kinases (Figure 1). One pathway utilizes the second messenger, cyclic adenosine monophosphate (cAMP), whereas the other employs two synergistic bifurcating signals, inositol 1,4,5-triphosphate (IP_3) and diacylglycerol (DG). It is known that the transducing proteins involved in these two pathways are a highly conserved family of G proteins which bind guanosine triphosphate (GTP).[96,97] The G protein has enzymatic activity and converts GTP into guanosine diphosphate (GDP) + Pi. In the case of the adenylate cyclase (AC) pathway, the G protein interacts with AC and converts adenosine 5'-triphosphate (ATP) to cAMP. In the other pathway, phospholipase C (PL-C) is also acted upon by a G protein,[98] which increases the enzymatic conversion of the membrane lipid phosphatidylinositol 4,5-biphosphate (PIP_2) into IP_3 and DG.[95] Considerable evidence implicates the cyclic nucleotides, cAMP and cyclic guanosine monophosphate (GMP) (cGMP) as playing regulatory roles in the immune response. For example, cGMP is associated with promotion of proliferation, cytotoxicity, and lymphokine secretion; however, cAMP is associated with inhibition of these functions.[99-101] An intracellular cGMP increase by an indirect activation of guanylate cyclase has been found to be associated with mitogen-induced T cell proliferation,[100] but evidence for changes in cAMP level in the mitogen-activated T cells remains controversial.[101] Recently, al-

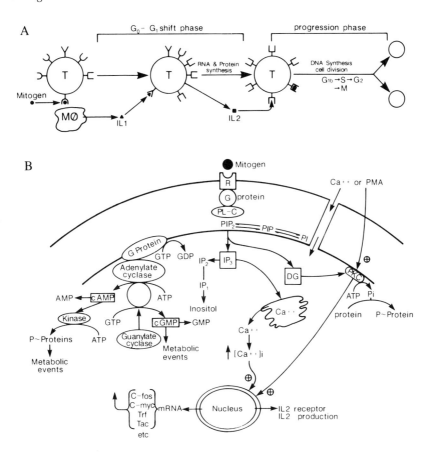

FIGURE 1. Model depicts a possible mechanism by which alcohol could affect the events of the signal transduction cascade involved in mitogen-stimulated T cell activation. (A) The binding of T cell receptor (TCR) complex by mitogen plus accessory signals provided by macrophages activate the resting T cells to leave G_0 phase and enter cycling phase in the presence of T cell growth factors, and then receptors expressed. (B) Binding of mitogen and the TCR complex leads to activation of the known second message pathway (phospholipase C pathway). Phospholipase C (PL-C) hydrolyzes polyphosphoinositol (PIP_2) to yield diacylglycerol (DG) and inositol 1,4,5 triphosphate (IP_3). The second messengers mediate the mobilization of extracellular and intracellular Ca^{++} (from the endoplasmic reticulum), and activation of protein kinase C (PKC). Thus, the signals generated then are transduced to the nucleus to activate expression of genes, (i.e., IL-2, IL-2R, and oncogenes, etc.) required for T cells to grow. Alcohol could affect one or more of these events mentioned above. In addition, alcohol could also suppress T cell proliferation by inhibiting the accessory signals generated by macrophages.

tered adenosine receptor-stimulated cAMP production has been observed in alcoholic patients;[102,103] however, the role of adenylate cyclase in T cell activation of these alcoholic subjects is unclear. Because (1) the ability of mitogen to affect the cellular concentration of cAMP in T cells remains controversial, (2) changes in the levels of cyclic nucleotides (both cAMP and cGMP) in T cells stimulated by mitogen appear to be earlier events occurring in the $G_0 \rightarrow G_1$ shift phase, and (3) our previous results demonstrated that cycling T cells ($G_1 \rightarrow S \rightarrow G_2 \rightarrow M$) are likely affected most by alcohol,[32,34,91] we believe that hydrolysis of the inositol phospholipid (PL-C) signal transduction pathway, rather than the adenylate cyclase system using the second messenger, cAMP, or the T cell receptors (TCR) phosphorylation pathway, should be one of the better target systems to study mechanisms of the immunosuppressive effects of alcohol on T cell proliferation.

V. SUMMARY

Attempts were made to obtain general information on the effect of alcohol exposure *in vivo* and *in vitro* on the immune responses of young and old mice, and to provide an animal model for studying mechanisms of alteration of both cellular and humoral responses caused by chronic alcoholism. The results demonstrated that both T cell proliferation induced by plant lectin and the T cell-dependent antibody response are impaired in young and old mice subjected to both extended alcohol consumption and alcohol exposure *in vitro*. This impaired T cell proliferation induced by alcohol appears to result from a decrease in the responsiveness to IL-2, but not production of IL-2. However, the age-related decline in the proliferative activities of splenic cells from all three different diet-fed mice is due in part to a decrease in the production of IL-2 and the responsiveness to IL-2. Furthermore, the magnitude of alcohol-mediated suppression of T cell proliferation induced by PMA/ionomycin was comparable to that induced by ConA. Based on the findings generated by our laboratory and others, we therefore proposed the hypothesis that alcohol suppresses the proliferative capacity of murine T cells by affecting their transmembrane signal transduction events which lead into the DNA synthesis of the cycling phase. An extension of these studies may provide a better understanding of mechanisms of the immunosuppressive action of alcohol.

ACKNOWLEDGMENTS

The authors thank Dr. A. N. Taylor for critically reading the manuscript, and Mr. J. Sproul for his secretarial help.

REFERENCES

1. **Makinodan, T. and Kay, M. M. B.,** Age influence on the immune system, *Adv. Immunol.,* 29, 287, 1980.
2. **Thoman, M. L. and Weigle, W. O.,** Lymphocytes and aging, Interleukin-2 production and activity in aged animals, *J. Immunol.,* 127, 2102, 1981.

3. **Miller, R. A. and Stutman, O.,** Decline, in aging mice, of the anti-2,4,6,-trinitrophenyl (TNP) cytotoxic T cell response attributable to loss of Lyt 2, interleukin 2-producing helper cell function, *Eur. J. Immunol.,* 11, 751, 1981.

4. **Thoman, M. L. and Weigle, W. O.,** Cell-mediated immunity in aged mice: an underlying lesion in IL2 synthesis, *J. Immunol.,* 128, 2358, 1982.

5. **Joncourt, F., Wang, F., Kristensen, F., and De Weck, A. L.,** Aging and immunity: decrease in interleukin-2 production and interleukin-2-dependent RNA synthesis in lectin-stimulated murine spleen cells, *Immunobiology,* 163, 521, 1982.

6. **Chang, M.-P., Makinodan, T., Peterson, W. J., and Strehler, B. L.,** Role of T cells and adherent cells in age-related decline in murine interleukin-2 production, *J. Immunol.,* 129, 2426, 1982.

7. **Miller, R. A. and Stutman, O.,** Limiting dilution analysis of IL2 production: studies of age, genotype, and regulatory interactions, *Lymphokine Res. News,* 3, 79, 1982.

8. **Inamizu, T., Chang, M.-P., and Makinodan, T.,** Decline in interleukin(IL)-1 production with age, *Gerontologist,* 23, 249, 1983.

9. **Bruley-Rosset, M. and Vergnon, I.,** Interleukin-1 synthesis and activity in aged mice, *Mech. Ageing Dev.,* 24, 247, 1984.

10. **Inamizu, T., Chang, M.-P., and Makinodan, T.,** Influence of age on the production and regulation of interleukin-1 in mice, *Immunology,* 33, 447, 1985.

11. **Chang, M.-P., Utsuyama, M., Hirokawa, K., and Makinodan, T.,** Decline in the production of interleukin-3 with age in mice, *Cell. Immunol.,* 15, 1, 1988.

12. **Fong, T. C. and Makinodan, T.,** Preferential enhancement by 2-mercaptoethanol of IL-2 responsiveness of T blast cells from old over young mice is associated with potentiated protein kinase C translocation, *Immunol. Lett.,* 30, 149, 1989.

13. **Fong, T. C. and Makinodan, T.,** *In situ* hybridization analysis of the age-associated decline in IL-2 mRNA expressing murine T cells, *Cell. Immunol.,* 118, 199, 1989.

14. **Kennes, B., Hubert, C. I., Brohee, D., and Neve, P.,** Early biochemical events associated with lymphocyte activation in ageing. I. Evidence that Ca^{2+} dependent processes induced by PHA are impaired, *Immunology,* 42, 119, 1981.

15. **Miller, R. A., Jacobson, B., Weil, G., and Simons, E. R.,** Diminished calcium influx in lectin-stimulated T cells from old mice, *J. Cell. Physiol.,* 132, 337, 1987.

16. **Proust, J. J., Filburn, C. R., Harrison, S. A., Buchholz, M. A., and Nordin, A. A.,** Age-related defect in signal transduction during lectin activation of murine T lymphocytes, *J. Immunol.,* 139, 1472, 1987.

17. **Hsu, C. C. S. and Leevy, C. M.,** Inhibition of DNA-stimulated lymphocyte transformation by plasma from patients with advanced alcoholic cirrhosis, *Clin. Exp. Immunol.,* 8, 749, 1971.

18. **Glassman, A. B. and Bennett, C. E.,** B and T lymphocytes, quantitation, function, and clinical applicability, *Ann. Clin. Lab. Sci.,* 10, 455, 1980.

19. **Kaplan, D. R.,** A novel mechanism of immunosuppression mediated by ethanol, *Cell. Immunol.,* 102, 1, 1986.

20. **Roselle, G. A. and Mendenhall, C. L.,** Ethanol-induced alterations in lymphocyte function in the guinea pig, *Alcohol.: Clin. Exp. Res.,* 8, 62, 1984.

21. **Mutchnic, M. G. and Lee, M. H.,** Impaired lymphocyte proliferative response to mitogen in alcoholic patients. Absence of a relation to liver disease activity, *Alcohol.: Clin. Exp. Res.,* 12, 155, 1988.

22. **Jerrells, T. R., Peritt, Marrietta, C., and Eckardt, M. J.,** Mechanisms of suppression of cellular immunity induced by ethanol, *Alcohol.: Clin. Exp. Res.,* 13, 490, 1989.

23. **Grossman, C. J., Mendenhall, C. L., and Roselle, G. A.,** Alcohol and immune regulation. I. *In vivo* effect of ethanol on concanavalin A sensitive thymic lymphocyte function, *Int. J. Immunopharmacol.,* 10, 187, 1988.

24. **Bagasra, O., Howeedy, A., Dorio, R., and Kajdacsy-Balla, A.,** Functional analysis of T cell subsets in chronic experimental alcoholism, *Immunology,* 61, 63, 1987.

25. **Jerrells, T. R., Marietta, C. A., Majchrowicz, M. J., and Weight, F. F.**, Effects of ethanol administration on parameters of immunocompetency, *J. Leuk. Biol.*, 39, 499, 1986.

26. **Roselle, G. and Mendenhall, C.**, Alteration of *in vitro* human lymphocyte function by ethanol, acetaldehyde, and acetate, *J. Clin. Lab. Immunol.*, 9, 33, 1982.

27. **Glassman, A. B. and Bennett, C. E.**, B and T lymphocytes: quantitation, function, and clinical applicability, *Ann. Clin. Lab. Sci.*, 10, 455, 1980.

28. **Gilhus, N. E. and Matre, R.**, *In vitro* effect of ethanol on subpopulations of human blood mononuclear cells, *Int. Arch. Allergy Appl. Immunol.*, 68, 382, 1982.

29. **Lundy, J., Raaf, J. H., Deakins, S., Wanebo, H.-J., Jacobs, J. D. A., Lee, T. D., Jacobowitz, D., Spear, C., and Oettgen, H. F.**, The acute and chronic effects of alcohol on the human immune system, *Surgery Gynec. Obstet.*, 141, 212, 1975.

30. **Dehne, M., Mendenhall, C., Grossman, C., Roselle, G., and Ghosn, S.**, The effect of acute ethanol consumption on *in vitro* cellular function, *Fed. Proc. Am. Soc. Exp. Biol.*, 46 (Abstr.), 2313, 1987.

31. **Chang, M.-P., Yamamura, R. H., Castle, S., and Norman, D. C.**, Suppressive effect of ethanol on immune response of T and B cells from young and old mice, *Gerontologist*, 38, 228A, 1988.

32. **Chang, M.-P. and Norman, D. C.**, Immunotoxicity of alcohol in young and old mice. I. *In vitro* suppressive effects of ethanol on the immune response of T and B immune cells of aging mice, *Alcohol.: Clin. Exp. Res.*, 14(2), 210, 1990.

33. **Roselle, G. A., Mendenhall, C. L., and Grossman, C. J.**, Age-dependent alterations of host immune response in the ethanol-fed rat, *J. Clin. Lab. Immunol.*, 29, 99, 1989.

34. **Chang, M.-P. and Norman, D. C.**, Immunotoxicity of alcohol in young and old mice. II. Impaired T cell proliferation and T cell-dependent antibody responses of young and old mice fed ethanol-containing liquid diet, *Mech. Ageing Dev.*, 57, 175, 1991.

35. **Gilman, S. C., Rosenberg, J. S., and Feldman, J. D.**, T lymphocytes of young and aged rates. II. Functional defects and the role of interleukin-2, *J. Immunol.*, 128, 644, 1982.

36. **Grossman, A., Ledbetter, J. A., and Rabinovitch, P. S.**, Reduced proliferation in T lymphocytes in aged humans is predominantly in the CD8 + subset, and is unrelated to defects in transmembrane signaling which are predominantly in the CD4 + subset, *Exp. Cell. Res.*, 180, 367, 1989.

37. **Lustyik, G. Y. and O'Leary, J. J.**, Aging and intracellular free calcium response in human T cells after stimulation by phytohemagglutinin, *J. Gerontol.*, 44, 1330, 1989.

38. **Rabinowe, S. L., Nayak, R. C., Kirsch, K., George, K. L., and Eisenbarth, G. S.**, Aging in man. Linear increase of novel T cell subset defined by antiganglioside monoclonal antibody 3G5, *J. Exp. Med.*, 165, 1436, 1987.

39. **Sidman, C. L., Luther, E. A., Marshall, J. D., Nguyen, K. A., Roopenian, D. C., and Worthen, S. M.**, Increased expression of major histocompatibility complex antigens on lymphocytes from aged mice, *Proc. Natl. Acad. Sci. U.S.A.*, 84, 7624, 1987.

40. **Bender, B. S., Chrest, F. J., Nagel, J. A., and Adler, W. H.**, Peripheral blood CD8 + subsets in young and elderly adults: enumeration by two-color immunofluorescence and flow cytometry, *Aging: Immunol. Infect. Dis.*, 1, 23, 1988.

41. **Moody, C. E., Innes, J. B., Staiano-Coico, L., Incefy, G. S., Thaler, H. T., and Weksler, M. E.**, Lymphocyte transformation induced by autologous cells. XI. The effect of age on the autologous mixed lymphocyte reaction, *Immunology*, 44, 431, 1981.

42. **Nagel, J. E., Chrest, F. J., and Adler, W. H.**, Enumeration of T lymphocyte subsets by monoclonal antibodies in young and aged humans, *J. Endocrinol.*, 127, 2086, 1981.

43. **Ceuppens, J. L. and Goodwin, J. S.**, Regulation of immunoglobulin production in pokeweed mitogen-stimulated cultures of lymphocytes from young and old adults, *J. Immunol.*, 128, 2429, 1982.

44. **Mascart-Lemone, F., Delespesse, G., Servais, G., and Kuntsler, M.**, Characterization of immunoregulatory T lymphocytes during ageing by monoclonal antibodies, *Clin. Exp. Immunol.*, 48, 148, 1982.

45. **Thompson, J. S., Wekstein, D. R., Rhoades, J. L., Kirkpatrick, C., Brown, S. A., Roszman, T., Straus, R., and Tietz, N.,** The immune status of health centenarians, *J. Am. Geriatr. Soc.,* 32, 274, 1984.

46. **Ernst, D. N., Weigel, W. D., McQuitty, D. N., Rothermel, A. L., and Hobbs, M. V.,** Stimulation of murine T-cell subsets with anti-CD3 antibody. Age-related defects in the expression of early activation molecules, *J. Immunol.,* 142, 1413, 1989.

47. **Hori, Y., Perkins, E. H., and Halsall, M. D.,** Decline in phytohemagglutinin responsiveness of spleen cells from aging mice, *Proc. Soc. Exp. Biol. Med.,* 144, 48, 1973.

48. **Kay, M. M. B., Mendoza, J., Diven, J., Denton, T., Union, N., and Lajiness, M.,** Age-related changes in the immune system of mice of 8 medium and long-lived strains and hybrids. I. Organ, cellular and activity changes, *Mech. Ageing Dev.,* 11, 295, 1979.

49. **Walters, C. S. and Claman, H. N.,** Age-related changes in cell-mediated immunity in BALB/c mice, *J. Immunol.,* 115, 1438, 1975.

50. **Schwab, R., Hausman, P. B., Rinnooy-Kan, E., and Weksler, M. E.,** Immunological studies of aging. X. Impaired T lymphocytes and normal monocytes response from elderly humans to the mitogenic antibodies OKT3 and Leu 4, *Immunology,* 55, 677, 1985.

51. **Kishimoto, S., Tomino, S., Inomata, K., Kotegawa, S., Saito, T., Kuroki, M., Mitsuya, H., and Hisamitsu, S.,** Age-related changes in the subsets and functions of human T lymphocytes, *J. Immunol.,* 121, 1773, 1978.

52. **Bach, M. A.,** Lymphocyte-mediated cytotoxicity: effects of ageing, adult thymectomy and thymic factor, *J. Immunol.,* 119, 641, 1977.

53. **Bach, M. A.,** Influence of aging on T cell subpopulations involved in the *in vitro* generation of allogeneic cytotoxicity, *Clin. Immunol. Immunopathol.,* 13, 220, 1979.

54. **Callard, R. E. and Basten, A.,** Immune functions in aged mice. IV. Loss of T cells and B cell functions in thymus-dependent antibody response, *Eur. J. Immunol.,* 8, 552, 1978.

55. **Krogsrud, R. L. and Perkins, E. H.,** Age-related changes in T cell function, *J. Immunol.,* 118, 1607, 1977.

56. **Goodman, S. A. and Makinodan, T.,** Effect of age on cell-mediated immunity in long-lived mice, *Clin. Exp. Immunol.,* 19, 533, 1975.

57. **Nagel, J. E., Chopra, R. K., Chrest, F. J., McCoy, M. T., Schneider, E. L., Holbrook, N. J., and Adler, W. H.,** Decreased proliferation, interleukin 2 synthesis, and interleukin 2 receptor expression are accompanied by decreased mRNA expression in phytohemagglutinin-stimulated cells from elderly donors, *J. Clin. Invest.,* 81, 1096, 1988.

58. **Gillis, S., Kozak, R., Durante, M., and Weksler, M. E.,** Immunological studies of aging. Decreased production of and response to T cell growth factor by lymphocytes from aged humans, *J. Clin. Invest.,* 67, 937, 1981.

59. **Kariv, I., Ferguson, F. G., and Garman, C.,** Age and gender-associated effects on the kinetics of interleukin-2 and interleukin-2 receptor expression in mice, *Aging: Immunol. and Infect. Dis.,* 2, 261, 1990.

60. **Cheung, H. T., Twu, J. S., and Richardson, A.,** Mechanism of the age-related decline in lymphocyte proliferation: role of IL-2 production and protein synthesis, *Exp. Gerontol.,* 18, 451, 1983.

61. **Bruley-Rosset, M. and Payelle, B.,** Deficient tumor-specific immunity in old mice: *in vivo* mediation by suppressor cells, and correction of the defect by interleukin 2 supplementation *in vitro* but not *in vivo, Eur. J. Immunol.,* 17, 307, 1987.

62. **Thoman, M. L. and Weigle, W. O.,** Reconstitution of *in vivo* cell-mediated lympholysis responses in age mice with interleukin 2, *J. Immunol.,* 134, 949, 1985.

63. **Gottesman, S. R. S., Walford, R. L., and Thorbecke, G. J.,** Proliferative and cytotoxic immune functions in aging mice. III. Exogenous interleukin-2 rich supernatant only partially restores alloreactivity *in vitro, Mech. Ageing Dev.,* 31, 103, 1983.

64. **Miller, R. A.,** Age-associated decline in precursor frequency for different T cell-mediated reactions, with preservation of helper or cytotoxic effect per precursor cell, *J. Immunol.,* 132, 63, 1984.

65. **Negoro, S., Hara, H., Miyata, S., Saiki, O., Tanaka, T., Yoshizaki, K., Igarishi, T., and Kishimoto, S.,** Mechanisms of age-related decline in antigen-specific T cell proliferative response: IL-2 receptor expression and recombinant IL-2 induced proliferative response of purified TAC-positive T cells, *Mech. Ageing Dev.,* 36, 223, 1986.
66. **Nordin, A. A. and Collins, G. D.,** Limiting dilution analysis of alloreactive cytotoxic precursor cells in aging mice, *J. Immunol.,* 131, 2215, 1983.
67. **Vie, H. and Miller, R. A.,** Decline, with age, in the proportion of mouse T cells that express IL-2 receptors after mitogen stimulation, *Mech. Ageing Dev.,* 33, 313, 1986.
68. **Froelich, C. J., Burkett, J. S., Guiffaut, S., Kingsland, R., and Brauner, D.,** Phytohemagglutinin induced proliferation by aged lymphocytes: reduced expression of high affinity interleukin-2 receptors and interleukin-2 secretion, *Life Sci.,* 43, 1583, 1988.
69. **Abraham, C., Tal, Y., and Gershon, H.,** Reduced *in vitro* response to concanavalin A and lipopolysaccharide in senescent mice: a function of reduced number of responding cells, *Eur. J. Immunol.,* 7, 301, 1977.
70. **Inkeles, B., Innes, J. B., Kuntz, M. M., Kadish, A. S., and Weksler, M. E.,** Immunological studies of aging. III. Cytokinetic basis for the impaired response of lymphocytes from aged humans to plant lectins, *J. Exp. Med.,* 145, 1176, 1977.
71. **Joncourt, F., Bettens, F., Kristensen, F., and DeWeck, A. L.,** Age-related changes in mitogen responsiveness in different lymphoid organs from outbred NMRI mice, *Immunobiology,* 158, 439, 1981.
72. **Kubbies, M., Schindler, D., Hoehn, H., and Rabinovitch, P. S.,** BrdU-Hoechst flow cytometry reveals regulation of human lymphocyte growth by donor-age-related growth fraction and transition rate, *J. Cell. Physiol.,* 125, 229, 1985.
73. **Staiano-Coico, L., Darzynkiewicz, Z., Melamed, M. R., and Weskler, M. E.,** Immunological studies of aging. IX. Impaired proliferation of T lymphocytes detected in elderly humans by flow cytometry, *J. Immunol.,* 132, 1788, 1984.
74. **Sohnle, P. G., Collins-Lech, C., and Huhta, K. E.,** Age-related effects on the number of human lymphocytes in culture initially responding to an antigenic stimulus, *Clin. Exp. Med.,* 47, 138, 1982.
75. **Hefton, J. M., Darlington, G. J., Casazza, B. A., and Weksler, M. E.,** Immunologic studies of aging. V. Impaired proliferation of PHA responsive human lymphocytes in culture, *J. Immunol.,* 125, 1007, 1980.
76. **Tice, R. R., Schneider, E. L., Kram, D., and Thorne, P.,** Cytokinetic analysis of the impaired proliferative response of peripheral lymphocytes from aged humans to phytohemagglutin, *J. Exp. Med.,* 149, 1029, 1979.
77. **Miller, R. A.,** Immunodeficiency of aging: restorative effects of phorbol ester combined with calcium ionophore, *J. Immunol.,* 137, 805, 1986.
78. **Lerner, A., Philosophe, B., and Miller, R. A.,** Defective calcium influx and preserved inositol phosphate generation in T cells from old mice, *Aging: Immunol. Infect. Dis.,* 1, 149, 1988.
79. **Miller, R. A., Philosophe, B., Ginis, I., Weil, G., and Jacobson, B.,** Defective control of cytoplasmic calcium concentration in T lymphocytes from old mice, *J. Cell. Physiol.,* 138, 175, 1989.
80. **Thoman, M. L. and Weigle, W. O.,** Partial restoration of ConA-induced proliferation, IL-2 receptor expression, and IL-2 synthesis in aged murine lymphocytes by phorbol myristate acetate and ionomycin, *Cell. Immunol.,* 114, 1, 1988.
81. **Buckler, A., Vie, H., Sonensheim, G., and Miller, R. A.,** Defective T lymphocytes in old mice: diminished production of mature c-myc RNA after mitogen exposure not attributable to alterations in transcription or RNA stability, *J. Immunol.,* 140, 2442, 1988.
82. **Gamble, D. A.,** Analysis of c-myc Gene Expression in Relationship to Proliferative Capacity in Human Lymphocytes and the Effect of Aging, Ph.D. thesis, Cornell University Medical College, New York, 1987.

83. **Norman, D. C., Chang, M.-P., Castle, S. C., Van Zuylen, J. E., Taylor, A. N.,** Diminished proliferative response of ConA-blast cells to interleukin 2 in rats exposed to ethanol *in utero, Alcohol.: Clin. Exp. Res.,* 13, 69, 1989.

84. **Ewald, S. J. and Frost, W. W.,** Effect of prenatal exposure to ethanol on development of the thymus, *Thymus,* 9, 211, 1987.

85. **Menjan, A. A. and Mandell, W.,** Fetal alcohol and immunity: depression of mutagen-induced lymphocyte blastogenesis, *Neurobiobehav. Toxicol.,* 2, 213, 1980.

86. **Ewald, S.,** T lymphocyte populations in fetal alcohol syndrome, *Alcohol.: Clin. Exp. Res.,* 13, 485, 1989.

87. **Norman, D. C., Chang, M.-P., Wong, C. M. K., Branch, B. J., Castle, S., and Taylor, A. N.,** Changes with age in the proliferative response of splenic T cells from rats exposed to ethanol in utero, *Alcohol.: Clin. Exp. Res.,* 15, 428, 1991.

88. **Johnson, R. D. and Williams, R.,** Immune responses in alcoholic liver disease, *Alcohol.: Clin. Exp. Res.,* 10, 471, 1986.

89. **Bagasra, O., Howeedy, A., Kajdacsy-Balla, A.,** Macrophage function in chronic experimental alcoholism. I. Modulation of surface receptors and phagocytosis, *Immunology,* 65, 405, 1988.

90. **Makinodan, T., Chang, M.-P., and Kinohara, N.,** Influence of age on cellular differentiation: a T cell model, *Exp. Gerontol.,* 21, 241, 1986.

91. **Chang, M.-P. and Norman, D. C.,** Mechanism of ethanol-mediated immunosuppression in mice: ethanol suppresses T cell proliferation without affecting IL2 production and IL2 receptor expression, *Int. J. Immunopharmacol.,* 14, 707, 1992.

92. **Jerrells, T. R., Perritt, D., Eckardt, M. J., and Marietta, C. A.,** Alterations in interleukin-2 utilization by T cells from rats treated with ethanol-containing diet, *Alcohol.: Clin. Exp. Res.,* 14, 245, 1990.

93. **Alemseged, T., Albert, F., Golstein, P., and Schmitt-Verhulst, A. M.,** Early steps of lymphocyte activation bypassed by synergy between calcium ionophores and phorbol ester, *Nature (London),* 313, 318, 1985.

94. **Nishizuka, Y.,** The role of protein kinase C in cell surface signal transduction and tumor promotion, *Nature (London),* 308, 693, 1984.

95. **Berridge, M. J. and Ervine, R. F.,** Inositol triphosphate, a novel second messenger in cellular signal transduction, *Nature (London),* 312, 315, 1984.

96. **Gilman, A. G.,** G proteins: transducers of receptor-generated signals, *Annu. Rev. Biochem.,* 56, 615, 1987.

97. **Chedid, M., Shirakawa, I., Naylor, P., and Mizel, S. B.,** Signal transduction pathway for IL-1: involvement of a pertussis toxin-sensitive GTP-binding protein in the activation of adenylate cyclase, *J. Immunol.,* 142, 4301, 1989.

98. **Cockcroft, S. and Gomperts, B. D.,** *Nature (London),* 285, 167, 1980.

99. **Hadden, J. W. and Coffey, R. G.,** Cyclic nucleotides in mitogen-induced lymphocyte proliferation, *Immunol. Today,* 3, 299, 1982.

100. **Hadden, J. W., Coffey, R. G., and Hadden, E. M.,** Cyclic nucleotides and calcium in lymphocyte regulation and activation, *Ann. N.Y. Acad. Sci.,* 76, 241, 1979.

101. **Parker, C. W.,** Role of cyclic nucleotides in regulating lymphocytes, *Ann. N.Y. Acad. Sci.,* 76, 255, 1979.

102. **Diamond, I., Wrubell, B., Estrin, W., and Gordon, A.,** Basal and adenosine receptor-stimulated levels of cAMP are reduced in lymphocytes from alcohol patients, *Proc. Natl. Acad. Sci. U.S.A.,* 84, 1413, 1987.

103. **Nagy, L., Diamond, I., and Gordon, A.,** Cultured lymphocytes from alcoholic subjects have altered cAMP signal transduction, *Proc. Natl. Acad. Sci. U.S.A.,* 85, 6973, 1988.

104. **Chang, M.-P. and Norman, D. C.,** Diminished T cell proliferative response from ethanol-fed mice is not due to loss of IL-2 binding affinity and the number of binding sites, submitted.

Chapter 4

MODULATION OF NATURAL KILLER CELL ACTIVITY BY ALCOHOL

Gary G. Meadows and Sally E. Blank

TABLE OF CONTENTS

5761-6/93/$0.00 + $.50

I. INTRODUCTION

Natural killer (NK) cells are a group of distinct lymphocytes distributed among various lymphoid and nonlymphoid tissues that play an important role in the pathogenesis and progression of various infectious diseases, autoimmune diseases, and cancer in animals and humans. NK cells in humans represent a heterogeneous group of cells defined as large granular lymphocytes (LGL), that do not express surface CD3 or CD5 antigen, or any of the known T cell receptor chains, and are characterized by their expression of CD16 (Leu11), CD56 (NKH-1, Leu 19), and CD57 (HNK-1, Leu 7) surface markers.[1] In mice, NK cells are characterized by expression of either NK 1.1, NK 2.1, or NK 3.1 alloantigens, depending on the strain, and more recently by the LGL-1 antigen, which exhibits more universal expression on murine NK cells.[2] In contrast to human NK cells, about one-half of the LGL-1$^+$ cells express CD3 antigen, and all murine NK cells express CD5 antigen. Rat NK cells are asialo-GM$_1^+$, do not express T cell antigens, and express CD8 (OX8) antigen.[1] Several recent reviews discuss in detail the characteristics, biology, and role of NK cells in these diseases.[1,3,4] This chapter will concentrate solely on what is known to date about the effects of alcohol and its metabolites on NK cell activity. In addition, since NK cells can participate in antibody-dependent cell-mediated cytotoxicity (ADCC), this function is also discussed. As the reader will recognize, ethanol is reported to have no effect on, to increase, or to decrease NK cytolytic activity. An additional aim of this chapter is to point out variables that could contribute to the disparity in the literature which make it difficult to compare one study with another.

II. *IN VITRO* EFFECTS OF ETHANOL AND ITS METABOLITES

The effects of ethanol on *in vitro* NK cytolytic activity have not been consistent, and ethanol appears to modulate human peripheral blood mononuclear cells (PBMC) differently than splenic lymphocytes from rodents. The majority of investigations report, however, that ethanol, when present in the assay media during analysis, inhibits both human and rodent NK cell activity. These effects have been observed at physiologically attainable ethanol concentrations ranging from 11 to 110 mM (0.05 to 0.5% w/v).[5] At these concentrations, all studies show no effect of ethanol on cell viability. Determination of a physiological blood concentration of acetaldehyde that modulates NK cell activity has been difficult because of the inherent volatility and reactivity of this metabolite of ethanol; however, a concentration of 15 μM (0.05% w/v) is physiologically attainable.[6]

A. HUMAN NATURAL KILLER CELLS

The lack of consistency regarding the effect of ethanol added *in vitro* to human peripheral blood lymphocytes on NK cytolytic activity largely reflects differences in experimental conditions (Table 1). Four studies report inhibition,[7-10] and one study reports enhancement[11] when ethanol is added to the assay. Another[12] states that ethanol added directly to effector and target cells inhibits NK cell activity. When ethanol was added directly to the assay, inhibition was observed at ethanol concentrations as low as 11 mM (0.05% w/v). Higher concentrations consistently inhibited cytolytic activity in a dose-dependent fashion. Inhibition of NK cell activity by ethanol was not reversed when monocytes were removed from the assay medium. Monocytes can suppress NK cell function.[8] The effects of ethanol in the collective *in vitro* experiments were not target specific; inhibition was observed against three different target cells.[7,8] Effector to target binding, when determined, was not affected by ethanol (see Table 1).

Another approach to studying the effect of ethanol *in vitro* has been to pretreat the effector and/or target cells prior to assay. Thus, the determination of cytolytic activity is not conducted in the presence of ethanol. Two studies reported enhancement,[10,13] and one study reported no effect at low levels of ethanol. Another reported inhibition of cytolytic activity at high, but physiologically attainable concentrations, when effector cells were preincubated with ethanol before assay.[12] Enhancement was observed when the effector cells were preincubated for 1 to 24 h before assay; whereas, inhibition required incubation with ethanol for 72 h. The increase in cytolytic activity was observed after 1 h of incubation with as little as 2.2 nM ethanol.[13] Thus, the effect of ethanol may be biphasic: stimulating NK cell activity at low concentrations and inhibiting at high concentrations.

In an investigation by Nair et al.[12] (Table 1), slight enhancement (not statistically significant) was observed at the low (17 to 35 mM) ethanol concentrations against K562 and HSB target cells, but higher concentrations were inhibitory to K562, HSB, and U937 target cells. Purified preparations of LGL were inhibited at 70 and 103 mM ethanol against K562 targets.[12] Pretreatment of PBMC with 70 or 103 mM ethanol for 72 h in the presence of ethanol followed by washout of the ethanol, and further treatment with 500 U/ml of interferon (IFN)-α exhibited cytotoxicity levels similar to control effector cells without IFN treatment; however, cytotoxicity levels were 46% higher in untreated cells compared to untreated control PBMC. These investigators found that nicotine added directly to mixtures of effector and target cells, significantly inhibited NK activity at concentrations of 5 and 10 μg/ml. Nicotine (2 μg/ml) and ethanol at noninhibitory concentrations (1.7 mM, 17 mM, and 35 mM) showed significant suppression of NK activity when combined. This finding is important, since tobacco use is known to suppress NK cell activity *in vivo*,[14] and would appear to be an important variable to control when selecting subjects for both *in vitro* and *in vivo* studies.

Little is known concerning the possible mechanisms of enhancement or inhibition of NK cell activity, and more studies are needed in this area. Effector to target binding and conjugate formation was not different in the studies

TABLE 1
Summary of Investigations Showing Significant Effects of Ethanol *In Vitro* on Human NK Cell Cytolytic Activity

Subjects	Effector cells (E)[a]	Target cells (T)	Ethanol concentration mM (%)[b]	Response in NK cell activity	Comments	Ref.
Not identified	PBMC[a]	Molt-4 K562	80 (0.37)	50% inhibition	3 h ^{51}Cr release assay No effect on E:T binding Ethanol added to assay Statistical significance not indicated Ethanol concentration in media not determined	7
Healthy adults	PBMC depleted of monocytes	K562	18 (0.08) 52 (0.24) 87 (0.40) 174 (0.80)	29% inhibition 49% inhibition 61% inhibition 100% inhibition	4 h ^{51}Cr release assay 40–50% loss of ethanol after 4 h incubation period Ethanol added to assay 20 h ^{51}Cr release assay Ethanol added to assay Ethanol concentration not determined after 20 h incubation period	8
		Chang liver cells	18 (0.08) 52 (0.24) 87 (0.40) 174 (0.80)	12% inhibition 23% inhibition 32% inhibition 64% inhibition		
Normal adult males (20–31 years of age); subjects included abstainers and drinkers consuming 10–15 g of alcohol per week	PBMC	K562	(0.10)[c] (0.20) (0.50) (1.00) (2.00) (5.00)	25% enhancement 350% enhancement 280% enhancement 300% enhancement 290% enhancement 100% inhibition	4 h ^{51}Cr release assay Responses estimated at 10:1 E:T Ethanol added to assay Ethanol concentration not determined in assay media	11

Subjects	Effector cells	Target cells	Ethanol mM (%)	Effect	Comments	Ref.
Not identified	PBMC	K562	11 (0.05) 88 (0.40)	Inhibition[d] 60% inhibition	Ethanol added to assay Target binding capacity not altered in presence of ethanol Ethanol concentration not determined in assay media Statistical significance not indicated	9
Normal donors	PBMC	K562	54 (0.25) 110 (0.51)	190% enhancement 220% enhancement	PBMC incubated 16–24 h with ethanol and then washed prior to 4 h ^{51}Cr release assay 20% loss of ethanol during 16–24 h incubation period	10
			22 (0.10) 110 (0.50)	Minimal inhibition 50% inhibition	Ethanol added to 4 h ^{51}Cr release assay	
Healthy nonsmoking adults; moderate to low drinkers who abstained for alcohol for at least 1 week before testing	PBMC depleted of monocytes	K562	17 (0.08) 35 (0.16) 70 (0.32) 103 (0.47)	No effect No effect 63% inhibition 73% inhibition	Effector cells incubated with ethanol for 72 h washed and then used in a 4 h ^{51}Cr release assay Evaporation was 39% after 24 h, 48% after 48 h, and 59% at end of 72 h incubation E:T binding inhibited by 38% at 70 mM and by 47% at 103 mM ethanol	12
		HSB	17 (0.08) 35 (0.16) 70 (0.32) 103 (0.47)	No effect No effect 53% inhibition 54% inhibition	HSB is an NK-sensitive T cell leukemia	
		U937	17 (0.08) 35 (0.16) 70 (0.32) 103 (0.47)	No effect No effect No effect 36% inhibition	U937 is an NK-sensitive histiocytic lymphoma cell line	

TABLE 1 (continued)
Summary of Investigations Showing Significant Effects of Ethanol *In Vitro* on Human NK Cell Cytolytic Activity

Subjects	Effector cells (E)	Target cells (T)	Ethanol concentration mM (%)[b]	Response in NK cell activity	Comments	Ref.
	LGL[c]	K562	17 (0.08) 70 (0.16) 103 (0.47)	No effect 46% inhibition 50% inhibition		
Normal volunteers	PBMC depleted of monocytes	K562	2.2 (0.01)	40% enhancement	Enhancement seen when ethanol added to 3 h ^{51}Cr release assay, when effector and target cells incubated separately for 1 h before assay, and when preincubated effector and target cells were combined Enhancement also observed when effector cells incubated for 1 h with 0.22 µM and 2.2 nM ethanol	13

a   PBMC, peripheral blood mononuclear cells.

b   %, w/v.

c   %, w/v or v/v not specified.

d   Percentage inhibition not specified.

e   LGL, PBMC depleted of monocytes and fractionated on a discontinuous density gradient of Percoll. The fraction of lymphocytes banding at the 37.5% Percoll interface were used. About 75–80% of the cells in this fraction were positive to staining with HNK1 monoclonal antibody.

showing enhancement.[10,13] However, binding was inhibited by ethanol in a study[12] reporting decreased cytolytic activity, and was not affected in another.[9] Enhancement reportedly is due to an increased rate of killing by NK cells.[10,13] Rice, et al.[10] observed that enhancement was limited to the first hours of NK assay when NK cells exhibited decreased sensitivity to the proteinase substrate, acetyl tyrosine ethyl ester. The data were interpreted by the authors as being consistent with either enhanced *de novo* synthesis and/or increased storage of a chymotrypsin-like enzyme or its natural substrate; however, no concomitant increase in protein synthesis was detected with ethanol treatment. Whereas Rice et al.[10] found that recruitment of effector cells was enhanced by ethanol, Kendall and Targan[13] observed the opposite effect. They demonstrated that PBMC depleted of monocytes and exposed to 0.01 to 1 μM prostaglandin (PGE$_2$) solubilized in media, exhibited enhanced cytotoxicity.[13] However, inhibition was observed when K562 and PBMC target-cell conjugates were exposed to PGE$_2$.[13] Pretreatment of effector cells with a combination of 1 μM PGE$_2$ and 2.2 mM ethanol activated NK cytolytic activity, but was inhibitory when present during the assay. These results indicate the complexity of PGE$_2$ and ethanol on the cytolytic process, and demonstrate that modulation by PGE$_2$ could be both stimulatory and inhibitory. Another study[15] indicated that 1.0% ethanol incubated with PBMC for 48 h at 37°C *in vitro,* resulted in a twofold reduction of the CD16$^+$ NK cell marker on lymphocytes. The effect of lower, more physiological levels of ethanol, on the numbers of CD16$^+$ lymphocytes is not known.

The effects of ethanol in interleukin-2 (IL-2) production and receptor expression in human NK cells is not specifically known. Nair et al.[12] examined the effect of ethanol on activation of PBMC by IL-2. In this study, PBMC were precultured with 5 to 10 IU/ml of human recombinant IL-2, with or without ethanol concentrations ranging from 17 to 103 mM, for five to six days. Activity of the washed-effector cells against both NK-sensitive HSB and NK-resistant SB (a B cell leukemia line) target cells was inhibited at 70 and 103 mM ethanol. Relevant to this finding is a study by Kaplan,[16] demonstrating that PBMC incubated in the presence of 10 to 160 mM ethanol did not inhibit IL-2 production or the acquisition of IL-2 receptors (assessed by staining with monoclonal anti-Tac antibody). It is important to remember that these PBMC were not depleted of monocytes, and that the major cell type present in PBMC is the T lymphocyte. Additionally, ethanol suppressed the capacity of exogenously supplied IL-2 to stimulate proliferation of T lymphocytes that had previously acquired IL-2 receptors in a dose-dependent fashion.

NK cells can also express ADCC. Two investigations examined the effects of ethanol exposure on ADCC, and both report similar dose-dependent inhibition. Stacey[8] found that ADCC of PBMC depleted of monocytes was inhibited when ethanol was added to the assay media between 52 to 174 mM ethanol, and Nair et al.,[12] that activity was inhibited in lymphocytes previously incubated for 72 h at 70 and 103 mM, but not at 17 and 35 mM.

The effects of acetaldehyde on human PBMC have also been examined. At the nominal concentration of 0.01%, Prabhala and Watson[15] showed a fourfold decrease in CD16$^+$ NK cells attributable to acetaldehyde incubated with PBMC for 48 h. Stacey[8] examined the effects of acetaldehyde alone, and in combination with ethanol, on both NK cytolytic activity and ADCC. Acetaldehyde alone, when added to the assays at concentrations ranging from 17 to 170 μM (0.00008 to 0.0008% w/v), did not inhibit either NK or ADCC activity. Inhibition of NK cell activity was observed against both K562 and Chang liver cells at 1.7 mM (0.008% w/v) acetaldehyde. The measured concentration after a 4 h incubation period was 0.15 mM (0.00067% w/v): a loss of 91%, indicating the difficulty of insuring an effective concentration of this more volatile metabolite of ethanol. The effect of combined ethanol and acetaldehyde resembled the effects of ethanol alone.

B. RODENT CELLS

Studying the effects of ethanol *in vitro* on rodent NK cell activity has several advantages relative to the use of human cells, since the age, stress, and nutritional and infectious disease status can be more carefully controlled and monitored. Legitimate and illegitimate use of drugs, which may be immunomodulatory, can also be eliminated as contributory factors. However, there are many examples in the literature of different immune responses observed in rodents compared to their human counterpart. Nevertheless, studies on the effects of ethanol in rodents are important because of the advantages listed above. All reports to date have shown that ethanol inhibits NK cell activity when added directly to the assay of rat and mouse effector spleen cells (Table 2). Ethanol added to the assay media inhibited the binding of effector to target cells in C57BL/6 mice and BDIX rats.[17] Additionally, the effects were reversible, and NK cell cytolytic activity returned to normal when ethanol was removed. In the study by Walia et al.,[18,19] inhibition of NK activity was reversible when ethanol was removed after 2 or 4 h of preincubation. The inhibitory effects were abolished when either effector or target cells were preincubated individually for 1 h, washed, and then assayed.[17] Inhibition was observed in spleen cells not depleted of macrophages, in spleen cells partially depleted of B cells and macrophages by nylon wool passage, and in LGL cells obtained after further Percoll fractionation of nylon wool nonadherent (NWNA) spleen cells. The inhibition was less pronounced in NWNA cells, and LGL appeared to be more resistant to the effects of low (18 to 35 mM) ethanol concentrations.[20] These data suggest that macrophages may play some, but not an exclusive, role in inhibition of NK cell activity by ethanol. Yeralan and Jones[20] also reported that spleen cells from rats injected intraperitoneally (i.p.) with 250 μg polyriboinosinic-polyribocytodylic acid (poly IC) were less inhibited at 70 mM ethanol than unstimulated NK cells. They also found that NK activity in spleen cells was not stimulated by recombinant rat IFN-γ within the 4 h incubation period; however, splenocytes did respond to purified IFN-α + β. Spleen cells incubated with physiological amounts of ethanol and interferon α + β (10^2 to 10^4 units/microwell) were unresponsive to stimulation.

Ethanol inhibited ADCC at 44, 88, and 176 mM when added to the assay media.[19] Preincubation of target cells with 88 mM ethanol and then washed before adding to the ADCC assay did not alter target lysis.[18] Walia et al.[18] further suggest that the ox erythrocytes used as target cells in the ADCC assay, when preincubated with ethanol, exhibited increased maximum lysis compared to control target cells. When ethanol was present during the assay, the inhibitory effect of ethanol made the target cells more resistant to lysis. Ethanol did not inhibit the antibody sensitization step. The inhibition by ethanol added to the assay at 88 and 176 was partially restored after addition of 1 μM calcium ionophore A23187. The inhibition of ADCC by 44, 88, and 176 mM ethanol was completely reversed by the addition of 16 mM Ca^{++}. No toxicity was observed at the concentrations of calcium and calcium ionophore used in this study. Thus, these data suggest that ethanol may inhibit ADCC at a calcium-dependent step.

A study by Yeralan and Jones[20] utilizing rat spleen cells indicated that acetaldehyde in concentrations ranging between 0.3 to 15 mM (0.0013 to 0.067% w/v) inhibited NK activity of NWNA spleen cells from untreated rats when added to the assay. LGL were not inhibited at 1.5 mM (0.0067% w/v); whereas, spleen cells and NWNA cells were inhibited by 25% and 20% respectively.[20] Walia et al.[19,21] also showed inhibition of NK cell activity of C3H murine spleen cells at initial concentrations of 10 mM and 40 mM of acetaldehyde. The final concentrations of acetaldehyde in the media after the 4 h incubation assay were 1.3 mM and 5 mM respectively.[21] NK cell activity was not inhibited after a 2 h preincubation of spleen cells with acetaldehyde at 1 mM and 10 mM, suggesting that acetaldehyde, when added to the assay media, was inhibiting NK cell activity at the level of the effector cells, and that the inhibition was reversible when acetaldehyde was not present.[21] Acetaldehyde at a 40 mM decreased spleen cell viability by 30% after 4 h, and acetaldehyde inhibition of NK cell activity was not reversed after preincubation of effector spleen cells at this concentration.

Experiments on the effects of acetaldehyde on ADCC in rodent cells are limited. At initial concentrations up to 100 μM added to the assay, ADCC of spleen cells from C3H mice was potentiated at 18 h, but not after 4 h.[21] Acetaldehyde treatment at 10 mM for 15 min, however, potentiated ADCC. Thus, the effect of acetaldehyde was concentration- and time-dependent. ADCC, like NK cell activity, was inhibited at 10 mM and 40 mM acetaldehyde in the typical 18 h assay. Spleen cell preparations depleted of macrophages exhibited similar effects compared to unfractionated spleen cells. The sensitized-ox red blood cells used as targets were not susceptible to the effects of acetaldehyde at initial concentrations between 40 μM and 40 mM. Preincubation for 2 h of effector cells did not affect ADCC at concentrations of

TABLE 2
Summary of Studies Showing Significant Effects of Ethanol *In Vitro* on Rodent NK Cell Cytolytic Activity

Subjects	Effector cells (E)	Target cells (T)	Ethanol concentration mM (%)[a]	Response in NK cell activity	Comments	Ref.
Male F344 rats 6 to 8-weeks old	Spleen cells	Yac	18 (0.08) 35 (0.16) 70 (0.32)	36% inhibition 41% inhibition 63% inhibition	Ethanol added to assay 4 h ^{51}Cr release assay Responses evaluated at 50:1 E:T Ethanol concentration in assay media not determined	20
	NWNA[b]		18 (0.08) 35 (0.16) 70 (0.32)	No effect 32% inhibition 50% inhibition		
	LGL[c]		18 (0.08) 35 (0.16) 70 (0.32)	No effect No effect 28% inhibition	LGL exhibited approximately a fourfold increase in NK activity compared to unfractionated spleen cells LGL populations studied contained 30–50% T cells but <10% B cells or macrophages	
Adult C3H/HEN male and female mice	Spleen cells	Yac	22 (0.10) 88 (0.40) 176 (0.80)	No effect 43% inhibition 78% inhibition	Ethanol added to assay 4 h ^{51}Cr release assay Responses evaluated at 128:1 E:T Ethanol concentration not determined in assay media Total ethanol loss was 6.24% per h	18, 19

C57BL/6 mice	NWNA	Yac	13 (0.06)	No effect	Ethanol added to assay	17
			26 (0.12)	22% inhibition	4 h ^{51}Cr release assay	
			52 (0.24)	32% inhibition	Responses estimated at 50:1 E:T	
			103 (0.47)	60% inhibition	Ethanol concentration not determined in assay media	
			206 (0.95)	80% inhibition		
BDIX rats	NWNA	Yac	13 (0.06)	No effect	Same conditions as for C57BL/6 mice	
			52 (0.24)	38% inhibition		
			103 (0.47)	48% inhibition		
			206 (0.95)	60% inhibition		

[a] %, w/v.

[b] NWNA, nylon wool nonadherent cells.

[c] LGL, NWNA cells further purified on Percoll gradients.

acetaldehyde up to 1 mM, but ADCC was severely inhibited at 10 mM and 40 mM.

III. *IN VIVO* EFFECTS OF ALCOHOL CONSUMPTION

A. FACTORS INFLUENCING NATURAL KILLER CELL ACTIVITY

There are many important variables that influence NK cell activity and can complicate the design and interpretation of the role of ethanol on this activity. NK function is influenced by age,[1,3] gender,[3] exercise,[3,22,23] emotional status,[3,24,25] and is susceptible to circadian variation.[3] In rodents, there is a significant interaction of ethanol and stress, leading to alterations in adrenocorticotropin, corticotropin releasing factor, β-endorphins, and catecholamines.[26-30] Corticosterone concentration increases during ethanol consumption.[27,31-33] Glucocorticoids are known to modulate both human and rodent lymphocytes, which could directly or indirectly modulate NK cell activity.[34-38] In fact, Tabakoff et al.[33] suggest that "stress related to ethanol consumption may be of greater importance than the circulating ethanol concentration in producing the elevation in plasma glucocorticoids". Elevated plasma catecholamines during long-term alcohol ingestion[39] are correlated with suppression of NK cell activity in rats.[40] Corticotropin-releasing factor, through its effect on the autonomic nervous system, also reduces NK cell activity.[41]

Interpretation of the effects of ethanol and its metabolites on NK cell function in humans and animals is complicated by the wide variety of factors that can, in addition to alcohol consumption, influence activity. In humans, alcoholics may have varying degrees of liver damage, and are frequently malnourished. Nonalcoholic patients with primary biliary cirrhosis exhibit low NK and ADCC activity, while patients with chronic active hepatitis that were hepatitis B surface antigen-negative had normal NK and ADCC responses.[42] In another investigation,[43] NK cell activity was significantly reduced in patients with chronic active hepatitis. Killer (K) cells, defined as PBMC that were surface-immunoglobulin negative and formed rosettes with IgG sensitized chicken erythrocytes, were reduced in patients with primary biliary cirrhosis, but not in patients with chronic active hepatitis. The reduction in K cells was accompanied by a parallel decrease in ADCC.[44] In autoimmune liver disease, however, NK activity may be elevated.[45] Reduction in the number of K cells has been associated with the decrease in ADCC in patients with primary biliary cirrhosis.[44] A number of reports indicate enhanced cytotoxicity of peripheral blood lymphocytes from patients with alcoholic liver injury toward autochthonous liver cells or liver cell lines.[46-48] It is unknown what contribution NK cells play in this response. Additionally, intra-hepatic lymphocytes from biopsies of patients with alcoholic hepatitis have not demonstrated an increase of Fc receptor-positive (CD16$^+$) cells thought to be involved in ADCC.[49] Together with the observation that hepatocytes of alcoholic patients lack membrane-bound immunoglobulin, it is questionable whether ADCC plays an important role in hepatocyte injury.[48]

NK cells play an important role against many viral, bacterial, and fungal infections in humans.[1,3] The relevance to alcohol research is that concomitant infections can have both stimulatory and suppressive effects on NK cell cytolytic activity, and complicate interpretation of the direct effect of alcohol on NK activity. NK cells appear to be especially important in protection against cytomegalovirus, Epstein-Barr virus, and herpes simplex infections, since patients with immunosuppressed NK activity are more susceptible to these infections.[3,50,51] Patients with AIDS and AIDS-related complex also show abnormalities in NK cell function.[52] The link between alcohol and AIDS has been twofold. The first is that alcohol as a disinhibiting factor may lead to unsafe sexual behavior, and therefore unprotected exposure to HIV infection,[53] and the second is attributable to its actual immunosuppressive effect. The ability of fresh NK cells to lyse HIV-infected T cells or U937 target cells further supports a role for NK cells in retrovirus infections.[3]

In animals, NK cells also limit murine cytomegalovirus, Theiler's murine encephalitis virus, and possibly hepatitis virus infections.[54-57] Although the importance of NK cells in defense of mice against a number of other viruses is not completely known, it is well-established that NK cell activity is considerably boosted during acute infection with a number of important murine pathogens, including murine hepatitis virus, lymphocytic choriomeningitis virus, Maloney sarcoma virus, polyoma virus, Sendai virus, and mouse adenovirus.[58-60] Thus, it is extremely important that viral status is known when determining the effect of alcohol on immune response in both humans and rodent systems. It is quite likely that NK cell activity which would ordinarily be suppressed in the alcoholic or alcohol-consuming rodent would appear normal, or even stimulated, during viral infection.

Tobacco use is another important variable to control in humans studies, since NK cell activity in age- and gender-matched normal subjects is lower in smokers than in nonsmokers.[14] The concurrent use of other drugs of abuse and alcohol further complicates analysis on the effect of alcohol on NK cell function.[61]

Nutritional status is known to modulate NK cell activity, and can either stimulate or suppress immune responses. Severe starvation or protein-calorie malnutrition in humans and animals is associated with depressed NK cell activity.[62-65] Recently, we reported that undernourishing mice with dietary restriction without complete starvation also decreases NK cell activity.[66] Saxena et al.[64] also showed that reinstitution of a normal diet to starved mice resulted in a rebound effect to higher than normal levels of NK activity after three days of refeeding, returning to normal by eight days. Since mice during the first few days of ethanol consumption tend to decrease their intake of food,[67] determination of NK cell activity shortly after intake is resumed, may complicate interpretation of ethanol's capacity to modulate NK cell activity. Additionally, we previously showed that specific dietary restriction of tyrosine and phenylalanine decreased NK cell activity. Restriction of methionine stimulated NK cell activity.[68] The effects on NK cell activity of other amino acids modulated by ethanol are unknown.[69-71] Liver disease is also influenced by nutrients. Methionine and other lipotrope deficiencies appear in alcoholics, and further interact with alcohol in the development of cirrhosis.[72] In addition, liver cirrhosis is positively correlated with both alcohol and fat consumption.[73] The role of specific nutrients in the genesis of immunological abnormalities during alcohol consumption remains unclear, and is difficult to examine, whether immunological modulation results from generalized malnutrition, malabsorption of specific nutrients, or is the consequence of direct alcohol exposure.[70,74-76]

B. HUMAN INVESTIGATIONS

A few studies have specifically investigated NK cells from human alcoholics. The status of the patient and control groups is outlined in Table 3. Three investigations specifically evaluated NK cell numbers and function in patients with alcoholic liver disease. Charpentier et al.[77] found that NK cell activity of PBMC against two types of target cells was low in patients with inactive alcoholic cirrhosis, and that the defect was more pronounced in patients with severe malnutrition than in those with mild or moderate malnutrition. Decreased NK activity in patients with alcoholic cirrhosis was decreased against both K562 and MOLT 4 target cells. The murine P815 cell line, which is NK insensitive, was not lysed by normal cells or cells from cirrhotic patients. No relationship was observed between decreased NK activity and hepatocellular function. Impaired NK activity in alcoholic cirrhosis patients was not due to modification of kinetic activity, inhibitory factors in serum, or to suppressive effects of other lymphocytes and macrophages. Patients with alcoholic cirrhosis responded with enhancement of NK cell activity when their lymphocytes were preincubated for 1 to 3 h with 1000 or 2000 IU/ml of purified human fibroblast interferon; however, the response was not as strong as in control subjects.

Jovanovic et al.[78] reported differences in the number and percentages of CD57+ NK/K cells in the blood of alcoholics with normal liver or steatosis, and also found that these cell numbers were related to the drinking status of the patients. A higher number of these cells, but not T cell subsets, was seen in active alcoholics, compared to those abstinent patients who refrained from alcohol use for a period of two weeks to four years. Two of three patients observed at the time of hospitalization and ten days after detoxification, exhibited an 18 and 38% decrease in the number of CD57+ cells. Because CD57 is co-expressed on NK and K cells, and because these cells were increased in alcoholic hepatitis and cirrhosis, it would be difficult to clearly determine the relative contribution of K and NK cells to the increased

TABLE 3
Characteristics of Subjects Used for NK Investigations in Humans

Alcohol consuming subjects	Liver status (no. patients)	Alcohol use	Control group and comments	Ref.
59 patients with alcoholic cirrhosis; Age range: 43–71 yr; Mean age: 57 yr; Nutritional status: 39-mild to moderate malnutrition 20-severe malnutrition; Tobacco/Drug use: unknown; Infectious Diseases: All were hepatitis B surface antigen and antibody negative	Steatosis (21) Hepatitis (24) No liver disease (12)	40 Patients >80 g/d for more than 10 yr 19 patients between 50–80 g/d. No recent history of massive intoxication before study	Age and gender matched blood donors apparently healthy and free from infectious disease	77
30 male alcoholic patients admitted for detoxification; Age range: 34–69 yr; Mean age: 50.5 yr; Nutritional status: unknown; Tobacco/Drug use: unknown; Infectious Diseases: unknown	Normal or steatosis (12) Hepatitis (7) Cirrhosis (11)	>80 g/d but 8 were abstinent for 15 d to 4 yr	20 healthy laboratory hospital and staff; 16 male, 4 women; Mean age: 36.8 yr (Age range 28–66) No history of liver disease or alcoholism	78
63 alcoholics Gender: not indicated Age: not indicated Nutritional status: not reported Tobacco/Drug use: unknown Infectious Diseases: unknown	Hepatitis (19) Hepatitis + cirrhosis (44)	Not reported	No control group Liver biopsies assayed for the presence of lymphocytes in alcoholics	79

TABLE 3 (continued)
Characteristics of Subjects Used for NK Investigations in Humans

Alcohol consuming subjects	Liver status (no. patients)	Alcohol use	Control group and comments	Ref.
5 alcoholics 2 male, 3 female Age: not indicated Nutritional status: Well-nourished Tobacco/Drug use: All taking disulfiram and chlordi-azepoxide Infectious Diseases: One with mild bacterial conjunc-tivitis	No cirrhosis, hepatitis, or pancreati-tis in history or indicated by phys-ical examination	History of 10 yr of consumption; 1 qt of alcohol per day no less than 1 mo before admission Each imbibed on the day of admis-sion Blood alcohol not determined	Immune status evaluated 72 h after admission 5 Gender matched volunteers used as control Did not consume alcohol or other medications within 72 h preceding assay	80
27 chronic alcoholics admitted for detoxification and 5 volunteers who were regular consumers 30 male, 2 female Mean age: 39.9 yr Age range: 18–61 Nutritional status: Adequate except in four subjects who consumed <1 meal per d Tobacco/drug use: 70% were smokers 5 were unspecified drug addicts Infectious diseases: Free of clinical evidence of bac-terial or viral infection	Hepatomegaly (4) Cirrhosis(1)	Volunteer users consumed 20–100 g alcohol per day Chronic alcoholics consumed 218 g/d (range: 20–400 g/d)	15 Control subjects 12 male, 3 female Mean age: 38.6 Age range: 30–70 Nutritional status: adequate No clinical illness or drug addi-tion None smoking All subjects evaluated between 1 and 7 d following admission	81

40 chronic alcoholics
32 male, 8 female
Age: 35.9 ± 10 (SD)
Nutritional status: unknown
Tobacco/Drug Use:
  Drug users excluded
  Nearly all smoked ≥25 cigarettes per day for at least 10 years
Infectious Diseases: unknown
	Unknown	Consumed ≥6 cans/bottles of beer, ≥5 glasses of wine or ≥5 drinks of hard liquor per day within last month
		Mean number of drinking days were:
		Beer — 14.7
		Wine — 3.7
		Liquor — 11.3
			Two control groups:
			Smokers:
			11 male, 17 female
			Age: 42 ± 15
			25 Years of heavy smoking by same criteria as alcoholics
			Mean number of drinking days by same criteria as alcoholic group were:
			Beer — 0.5
			Wine — 0.05
			Liquor — 0.6
			Nonsmokers:
			19 male, 21 female
			Age: 47 ± 12
			85% Never smoked or quit > 15 yrs ago
			Mean number of drinking days by same criteria as alcoholic group were:
			Beer — 0.3
			Wine — 0
			Liquor — 0.2
				Alcoholics with overt alcohol-related liver disease such as jaundice or esophageal varices were excluded
				γ-Glutamyltransferase elevated compared to control group
				Bilirubin decreased compared to control
					82

19 male alcoholics without depression Age: 44 ± 8 9 male alcoholics with depression Age: 44 ± 11 Nutritional status: Serum folate elevated compared to depressives		Alcoholics: 13 ± 9 drinks per drinking day during last 3 mo 25 ± 8 drinking days per mo Alcoholics + Depression: 13 ± 8 drinks per drinking d during last 3 mo 25 ± 7 drinks per drinking d during last 3 mo	Control subjects: 50 healthy drug free males Tobacco use: unknown Age: 42 ± 10 Alcohol consumption: 2 ± 1 drinks per drinking d during last 3 mo 11 ± 9 drinking d per mo		24

TABLE 3 (continued)
Characteristics of Subjects Used for NK Investigations in Humans

Alcohol consuming subjects	Liver status (no. patients)	Alcohol use	Control group and comments	Ref.
Tobacco/Drug use: Tobacco use unknown All were medication-free for >3 mo except 12 who were removed from chlordiazepoxide 3 wk before study Infectious Diseases: All were free of physical disease by examination, no history of recent (<2 wk) viral infections, nor disease-like autoimmunity, or cancer that would affect immune function			Subjects with Depression: 18 healthy drug free males Tobacco use: unknown Age: 47 ± 12 Alcohol consumption: 1 ± 2 drinks per drinking day during last 3 mo 4 ± 8 drinking days per mo Depression with history of alcoholism in remission: 26 healthy drug free males Tobacco use: unknown Age: 43 ± 10 Alcohol consumption: 4 ± 8 drinks per drinking day during last 3 mo 4 ± 7 drinking d per mo. Serum γ-glutamyltransferase elevated compared to control	

cytolytic activity. NK cell activity was not determined in this study. Neither age nor race correlated with the alterations in the numbers of CD57$^+$ cells.

Chedid and Mendenhall[79] surveyed alcoholic patients with hepatitis and cirrhosis to assess the lymphocyte profile in liver biopsies. The presence of NK cells was based on the staining for CD16 and CD57. No NK cells were present; however, anti-CD16 stained pigment-containing macrophages and anti-CD57 outlined the bile duct epithelium. Because of the irrelevant staining, these investigators caution against using flow cytometry on liver cells obtained by collagenase digestion. Their data suggest that NK cells do not play a major role in hepatocyte necrosis in alcoholic liver disease.

Ericsson et al.[80] found normal ADCC and NK cell cytotoxicity in well-nourished, recently sober chronic alcoholics that were free of underlying disease, including alcoholic hepatitis, pancreatitis, and cirrhosis. For their assays, ADCC and NK cell cytotoxicity were determined in NWNA PBMC against herpes simplex virus-infected Chang liver cells in an 18 h chromium release assay.

Saxena et al.[81] studied NK cell activity in PBMC against K562 target cells in a typical 4-h chromium release assay. The results of eleven separate experiments were reported, and in six experiments, NK activity was distinctly higher in the alcoholic subjects compared to the control population. Elevation was less marked in three experiments, and in one experiment, no apparent effect was observed. Marked individual variation among the cell donors and between individual experiments was reported, as evidenced by the range of target cell lysis: 12 to 52% for controls and 22 to 87% for alcoholic subjects. Depletion of macrophages did not alter the NK-stimulatory effects of ethanol.

NK cell activity and serum interferon levels were recently studied in alcoholics with known smoking status, and the study included the appropriate smoking and nonsmoking controls. In this study, Chadha et al.[82] report that NK cell activity of PBMC was not altered in the chronic alcoholics compared to controls. The heavy cigarette smokers exhibited about a 37% decrease in NK cell activity. Serum interferon levels were highest in the chronic alcoholics compared to both control groups which were not different. Interferon inactivators were low or not detectable in the serum of the nonsmoking control group, but were nearly fivefold higher in the heavy cigarette smokers, and 8.5-fold higher in the chronic alcoholics in comparison. The ability of PBMC from both chronic alcoholics and heavy cigarette smokers to produce IFN-α and IFN-γ exhibited about a three- to fourfold decrease compared to the nonsmoking control group. No significant differences were observed between the smoking and chronic alcoholic groups. Minority and gender differences were present in the test subjects; however, gender differences in the determination of serum interferon levels were low-to-moderate in magnitude. Differences between minorities, which included African-American and Hispanic subjects, were minimal compared to Americans of European extraction; however, the minority subjects had somewhat higher scores on serum interferon levels. Age was low-to-moderately correlated with the findings, but using age as a covariate in the analysis of variance, did not alter the findings between the three experimental groups. It is interesting that even though the chronic alcoholics were comprised primarily of heavy cigarette smokers, NK cell activity was not suppressed in this group. It is possible that the overall weaker interferon system among the chronic alcoholics could have increased susceptibility to infectious agents that augment NK cell activity to give the appearance of normal function. Since the infectious disease status was unknown, this remains a possibility.

Depression is also associated with decreased NK cell activity. In a study of Irwin et al.,[24] the independent and combined interaction between depression and alcohol abuse on NK cell cytotoxicity was examined. Primary alcoholics with and without secondary depression and depressed patients with and without histories of alcohol abuse were compared. Nutritional and other indicators of health status were relatively normal in this study. Whereas γ-glutamyltransferase was elevated in all active alcoholics, the values for alanine aminotransferase, aspartate aminotransferase, and alkaline phosphatase, which are indicative of liver damage, were statistically indistinguishable among the five experimental groups. These findings suggest that the alcoholics were free of severe liver disease. Even though folate levels were higher in the alcoholic patients compared to depressive patients, they were also similar to the control values. The total leukocyte count was higher in all four experimental groups, and the absolute number of lymphocytes and monocytes was greater in the alcoholics compared to controls. PBMC from all four patient groups had significantly lower NK cell activity at all four effector to target ratios (40:1, 20:1, 10:1, 5:1). Cytolytic activity expressed as lytic units was also lower in the patient groups compared to controls. Alcoholic patients with secondary depression had lower lytic activity than the alcoholics without depression, and the patients with depression and a history of alcoholism had lower NK cell activity than those depressive patients not exhibiting alcohol abuse. The values for lytic activity in the depressive and alcoholic subjects were about 50% of the activity in the control group. Reduced NK cell activity (in lytic units) was correlated with increased numbers of leukocytes and neutrophils and with age. Chlordiazepoxide therapy, and the levels of γ-glutamyltransferase, folate, and vitamin B_{12} were correlated with NK cell activity. Additionally, in eight depressive patients who had undergone a two-week antidepressant washout, NK lytic activity was similar to that found in depressive patients that were ≥90 days free of antidepressants. There was a trend between the total number of drinks per month, and reduced lytic activity and increased leukocyte count and neutrophil numbers. Depression significantly correlated with reduced NK cell activity and with increased leukocyte count, and neutrophil and monocyte numbers. The correlation between depression and NK cell activity was also significantly correlated with depressives having a history of alcoholism, but not with other groups. Also of importance is the finding that single levels of plasma cortisol levels did not correlate with NK cell activity in a subsample consisting of 107 subjects which confirmed an earlier study.[83]

C. ANIMAL INVESTIGATIONS

Experiments to examine the effect of alcohol consumption on NK cell activity in animals, and the studies have been limited to rats and mice. Low consumption of ethanol up to 17% of the total calories (12 to 19 g/kg body weight/day) are reported to have either no effect[68,84] or a stimulatory[85] effect on NK cell activity. Ethanol administered as 36% of the total caloric intake to rats did not effect NK cell activity.[11] However, when ethanol consumption ranged between 27 to 40% of the derived calories (22 to 38 g/kg body weight per day), NK cell activity was consistently suppressed in mice.[66,67,84,86]

Mufti et al.,[11] feeding the Lieber deCarli (1982) liquid diet formulation to male Sprague-Dawley weanling rats for 12 weeks, found no alteration in NK cell activity against K562 target cells in a 4 h chromium release assay. Rats obtained 36% of their total dietary caloric intake when ethanol was incorporated into the diet at 1 and 7% w/v. Pair-fed animals received isocaloric diets, so that total caloric intake and diet intake were identical. No differences in body weight, liver, or spleen weight were present compared to a pair-fed controls; however, thymus weight was decreased about 30% in ethanol-consuming animals.

Saxena et al.[85] studied the effect of acute and chronic low alcohol intake on NK cell activity. Eight-week-old female C57BL/6 mice were administered ethanol in the drinking water at 1.6, 3.2, 6.4, and 12.6% w/v over a two week period, and fed a pelleted diet. NK cell activity was determined in spleen cell suspensions against K562 targets in an 18 h chromium-release assay. Ethanol consumption ranged from 3.2 g/kg/day in mice given 1.6% ethanol, to 18.1 g/kg/day in mice consuming 12.6% ethanol. Food intake, body weight, spleen weight, and yield of spleen cells were not significantly different among the groups. Liquid intake and diet, however, were lower in the mice drinking 12.6% ethanol. NK cell activity was clearly enhanced in the mice consuming 6.4 and 12.6% ethanol, with the highest amount of stimulation in the 12.6% ethanol group. Little significant effect of ethanol at the 1.6 and 3.2% level was evident, even though NK cell activity tended to be higher in the ethanol-consuming mice. In another experiment, mice drinking 7.9% ethanol for two or eight days did not show enhanced NK activity; whereas, two- to threefold higher NK activity was observed in spleen cells from mice consuming this level of ethanol for four to six weeks. There was considerable variability in the time period required to see enhancement. In most experiments, a two to three week feeding period of 7.9% ethanol enhanced NK activity. But in some experiments, especially in older mice, the lag time was longer, and in one experiment, alcohol did not augment NK cell activity after a feeding period of six weeks. Anti-Thy 1 plus complement treatment, or nylon wool passage, did not alter the findings when mice were fed 7.9% ethanol for five weeks, and NK cell activity determined against both K562 in 18 h assays and Yac targets in a 4 h chromium release assay. Considerable variation in the lag phase before NK activation was observed in subsequent experiments, and in some mice, activation did not occur for up to two months.

We found no effect of ethanol on NWNA spleen cells from female C57BL/6 mice fed a nutritionally balanced diet and 10% w/v ethanol in the drinking water for two,[89] four,[68] and twelve[84] weeks, compared to pair-fed or *ad libitum* controls in 4 h chromium release assays against Yac lymphoma target cells. Ethanol intake averaged between 12 to 19 g/kg body weight per day, and no differences in body weight, food intake, spleen weight, thymus weight, or in the total cell number per spleen were observed. In addition, we also observed no differences in NK cell activity after preincubation for 18 to 24 h with 1000 IU/ml IL-2, which similarly boosted activity in control and ethanol-consuming groups. Blood ethanol levels determined in mice fed ethanol for four weeks were 4.0 mM (0.018% w/v).

NK cell activity is suppressed in female C57BL/6 mice administered 20% w/v ethanol in the drinking water for up to 70 days in NWNA splenocytes against Yac in a 4 h chromium release assay[66,67,84,86] (Table 4). Mice in all our studies were well-nourished and had maintained a normal range of food intake. Of additional importance in our studies is that sentinal mice have been examined and found negative for Sendai virus, pneumonia virus of mice, *Mycoplasma pulmonis,* minute virus of mice, mouse hepatitis virus, Reovirus-3, and Theiler's encephalomyelitis virus, for up to 70 days of ethanol consumption. We have not found differences between control and pair-fed animals, except in our initial study,[84] where NK cell activity was lower in pair-fed controls relative to *ad libitum*-fed mice. It is likely that this difference is, in part, associated with single housing mice in hanging wire cages, an additional stress to the mice. Therefore, all subsequent experiments were conducted with mice housed in polycarbonate cages, with hardwood shavings for bedding. In these studies, baseline NK cell activity was significantly reduced by 31 to 62% of control activity after acute (7 days) and chronic (up to 70 days) of ethanol exposure (Table 4). There was a trend toward lower NK cell activity one day after initiation of ethanol administration. Interpretation of these data is complicated, however, because mice given ethanol, decreased their food and fluid consumption, which resulted in rapid body weight loss. Mice typically resume normal food and fluid consumption by 3 days after initiation of ethanol feeding, such that there is no significant difference in body or spleen weight, or the number of splenocytes at 7 days (Table 5). We have observed decreased NK cell activity in mice exhibiting a mean blood alcohol concentration of 22 mM,[87] and also in mice with blood ethanol concentration at the time of assay ranging from 0 to 16 mM.[66,86] In these studies, blood ethanol concentration did not correlate with NK cell activity. We observed varying effects of ethanol on spleen and thymus weight;

TABLE 4
NK Cell Activity of Mice at Various Time
Periods of Ethanol Consumption

Consumption period (days)	% Inhibition of NK cell activity by ethanol relative to control	
	Baseline	IL-2-Stimulated
1	20.7	15.5
7	61.8[a]	29.7[a]
10	56.2[a]	ND[b]
14	33.1[a]	44.2[a]
14	31.2[a]	ND
30	49.3[a]	17.2
70	25.0[a]	ND
70	34.4[a]	40.5[a]

[a]   Inhibition significantly lower in ethanol-consuming group relative to control group.
[b]   Not determined.

however, both tended to be lower in ethanol-consuming mice. In some experiments, this was reflected in a significant decrease in splenocyte number (Table 5). When NK cell activity is expressed on the basis of lytic units per spleen, the reduction of activity is even more pronounced in these animals. It is important to note that in some experiments, splenocyte number was not different, and that splenocyte number did not correlate with NK cell activity.[66,86] We are currently examining the changes in splenocyte number relative to ethanol consumption, since it is possible that the decrease in NK cell activity could be partly explained by a decrease in the percentage of NK cells in the spleen. It is interesting that ethanol consumption tends to decrease thymus weight, which is sensitive to stress.[88] When this occurs, the stress due to ethanol administration may contribute to the decreased NK cell activity. We currently are examining the role of stress in modulation of NK cell activity in conjunction with our model of ethanol consumption.

Because nutritional status plays a critical role in modulation of the immune response, and because it remains unclear whether generalized malnutrition, malabsorption of essential nutrients, or the direct effects of ethanol exposure act independently or in concert, to modulate NK cell activity, we have begun to address these questions directly. Restriction of food intake by approximately 25 and 40% respectively, decreases baseline NK cell activity.[66,67] Furthermore, NWNA splenocytes from the undernourished mice were impaired in their ability to respond to IL-2 stimulation (18 to 24 h) compared to both diet unrestricted control and ethanol-consuming mice. Ethanol did not interact with undernourishment to further inhibit NK cell activity. Moreover, supplemental ethanol calories did not protect against the inhibitory effect of diet

TABLE 5
Changes in Host Parameters with Continuous Exposure to 20% w/v Ethanol

Ethanol consumption (days: group)	Ethanol intake (g/kg/d)	Body weight change (g)	Spleen weight (mg)	Thymus weight (mg)	Total cells per spleen (× 10⁷)	Splenocytes per mg spleen (× 10⁵)
1 C		-0.6 ± 0.1	65.0 ± 7.1	ND	3.3 ± 1.4	5.0 ± 2.1
E	21.5 ± 6.0	-1.6 ± 0.2^a	59.0 ± 8.2	ND	2.6 ± 1.0	5.0 ± 2.0
7 C		0.5 ± 0.6	55.5 ± 12.4	36.0 ± 10.2	2.1 ± 1.0	3.9 ± 1.8
E	35.0 ± 6.0	0.1 ± 0.6	52.7 ± 10.8	48.0 ± 23.3^b	2.8 ± 2.0	5.2 ± 3.6
10 C		-0.1 ± 0.5	62.0 ± 7.5	44.3 ± 11.5	11.6 ± 2.7	7.2 ± 1.4
E	26.2 ± 6.6	-0.8 ± 1.3	51.8 ± 6.5^a	29.3 ± 8.1^a	8.5 ± 1.6	4.4 ± 8.1^a
14 C		0.7 ± 1.3	55.1 ± 11.7	55.6 ± 26.6	2.5 ± 1.0	4.5 ± 1.6
E	27.1 ± 1.1	0.3 ± 1.1	50.7 ± 8.5	32.0 ± 10.3^a	1.6 ± 0.8^a	3.3 ± 2.0^a
14 C		7.8 ± 4.8	62.1 ± 3.1	44.3 ± 4.7	7.2 ± 0.6	11.6 ± 1.1
E	25.4 ± 1.6	2.2 ± 3.9	51.8 ± 2.7^a	29.3 ± 3.3^a	4.4 ± 0.3^a	8.5 ± 0.6^a
30 C		1.9 ± 1.4	56.4 ± 10.6	50.5 ± 10.8	3.3 ± 0.9	5.9 ± 1.4
E	29.8 ± 3.7	1.7 ± 1.5	52.2 ± 13.3	38.2 ± 17.4	2.5 ± 1.1	4.9 ± 1.9
70 C		2.5 ± 1.2	61.6 ± 11.2	ND	5.1 ± 1.5	8.4 ± 2.4
E	29.9 ± 2.7	2.0 ± 1.2	51.2 ± 9.2^a	ND	5.5 ± 0.7	11.5 ± 3.5^b
70 C		4.0 ± 1.1	72.3 ± 8.7	46.7 ± 8.5	6.5 ± 1.4	9.5 ± 2.8
E	37.9 ± 3.8	3.2 ± 1.1	58.5 ± 7.6	44.4 ± 12.2	5.5 ± 1.7	9.0 ± 1.8

Note: Values represent means ±SD. Range for number of mice used per experiment was 18 to 21. Mice (C, control, E, ethanol-consuming) at the time of assay ranged in age from 56 to 147 days old. ND, not determined.

[a] Significantly lower ($p < 0.05$) than controls. Body weight change = Final body weight − initial body weight.
[b] Significantly higher ($p < 0.05$) than controls.

restriction on NK cell activity. Spleen weight was not reduced by ethanol in unrestricted mice. However, marked reduction occurred with progressive undernutrition. Thymus weight was decreased by ethanol consumption in diet unrestricted mice; however, thymus weight loss was more marked in diet restricted mice. Interestingly, ethanol consumption partially protected against the decrease in spleen weight and thymus weight induced by diet restriction. Ethanol partially protected against loss in body weight which was primarily attributed to an increase in carcass lipid content. Body weight was not different in ethanol-fed mice that were food-restricted by 25% compared to unrestricted, ethanol-consuming mice. Therefore, adequate nutritional status cannot be assumed in ethanol-fed mice solely on the basis of body weight stability.

Various changes in host status related to ethanol consumption are presented in Table 5. Changes in body weight were similar in ethanol-consuming mice compared to control mice. The effects of ethanol on spleen weight, thymus weight, total spleen cells per spleen, and total spleen cells per mg spleen were variable, and did not correlate with inhibition of baseline NK cell activity. Additionally, blood ethanol concentration, and the percentage of food calories derived from ethanol were not good indicators of NK cell inhibition. The best correlation between NK cell activity and ethanol in our investigations has been the total amount of grams of ethanol consumed per day as a function of body weight (Figure 1). There may be a critical threshold of ethanol consumption (between 20 to 25 g/kg/day) that must be attained before NK cell activity is inhibited. From these data, it appears that suppression of NK cell activity is somewhat correlated to the total amount of ethanol consumed per kg of body weight (r = 0.78). This correlation is not related to the duration of ethanol consumption.

IV. SUMMARY AND CONCLUSIONS

The relationship between alcohol consumption and NK cells activity is complex and involves many interacting factors. It is clear from *in vitro* investigations using human and rodent cells that the sustained presence of a physiologically attainable blood ethanol concentration inhibits cytolytic activity of NK cells. Acetaldehyde in sufficient concentration is also inhibitory to NK cells *in vitro,* although it is more difficult to ascertain a physiologically or biologically relevant concentration.

The important question to be answered is what is the role of ethanol and its metabolites in modulation of NK cell activity *in vivo*? Our studies in which mice were administered ethanol in the drinking water have repeatedly shown inhibition of splenic NK cell activity when alcohol intake is above a threshold dose of 20 g/kg/day. NK cell activity in PBMC from human alcoholics is often normal, but elevated and reduced NK activity have also been reported. Moreover, it is not known whether NK activity is modulated differently by alcohol consumption in different body compartments, or whether alcohol

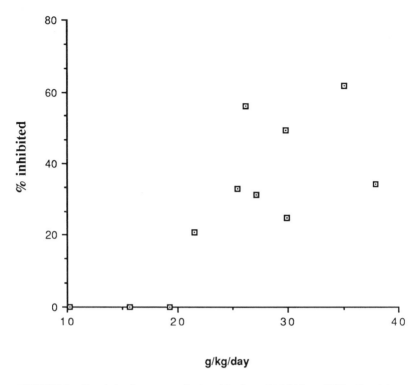

FIGURE 1.   Correlation between total ethanol intake and inhibition of NK cell activity.

consumption alters the kinetics and/or distribution of NK cells within these compartments. Alcoholics also often have varying degrees of liver damage. Since liver disease itself is immunomodulatory and because either one or more other important variables such as the amount of alcohol consumed, infectious disease status, nutritional state, and tobacco use have not always been controlled or reported in human experiments. It is also not clear whether alcohol has a direct effect on NK cell activity in the human. In contrast to the rodent experiments, most human investigations have utilized abstinent alcoholics. Thus, the question as to whether alcohol directly suppresses (or enhances) NK cell activity in humans remains to be answered. It is quite possible that NK cell activity is initially reduced by alcohol consumption in humans, and that this predisposes them to various viral, bacteria, and possible fungal disease. These diseases in turn are able to partially stimulate the suppressed NK cell to give the appearance of normal and even elevated cytolytic activity. The role of acetaldehyde in the immunomodulatory effects of alcohol consumption on NK cell activity *in vivo* is largely unknown. It is entirely possible that some inconsistencies in the findings, especially in humans, may be related to differences in ethanol metabolism. Although it appears that alcohol is a risk factor in development of cancer, the biological significance of the immunomodulation of NK cell activity to the carcinogenesis process and its effect on tumor progression is unknown and remains a challenge for future research.

ACKNOWLEDGMENTS

This work was supported by Research Grants AA07293, AA08386, and Research Scientist Development Award, AA00138, to Dr. Meadows from the National Institute on Alcohol Abuse and Alcoholism.

REFERENCES

1. **Trinchieri, G.,** Biology of natural killer cells, in *Advanced Immunology,* Vol. 47, Dixon, F. J., Ed., Academic Press, San Diego, 1991, 187.
2. **Mason, L., Giardina, S. L., Hecht, T., Ortaldo, J., and Mathieson, B. J.,** LGL-1: a non-polymorphic antigen expressed on a major population of mouse natural killer cells, *J. Immunol.,* 140, 4403, 1988.
3. **Whiteside, T. L. and Herberman, R. B.,** The role of natural killer cells in human disease, *Clin. Immunol. Immunopath.,* 53, 1, 1989.
4. **Storkus, W. J. and Dawson, J. R.,** Target structures involved in natural killing (NK): characteristics, distribution, and candidate molecules, *Crit. Rev. Immunol.,* 10, 393, 1990.
5. **Berkow, R. and Fletcher, A. J.,** *The Merck Manual,* 15th ed., Merck Sharp and Dohme Res. Lab., Rahway, NJ, 1987, 1479.
6. **Niemeiä, O., Israel, Y., Mizoi, Y., Fukunaga, T., and Eriksson, C. J. P.,** Hemoglobin-acetaldehyde adducts in human volunteers following acute ethanol ingestion, *Alcohol.: Clin. Exp. Res.,* 14, 838, 1990.
7. **Suthanthiran, M., Solomon, S. D., Williams, P. S., Rubin, A. L., Novogrodsky, A., and Stenzel, K. H.,** Hydroxyl radical scavengers inhibit human natural killer cell activity, *Nature (London),* 307, 276, 1984.
8. **Stacey, N. H.,** Inhibition of antibody-dependent cell-mediated cytotoxicity by ethanol, *Immunopharmacology,* 8, 155, 1984.
9. **Saxena, Q. B., Saxena, R. K., and Adler, W. H.,** Ethanol and natural killer activity, in *NK Cells and Other Natural Effector Cells,* Herberman, R. B., Ed., Academic Press, New York, 1982, 651.
10. **Rice, C., Hudig, D., Lad, P., and Mendelsohn, J.,** Ethanol activation of human natural cytotoxicity, *Immunopharmacology,* 6, 303, 1983.
11. **Mufti, S. I., Prabhala, R., Moriguchi, S., Sipes, I. G., and Watson, R. R.,** Functional and numerical alterations induced by ethanol in the cellular immune system, *Immunopharmacology,* 15, 85, 1988.
12. **Nair, M. P. N., Kronfol, Z. A., and Schwartz, S. A.,** Effects of alcohol and nicotine on cytotoxic functions of human lymphocytes, *Clin. Immunol. Immunopath.,* 54, 395, 1990.
13. **Kendall, R. A. and Targan, S.,** The dual effect of prostaglandin (PGE2) and ethanol on the natural killer cytolytic process: effector activation and NK-cell-target cell conjugate lytic inhibition, *J. Immunol.,* 125, 2770, 1980.
14. **Ferson, M., Edwards, A., Lind, A., Milton, G. W., and Hersey, P.,** Low natural killer-cell activity and immunoglobulin levels associated with smoking in human subjects, *Int. J. Cancer,* 23, 603, 1979.

15. **Prabhala, R. H. and Watson, R. R.,** Effects of various alcohols applied *in vitro* on human lymphocyte subtypes and mitogenesis, in *Prog. Biol. Res. Vol. 325. Alcohol, Immunomodulation, and AIDS,* Seminara, D., Watson, R. R., and Pawlowski, A., Eds., Alan R. Liss, New York, 1990, 155.

16. **Kaplan, D. R.,** A novel mechanism of immunosuppression mediated by ethanol, *Cell. Immunol.,* 102, 1, 1986.

17. **Ristow, S. S., Starkey, J. R., and Hass, G. M.,** Inhibition of natural killer cell activity *in vitro* by alcohol, *Biochem. Biophys. Res. Commun.,* 105, 1315, 1982.

18. **Walia, A. S., Pruitt, K. M., Rodgers, J. D., and Lamon, E. W.,** *In vitro* effect of ethanol on cell-mediated cytotoxicity by murine spleen cells, *Immunopharmacology,* 13, 11, 1987.

19. **Walia, A. S. and Lamon, E. W.,** *In vitro* effects of ethanol and acetaldehyde on cell-mediated cytotoxicity, in *Prog. Clin. Biol. Res. Vol. 325. Alcohol, Immunomodulation, and AIDS,* Seminara, D., Watson, R. R., and Pawlowski, A., Eds., Alan R. Liss, New York, 1990, 145.

20. **Yeralan, O. and Jones, J. M.,** Effects *in vitro* of ethanol and acetaldehyde on natural killer activity from rats, in *Prog. Biol. Res. Vol. 325. Alcohol, Immunomodulation, and AIDS,* Seminara, D., Watson, R. R., and Pawlowski, A., Eds., Alan R. Liss, New York, 1990, 165.

21. **Walia, A. S., Pruitt, K. M., Dillehay, D. L., Marshall, G. M., and Lamon, E. W.,** *In vitro* effect of acetaldehyde on cell-mediated cytotoxicity by murine spleen cells, *Alcohol.: Clin. Exp. Res.,* 13, 766, 1989.

22. **Berk, L. S., Nieman, D. C., Youngberg, W. S., Arabatzis, K., Simpson-Westerberg, M., Lee, J. W., Tan, S. A., and Eby, W. C.,** The effect of long endurance running on natural killer cells in marathoners, *Med. Sci. Sports Exerc.,* 22, 207, 1990.

23. **Simpson, J. R. and Hoffman-Goetz, L.,** Exercise stress and murine natural killer cell function, *Proc. Soc. Exp. Biol. Med.,* 195, 129, 1990.

24. **Irwin, M., Caldwell, C., Smith, T. L., Brown, S., Schuckit, M. A., and Gillin, J. C.,** Major depressive disorder, alcoholism, and reduced natural killer cell cytotoxicity, *Arch. Gen. Psychiatr.,* 47, 713, 1990.

25. **Khansari, D. N., Murgo, A. J., and Faith, R. E.,** Effects of stress on the immune system, *Immunol. Today,* 11, 170, 1990.

26. **Redei, E., Branch, B. J., and Taylor, A. N.,** Direct effect of ethanol on adrenocorticotropin (ACTH) release *in vitro, J. Pharmacol. Exp. Ther.,* 237, 59, 1986.

27. **Patel, V. A. and Pohorecky, L. A.,** Interaction of stress and ethanol: effect on b-endorphin and catecholamines, *Alcohol.: Clin. Exp. Res.,* 42, 785, 1988.

28. **Rivier, C. and Vale, W.,** Interaction between ethanol and stress on ACTH and b-endorphin secretion, *Alcohol.: Clin. Exp. Res.,* 12, 206, 1988.

29. **Rivier, C., Imaki, T., and Vale, W.,** Prolonged exposure to alcohol: effect of CRF mRNA levels, and CRF- and stress-induced ACTH secretion in the rat, *Brain Res.,* 520, 1, 1990.

30. **Guaza, C., Torrellas, A., and Borrell, S.,** Adrenocortical response to acute and chronic ethanol administration in rats, *Psychopharmacology,* 79, 173, 1983.

31. **Kakihana, R., Butte, J. C., Hathaway, A., and Noble, E. P.,** Adrenocortical response to ethanol in mice: modification by chronic ethanol consumption, *Acta. Endocrinol.,* 67, 653, 1971.

32. **Watson, R. R., Jackson, J. C., Hartmann, B., Sampliner, R., Mobley, D., and Eskelson, C.,** Cellular immune functions, endorphins, and alcohol consumption in males, *Alcohol.: Clin. Exp. Res.,* 9, 248, 1985.

33. **Tabakoff, B., Jaffe, R. C., and Ritzman, R. F.,** Corticosterone concentrations in mice during ethanol drinking and withdrawal, *J. Pharm. Pharmacol.,* 30, 371, 1978.

34. **Holbrook, N. J., Cox, W. I., and Horner, H. C.,** Direct suppression of natural killer activity in human peripheral blood leukocyte cultures by glucocorticoids and its modulation by interferon, *Cancer Res.,* 43, 4019, 1983.

35. **Nair, M. P. N. and Schwartz, S. A.,** Immunomodulatory effects of corticosteroids on natural killer and antibody-dependent cellular cytotoxic activities of human lymphocytes, *J. Immunol.,* 132, 2876, 1984.

36. **Nair, M. P. N. and Schwartz, S. A.,** Immunoregulation of human natural killer cells (NK) by corticosteroids: inhibitory effect of culture supernatants, *J. Allergy Clin. Immunol.,* 82, 1089, 1988.

37. **Hochman, P. A. and Cudkowicz, G.,** Suppression of natural cytotoxicity by spleen cells of hydrocortisone-treated mice, *J. Immunol.,* 123, 968, 1979.

38. **Cox, W. I., Holbrook, N. J., and Friedman, H.,** Mechanism of glucocorticoid action on murine natural killer cell activity, *J. Natl. Cancer Inst.,* 71, 973, 1983.

39. **Ogata, M., Mendelson, J. H., Mello, N. K., and Majchrowicz, E.,** Adrenal function and alcoholism II. catecholamines, *Psychosom. Med.,* 33, 159, 1971.

40. **Felton, D. L., Felten, S. Y., Bellinger, D. L., Carlson, S. L., Ackerman, K. D., Madden, K. S., Olschowki, J. A., and Livnat, S.,** Noradrenergic sympathetic neural interactions with the immune system: structure and function, *Immunol. Rev.,* 100, 225, 1987.

41. **Irwin, M., Hauger, R. L., Brown, M., and Britton, K. T.,** CRF activates autonomic nervous system and reduces natural killer cytotoxicity, *Am. J. Physiol.,* 255, R744, 1988.

42. **Vierling, J. M., Nelson, D. L., Strober, W., and Bundy, B. M.,** *In vitro* cell-mediated cytotoxicity in primary biliary cirrhosis and chronic hepatitis, *J. Clin. Invest.,* 60, 1116, 1977.

43. **Serdengecti, S., Jones, D. B., Holdstock, G., and Wright, R.,** Natural killer activity in patients with biopsy-proven liver disease, *Clin. Exp. Immunol.,* 45, 361, 1981.

44. **Sandilands, G. P., Macsween, R. N. M., Gray, K. G., Holden, R. J., Mills, P., Reid, F. M., Thomas, M. A., and Watkinson, G.,** Reduction in peripheral blood K cells and activated T cells in primary biliary cirrhosis, *Gut,* 18, 1017, 1977.

45. **Hirai, N., Kato, Y., Kobayashi, K., and Hattori, N.,** Natural killer (NK) cell activity and its *in vitro* response to interferon-a (Le) chronic liver diseases and hepatocellular carcinoma, *Liver,* 6, 212, 1986.

46. **Sorrell, M. F. and Leevy, C. M.,** Lymphocyte transformation and alcoholic liver injury, *Gastroenterology,* 63, 1020, 1972.

47. **Kaku, S. and Leevy, C. M.,** Lymphocyte cytotoxicity in alcoholic hepatitis, *Gastroenterology,* 72, 594, 1977.

48. **Zetterman, R. K. and Sorrell, M. F.,** Immunologic aspects of alcoholic liver disease, *Gasteroenterology,* 81, 616, 1981.

49. **Sanchez-Tapias, J., Thomas, H. C., and Sherlock, S.,** Lymphocyte populations in liver biopsy specimens from patients with chronic liver disease, *Gut,* 18, 472, 1977.

50. **Ho, M.,** Infection and organ transplantation, in *Anesthesia and Organ Transplantation,* Gelman, S., Ed., W. B. Saunders, Philadelphia, 1987, 49.

51. **Biron, C. A., Byron, K. S., and Sullivan, J. L.,** Severe herpes virus infections in an adolescent without natural killer cells, *New Eng. J. Med.,* 320, 1731, 1989.

52. **Sirianni, M. C., Tagliaferri, F., and Aiuti, F.,** Pathogenesis of the natural killer cell deficiency in AIDS, *Immunol. Today,* 11, 81, 1990.

53. **Leigh, B. C.,** Alcohol and unsafe sex: an overview of research and theory, in *Prog. Clin. Biol. Res., Vol. 325, Alcohol, Immunomodulation and AIDS,* Seminara, D., Watson, R. R., and Pawlowski, A., Eds., Alan R. Liss, New York, 1990. 35.

54. **Bukowski, J. F., Woda, B. A., Habu, S., Okumura, K., and Welsh, R. M.,** Natural killer cell depletion enhances virus synthesis and virus-induced hepatitis *in vivo, J. Immunol.,* 131, 1531, 1983.

55. **Bancroft, G. J., Shellam, G. R., and Chalmer, J. E.,** Genetic influences on augmentation of natural killer (NK) during murine cytomegalovirus infection: correlation with patterns of resistance, *J. Immunol.,* 126, 988, 1981.

56. **Paya, C. V., Patrick, A. K., Leibson, P. J., and Rodriguez, M.,** Role of natural killer cells as immune effectors in encephalitis and demyelination induced by Theiler's virus, *J. Immunol.,* 143, 95, 1989.

57. **Okada, M. and Minamishima, Y.,** The efficacy of biological response modifiers against murine cytomegalovirus infection in normal and immunodeficient mice, *Microbiol. Immunol.,* 31, 45, 1987.

58. **Schindler, L., Engler, H., and Kirchner, H.,** Activation of natural killer cells and induction of interferon after injection of mouse hepatitis virus type 3 in mice, *Infect. Immun.,* 35, 869, 1990.

59. **Herberman, R. B., Nunn, M. E., Holden, H. T., Staal, S., and Djeu, J. Y.,** Augmentation of natural cytotoxic reactivity of mouse lymphoid cells against syngeneic and human allogeneic target cells, *Int. J. Cancer,* 19, 555, 1977.

60. **Biron, C. A., Turgiss, L. K., and Welsh, R. M.,** Increase in NK cell number and turnover rate during acute viral infection, *J. Immunol.,* 131, 1539, 1983.

61. **Klimas, N. G., Morgan, R., Blaney, N. T., Chitwood, D., Page, J. B., Milles, K., and Fletcher, M. A.,** Alcohol and immune function in HIV-1 seronegative, HTLV — I/II seronegative and positive men on methadone, in *Prog. Clin. Biol. Res. Vol. 325. Alcohol, Immunomodulation, and AIDS,* Seminara, D., Watson, R. R., and Pawlowski, A., Eds., Alan R. Liss, New York, 1990, 103.

62. **Salimonu, L. S., Ojo-Amaize, E., Williams, A. I. O., Johnson, O. K., Cooke, A. R., Adekunle, F. A., Alm, G. V., and Wigzell, H.,** Depressed natural killer cell activity in children with protein-calorie malnutrition, *Clin. Immunol. Immunopath.,* 24, 1, 1982.

63. **Saxena, R. K., Saxena, Q. B., and Adler, W. H.,** Decline of murine natural killer activity in response to starvation, hypophysectomy, tumor growth, and beige mutation: a comparative study, in *NK cells and other natural effector cells.,* Herberman, R. B., Ed., Academic Press, New York, 1982, 645.

64. **Saxena, R. K., Saxena, Q. B., and Adler, W. H.,** Regulation of natural killer activity *in vivo:* part I — loss of natural activity during starvation, *Ind. J. Exp. Biol.,* 18, 1383, 1980.

65. **Cooper, W. C., Good, R. A., and Mariani, T.,** Effect of protein insuficiency on immune responsiveness, *Am. J. Clin. Nutr.,* 27, 647, 1974.

66. **Blank, S. E., Duncan, D. A., and Meadows, G. G.,** Suppression of natural killer cell activity by ethanol consumption and food restriction, *Alcohol.: Clin. Exp. Res.,* 15, 16, 1991.

67. **Meadows, G. G., Blank, S. E., and Duncan, D. A.,** Modulation of natural killer cell activity by alcohol consumption and nutritional status, in *Prog. Clin. and Biol. Res. Vol. 325. Alcohol, Immunosuppression and AIDS,* Seminara, D., Watson, R. R., and Pawlowski, A., Eds., Alan R. Liss, New York, 1990, 181.

68. **Abdallah, R. M., Starkey, J. R., and Meadows, G. G.,** Alcohol and related dietary effects on mouse natural killer-cell activity, *Immunology,* 50, 131, 1983.

69. **Eriksson, T., Carlsson, A., Liljequist, S., Hagman, M., and Jagenburg, R.,** Decrease in plasma amino acids in rat after acute administration of ethanol, *J. Pharm. Pharmacol.,* 32, 512, 1980.

70. **Shaw, S. and Lieber, C. S.,** Plasma amino acid abnormalities in the alcoholic: respective role of alcohol, nutrition and liver injury, *Gastroenterology,* 74, 677, 1978.

71. **Siegel, F. L., Roach, M. K., and Pomeroy, L. R.,** Plasma amino acid patterns in alcoholism: the effects of ethanol loading, *Proc. Natl. Acad. Sci. U.S.A.,* 51, 605, 1964.

72. **Rodgers, A. E., Fox, J. G., and Murphy, J. C.,** Ethanol and diet interactions in male Rhesus monkeys, *Drug-Nutr. Interactions,* 1, 3, 1981.

73. **Rotily, M., Durbec, J.-P., Sarles, P. B., and Sarles, H.,** Nutrition and alcohol in liver cirrhosis; a case-control study, *Crit. Rev. Acad. Sci.,* 3, 247, 1990.

74. **Yew, M. S., Moore, S., and Biesele, M. M.,** Effects of chronic ''moderate'' alcohol consumption on vitamins A and C status of male Sprague-Dawley rats, *Nutr. Rep. Int.,* 23, 427, 1981.

75. **Neville, J. N., Eagles, J. A., Samson, G., and Olson, R. E.,** Nutrition status of alcoholics, *Am. J. Clin. Nutr.,* 21, 1329, 1968.
76. **Guthrie, G. D., Myers, K. J., Gesser, E. J., White, G. W., and Koehl, J. R.,** Alcohol as a nutrient: interactions between ethanol and carbohydrate, *Alcohol.: Clin. Exp. Res.,* 14, 17, 1990.
77. **Charpentier, B., Franco, D., Paci, L., Charra, M., Martin, B., Vuitton, D., and Fries, D.,** Deficient natural killer cell activity in alcoholic cirrhosis, *Clin. Exp. Immunol.,* 58, 107, 1984.
78. **Jovanovic, R., Worner, T., Lieber, C. S., and Paronetto, F.,** Lymphocyte subpopulations in patients with alcoholic liver disease, *Dig. Dis. Sci.,* 31, 125, 1986.
79. **Chedid, A. and Mendenhall, C. L.,** Cell-mediated immunity in alcoholic liver disease, in *Prog. Biol. Res. Vol. 325. Alcohol, Immunomodulation, and AIDS,* Seminara, D., Watson, R. R., and Pawlowski, A., Eds., Alan R. Liss, New York, 1990, 321.
80. **Ericsson, C. D., Kohl, S., Pickering, M. D., Davis, J., Glass, G. S., and Faillace, L. A.,** Mechanisms of host defense in well nourished patients with chronic alcoholism, *Alcohol.: Clin. Exp. Res.,* 4, 261, 1980.
81. **Saxena, Q. B., Mezey, E., and Adler, W. H.,** Regulation of natural killer activity *in vivo.* II. The effect of alcohol consumption on human peripheral blood natural killer activity, *Int. J. Cancer,* 26, 413, 1980.
82. **Chadha, K. C., Whitney, R. B., Cummings, M. K., Norman, M., Windle, M., and Stadler, I.,** Evaluation of interferon system among chronic alcoholics, in *Prog. Clin. Biol. Res., Vol. 325. Alcohol. Immunomodulation, and AIDS,* Seminara, D., Watson, R. R., and Pawlowski, A., Eds., Alan R. Liss, New York, 1990, 123.
83. **Irwin, M., Daniels, M., Risch, S. C., Bloom, E., and Weiner, H.,** Plasma cortisol and natural killer cell activity during bereavement, *Biol. Psychiatr.,* 24, 173, 1988.
84. **Abdallah, R. M., Starkey, J. R., and Meadows, G. G.,** Toxicity of chronic high alcohol intake on mouse natural killer cell activity, *Res. Commun. Chem. Pathol. Pharmacol.,* 59, 245, 1988.
85. **Saxena, Q. B., Saxena, R. K., and Adler, W. H.,** Regulation of natural killer activity *in vivo:* part IV — high natural killer activity in alcohol drinking mice, *Ind. J. Exp. Biol.,* 19, 1001, 1981.
86. **Meadows, G. G., Blank, S. E., and Duncan, D. D.,** Influence of ethanol consumption on natural killer cell activity in mice, *Alcohol.: Clin. Exp. Res.,* 13, 476, 1989.
87. **Glassman, A. B., Bennett, C. E., and Randall, C. L.,** Effect of ethyl alcohol on human peripheral lymphocytes, *Arch. Pathol. Lab. Med.,* 109, 540, 1985.
88. **Dougherty, T. F. and White, A.,** Functional alterations in lymphoid tissue induced by adrenal cortical secretion, *Am. J. Anat.,* 77, 81, 1945.
89. **Meadows, G. G. and Blank, S. E.,** unpublished observations.

Chapter 5

ALCOHOL AND CYTOKINE SECRETION

Bernhard Watzl and Ronald R. Watson

TABLE OF CONTENTS

5761-6/93/$0.00 + $.50
© 1993 by CRC Press, Inc.

I. INTRODUCTION

Cytokines are biologically active, glycosylated polypeptide products secreted by activated lymphocytes, monocytes, and various other cells. They stimulate target cells at extremely low concentrations of 10^{-10} to 10^{-15} mol/l.[1] Cytokines function as intercellular messengers in the regulation of the immune system. This includes regulation of local and systemic inflammatory responses, as well as augmentation of host cell blastogenesis. Cytokines modulate reactions of the host to foreign antigens or injurious agents by regulating growth, mobility, and differentiation of leukocytes and other cells.[1] Any perturbation of this very tightly controlled system can result in immune alterations, and ultimately in increased incidence of infections and cancer.

The physicochemical characteristics of alcohol (ethanol) allow it to interfere intensively with functions and metabolism of cytokine-producing cells. Alcohol is completely miscible with water, and is to some degree, fat soluble. It crosses membranes by diffusion across a concentration gradient. Alcohol ingestion exposes immune cells to high concentrations of alcohol, and a metabolite, acetaldehyde. Reviews suggest that the continuous exposure of immunocompetent cells to alcohol suppresses the immune system.[2-4] In addition, alcohol abusers have frequent and severe infections, particularly with Gram-negative bacteria.[5] Several immune responses which are suppressed *in vitro* and/or *in vivo* by alcohol are at least partially regulated by various cytokines. Polymorphonuclear neutrophils (PMN) from chronic alcoholics without liver disease showed a depressed chemotaxis, which improved on alcohol withdrawal.[6,7] The capacity of PMN to adhere to endothelial cells is also decreased by alcohol.[8] Granulocytopenia is a further PMN disorder which is observed in alcoholics and in *in vitro* systems with alcohol.[9,10] The activation of PMN is critically dependent on the presence of interleukin-1 (IL-1) and tumor necrosis factor alpha (TNFα), especially with regard to functions such as hematopoiesis, chemotaxis, and adherence.[11] Phagocytosis by alveolar and peritoneal macrophages in animals and the particle clearance by mononuclear phagocytes in humans, a process which is activated by TNFα,[11] is reduced by alcohol.[12-14] In addition, interleukin-2 (IL-2)-dependent immune responses such as mitogen-stimulated lymphocyte transformation can be suppressed[15,16] and stimulated[17] by alcohol. However, there is a paucity of information available regarding the extent to which cytokines mediate the immunomodulating effects of alcohol. This chapter will focus on data about the effects of alcohol on the production and secretion of cytokines, obtained from patients with alcoholic liver disease, alcoholics without liver disease, animal models, and *in vitro* studies.

II. CYTOKINES

A. INTERLEUKIN-1 (IL-1)

IL-1 consists of two different peptides, IL-1α and IL-1β, which have nearly identical activities and bind with equal affinity to the same cell surface receptor. IL-1 is produced primarily by activated monocytes and macrophages, but also by a variety of other cell types.[1] IL-1α is mostly cell membrane-associated, while IL-1β represents the released form of IL-1. However, the exact mechanism by which IL-1 is secreted from the cells is still incompletely understood.

McClain et al.[18] were the first to publish data about serum IL-1 activity in six male patients with alcoholic hepatitis. Using the standard thymocyte costimulator assay, they measured a serum IL-1 activity in alcoholic hepatitis patients, which was up to ten times higher than in age and sex-matched controls. At the same time, they observed in these patients very low serum zinc and serum albumin concentrations, which are systemic effects of liver cells exposed to elevated IL-1 concentrations.[19] According to their hypothesis, alcohol ingestion increases intestinal permeability to a variety of macromolecules, including bacteria-derived endotoxin, which may chronically stimulate IL-1 release from hepatic Kupffer cells and other IL-1 secreting cells.[18] Preliminary data from another study[20,70] reported increased plasma IL-1 levels in patients with acute alcoholic hepatitis and in nondrinking patients with alcoholic cirrhosis, when compared to alcoholics with no liver disease and to controls. Patients with liver disease further showed increased numbers of activated cytotoxic T cells in the peripheral blood, while monocyte expression of the activation marker HLA-DR was not different between these groups. This study clearly demonstrated that alcohol ingestion itself did not modulate IL-1 secretion *in vivo*. Felver et al.[21] measured IL-1α and IL-1β on admission and after 30 days of hospitalization in plasma samples obtained from patients with severe alcoholic hepatitis. Plasma IL-1α content was higher in patients with alcoholic hepatitis (190 pg/ml) compared to controls (<50 pg/ml) and did not change during 30 days of hospitalization. Alcoholics without liver disease had normal plasma IL-1α levels (<50 pg/ml). In alcoholic cirrhosis, the plasma IL-1α concentration was not significantly different from controls. Plasma IL-1β concentration was not different between all the tested groups. Yokota et al.[22] isolated monocytes from patients with liver cirrhosis (alcoholic and nonalcoholic) and measured the capacity of these cells to secrete IL-1α and IL-1β after stimulation with lipopolysaccharide (LPS). Patients with liver cirrhosis secreted less IL-1 (no difference between IL-1α and β), but higher amounts of prostaglandin E_2 (PGE_2) than controls. The addition of indomethacin to monocyte cultures resulted in a significantly higher IL-1 release by monocytes of liver cirrhosis patients than by monocytes of controls. The mechanism of increased secretion of IL-1 and PGE_2 by monocytes of patients with liver cirrhosis was not clarified. However, increased IL-1 secretion *in vitro* correlated with enhanced secretion of acute phase reactants from the liver of these patients, which suggests a systemically elevated IL-1 release. Bird et al.[23] also investigated IL-1 secretion by monocytes of patients with acute alcoholic hepatitis and of patients with inactive alcoholic cirrhosis. IL-1 secretion did not differ between controls and alcoholic hepatitis patients, but was increased in patients with alcoholic cirrhosis. Alcohol also has effects on mucosal IL-1 secretion.[24] Intracolonic administration of alcohol resulted in mucosal IL-1 generation, presumably by the localization of PMN to the area, since leukotriene B4 (LTB$_4$), as well as myeloperoxidase activity, were increased in the mucosa.

Only preliminary data are available about the *in vitro* effects of alcohol on IL-1 secretion. Mitogen-activated peripheral blood mononuclear cells (PBMC) from healthy donors, incubated over 24 h with a range of various alcohol concentrations, showed a suppression of IL-1 secretion, which was independent of the applied alcohol dose.[25] A short-term treatment (60 min) of unstimulated rat Kupffer cells with alcohol suppressed messenger ribonucleic acid (mRNA) expression for IL-1α and IL-1β. However, if alcohol-exposed Kupffer cells were stimulated with LPS, they expressed mRNA for IL-1α and IL-1β in excess of that with LPS alone.[26] The authors concluded that chronic alcohol and endotoxin exposure may disrupt the normal immunoregulatory circuits of the liver.

These studies clearly show that patients with alcoholic hepatitis have elevated plasma IL-1 levels. Monocytes from patients with alcoholic cirrhosis have normal, increased as well as decreased, capacities to secrete IL-1, depending on the concentration of concomitantly secreted PGE$_2$. It is known that a highly significant positive correlation exists between IL-1 secretion and the severity of fibrosis in chronic hepatitis B virus infection,[27] suggesting that the increased plasma IL-1 activity found in alcoholic hepatitis patients may have caused the fibrotic process in the liver. The increased IL-1 secretion *in vivo* is probably not directly caused by alcohol itself, since alcoholics without liver disease demonstrate normal plasma IL-1 levels. Acetate, the metabolite which is produced of alcohol via the intermediate acetaldehyde, has been reported to enhance IL-1 production *in vitro* by human blood monocytes.[28] Elevated blood acetate levels are an indicator for alcohol ingestion in chronic alcoholics.[29] Therefore, alcohol-derived acetate could induce the increased plasma levels observed in patients with alcoholic hepatitis.[18,20,21] However, during 30 days of hospitalization and abstinence, plasma IL-1 levels in patients with alcoholic hepatitis did not decrease.[21]

B. TUMOR NECROSIS FACTOR (TNF)

TNF consists of two different peptides, TNFα and TNFβ, both exhibiting similar activities in regard to antitumor activity, immunomodulation, and inflammation. Despite the low degree of homology between TNFα and TNFβ at the amino acid level, they bind equally well to the same receptor.[1] TNFα is produced by monocytes/macrophages, but lymphocytes and NK cells are also able to produce TNFα. TNFα occurs in soluble form and in a membrane-associated form. Because of the major role of TNFα in the induction of the acute-phase response and the similarities between the alterations, which occur during the acute phase response and during the course of alcoholic liver disease,[30] several studies focused on TNFα secretion in alcoholic hepatitis and alcoholic cirrhosis patients.

Allen et. al.[20,31,32,70] measured plasma TNFα in patients with acute alcoholic hepatitis and in nondrinking patients with alcoholic cirrhosis. In alcoholic hepatitis and cirrhosis patients, plasma TNFα was significantly increased when compared to controls and to alcoholics without liver disease. The high TNFα levels correlated with the expression of lymphocyte activation markers, but not with monocyte activation markers. TNFα levels remained high in alcoholic hepatitis patients for the six month follow-up period. Since the peripheral blood monocytes were not activated, the authors speculated that nonparenchymal cells were the source of excess TNFα. Felver et al.[21] confirmed the elevated plasma TNFα in patients with alcoholic hepatitis. In their study, patients with alcoholic cirrhosis and alcoholic patients without clinically apparent liver disease had plasma TNFα levels comparable to non-alcoholic, healthy controls. PBMC from patients with alcoholic hepatitis spontaneously secrete significantly higher amounts of TNFα than healthy controls.[33] TNFα release by LPS-activated PBMC from patients with alcoholic hepatitis was 25.3 ± 3.7 U/ml compared to 10.9 ± 2.4 U/ml in controls. These results suggest that PBMC are contributing to the elevated plasma TNFα levels observed by others in alcoholic hepatitis patients.[20,31,32,70] Stahnke and Allen[32] extended their previous studies by measuring PBMC TNFα secretion in patients with alcoholic hepatitis and alcoholic cirrhosis. They did not observe differences in the spontaneous TNFα secretion, but the LPS-induced TNFα secretion was significantly increased in alcoholic hepatitis and alcoholic cirrhosis. It is important to note that these PBMC showed the same percentage of activation marker expression (HLA-DR) on the cell surface than control PBMC. *In vitro* exposure to alcohol of PBMC from patients with alcoholic hepatitis and from controls, resulted in decreased TNFα secretion,[33] which implies that alcohol itself is not a stimulus for increased PBMC TNFα release.

Animal studies investigating the effect of acute and chronic alcohol exposure on TNFα secretion have contributed further information to this field. Intravenous application of LPS caused comparable serum TNFα peaks after 90 min in both normal and chronic alcoholic rats.[34] In contrast, acute alcohol injections suppressed significantly serum TNFα levels in both groups. These results confirm the *in vitro* data,[33] that acute alcohol exposure suppresses TNFα release, independent of chronic alcohol exposure. In a further study, marked suppression of serum and bronchoalveolar fluid TNFα occurred after short-term alcohol exposure of rats.[35] D'Souza et al.[36] reported that the reduced-serum TNFα activity in rats after endotoxin challenge and *in vivo* exposure to various concentrations of alcohol was dose-dependent, with higher alcohol doses leading to higher suppression of serum TNFα activity. In contrast to the reported suppression of serum TNFα, one study observed after endotoxin challenge increased serum TNFα levels in chronically alcohol-fed rats.[37] However, a single alcohol administration followed by endotoxin, resulted in significantly lower serum TNFα level. Thus, it appears that rats respond differently to short-term and long-term alcohol exposure in regard to LPS-induced TNFα secretion. Hansen et al.[38] studied serum TNFα levels and expression of hepatic mRNA for TNFα in chronically alcoholic rats. The injection of LPS resulted in significantly higher serum TNFα levels in alcoholic rats compared to controls, but expression of mRNA for TNFα was induced in both groups. Kupffer cells from chronically alcohol-fed rats secreted lower amounts of TNFα than Kupffer cells from control rats.[39] Alcohol also affected TNFα gene expression in the HL-60 myeloid leukemia cell line.[40] TNFα transcripts were at low, but detectable, levels in untreated cells, while treatment with 86 and 172 mmol/L alcohol for 6 h was associated with an increase in the level of these transcripts. The secreted TNFα in culture supernatants was not measured.

C. INTERLEUKIN-6 (IL-6)

IL-6 is secreted by monocytes, lymphocytes, fibroblasts, and several other cell types.[1] The wide range of biological activities of IL-6 include stimulation of differentiation of B cells in mature immunoglobulin secreting cells. IL-6 is the only cytokine reported to date known to regulate acute-phase protein synthesis in human hepatocytes,[41] suggesting that it is involved in inflammatory liver processes observed in alcoholic hepatitis and cirrhosis.

Deviere et al.[42] studied serum IL-6 levels in patients with alcoholic cirrhosis. While IL-6 was undetectable in serum of healthy, nonalcoholic controls, alcoholic cirrhosis patients had serum IL-6 levels of 62.9 ± 24.1 U/ml. PBMC from these patients spontaneously secreted significantly higher amounts of IL-6 than PBMC from controls. The difference in LPS-induced PBMC IL-6 secretion was even more significant between these groups. There was a positive correlation between LPS-induced IL-6 secretion and IgA serum levels, but no significant correlation between IL-6 secretion and IgG serum levels. The authors further reported that LPS-induced IL-6 production by PBMC was also increased in nonalcoholic cirrhosis, but normal levels were found in alcoholics without liver disease or with fatty liver without cirrhosis. In another study,[31,70] patients with alcoholic hepatitis were found to exhibit higher plasma IL-6 levels than stable, nondrinking patients with alcoholic cirrhosis.[31] IL-6 concentrations correlated with the clinical status of the patients. Since PBMC from patients with increased IL-6 plasma levels did not express activation markers on the cell surface, the authors speculated that hepatic nonparenchymal cells were the source of excess IL-6.

Chronically alcohol-fed rats expressed IL-6 mRNA in liver cells 2 h after injection of LPS, while in control livers mRNA for IL-6 was not detectable. Without LPS, none of the livers from either group contained any mRNA for IL-6.[38] Thus, animal studies confirm the observations made in patients with alcoholic liver disease, that the combination of endotoxin and alcohol exposure results in high circulating IL-6 levels, which may partially mediate the hepatic inflammation observed in these patients.

D. INTERLEUKIN-2 (IL-2)

IL-2 exerts numerous immunologic effects by stimulating the proliferation of lymphocytes with subsequent amplification of immune responses.[1] Responsiveness of lymphocytes to IL-2 requires the expression of IL-2 receptors (IL-2R). Soluble IL-2R are released from activated cells, both *in vitro* and *in vivo*. IL-2 further enhances interferon-gamma production and augments killer cell activities. IL-2 is released from T cells by the pathway generally associated with secretory proteins.[43]

Patients with alcoholic cirrhosis demonstrate lower IL-2 secretion by stimulated PBMC than healthy, nonalcoholic controls.[42] There was a significant inverse correlation between IL-2 and IL-6 production. In a previous study, however, these authors reported a depression in the proliferation of T cells from patients with alcoholic cirrhosis compared to patients with alcoholic hepatitis and controls, while the capacity of T cells to secrete IL-2 was fully preserved.[44] Bird et al.[23] confirmed the reduced IL-2 secretion in this group of patients, but found also that PBMC from patients with nonalcoholic chronic liver disease had a lower capacity to release IL-2 after PHA stimulation in comparison with controls. Patients with alcoholic hepatitis showed the same intensity of IL-2 secretion by PBMC as controls. In contrast to these results, patients with alcoholic hepatitis, but not patients with alcoholic cirrhosis, expressed a reduced ability of PBMC to secrete IL-2.[45] PBMC from patients with alcoholic cirrhosis, but not from those with alcoholic hepatitis, responded to a co-stimulation with PHA and interferon-alpha (IFNα) by increasing IL-2 release. Nonalcoholic liver damage, such as chronic hepatitis B virus infection, is also known to cause a reduction in IL-2 secretion by PBMC,[27] which suggests that alcohol ingestion is not the primary cause for reduced IL-2 secretion in alcoholic liver disease. However, binge drinking in light-alcohol users resulted in a decreased ability of lymphocytes to produce IL-2, which persisted for four days.[46] *In vitro* exposure of PBMC from healthy volunteers to various concentrations of alcohol also decreased IL-2 secretion, independent of the applied alcohol dose, which suggests a direct suppressive effect of alcohol on IL-2 secretion.[25] In contrast to the results of this study, Kaplan[47] found no inhibition of IL-2 secretion with doses of alcohol ranging from 10 to 160 mmol/L. The major criticism in Kaplan's study is, however, that regular 96-well flat-bottom plates were used for 72 h incubations. Recent data have shown that in these microplates, alcohol evaporates from wells with high alcohol concentrations, and condenses immediately in adjacent wells with lower concentrations of alcohol.[48] Starting alcohol concentrations between 0 and 5% on one 96-well microplate resulted, after 72 h, in a nearly complete equilibrium in all the wells (final alcohol concentrations ranged between 0.31 and 0.49%). It is necessary to incorporate a barrier on each well to restrict diffusion. Therefore, diffusion of alcohol may have interfered with IL-2 secretion in Kaplan's study, equalizing exposure to alcohol of cells including controls.

The results from animal studies differ from data obtained in human alcoholics with liver disease. With the exception of intragastric alcohol infusion, chronic alcohol treatment in rats and mice does not result in liver damage beyond the stage of fatty liver, because of the natural aversion to alcohol in general, and the higher metabolic rate in these animals.[49] Human alcoholics obtain up to 50% of their calories from alcohol, compared with the maximum of 36% obtained by rodents. Human alcoholics are often malnourished, while alcohol-fed animals normally consume diets which supply nutrients several times beyond the actual requirements. As a consequence, alcohol effects on organ systems are more pronounced in humans than in rodents.

A four day alcohol administration by gastric intubation in rats did not result in a different IL-2 secretion by purified T lymphocytes when compared to T lymphocytes from control rats.[50] The alcohol treatment suppressed T lymphocyte proliferation, which could be explained by the decreased ability of blast cells from these animals to use IL-2. The high-affinity IL-2R expression was not decreased relative to controls. *In vitro* exposure of T cells from alcohol-treated rats and naive rats had no effect on IL-2 secretion.[17] There was also no difference between alcohol-treated and naive rats. It is not known if passive diffusion of alcohol from microwells was prevented in this study. T lymphocytes from three-month-old rats exposed *in utero* to alcohol were not significantly affected in their IL-2 secretion, as compared with T cells from offspring of pair-fed and normal diet groups.[51] T cells from young (3 months) and old (25 months) mice (BALB/c) treated *in vivo* with alcohol, showed normal IL-2 secretion.[52] The *in vitro* exposure of T cells from young and old BALB/c mice to alcohol had no effect on the secretion of IL-2.[53] Again, there is no mention of whether alcohol diffusion restriction covers were used to avoid well-to-well transfer, which again means that these data have to be analyzed cautiously. When alcohol diffusion was prevented, murine splenocytes from two- to three-week-old Swiss mice expressed an alcohol concentration-dependent inhibition of IL-2 secretion.[54] From these data it is not clear, whether the observed difference in IL-2 secretion between young mice is caused by the different strains of mice, by the age difference, by the prevention of alcohol diffusion, or by a combination of these factors.

E. INTERFERONS (IFN)

IFN are a heterogeneous group of polypeptides exhibiting potent antiviral and immunoregulatory activities. There are two types of IFN. Type I IFN consists of IFNα and IFNβ, both of which are induced *in vivo* by viral infections. IFNα is produced primarily by leukocytes and IFNβ by nonleukocytic cells. Type II IFN or IFNτ is produced during immune reactions by stimulated T lymphocytes or natural killer (NK) cells.[1] The immunomodulatory effects of IFN include activation of macrophages and neutrophils, stimulation of IL-1 secretion by monocytes/macrophages, and activation of NK cells. IFN also possess activities described as macrophage activating factor and monocyte migration inhibitory factor (MIF).

Mitogen-activated PBMC from patients with alcoholic cirrhosis release less IFNτ than activated PBMC from healthy subjects.[42] There was also a reduced IL-2 secretion in these patients, and the secretion of both lymphokines was inversely correlated with the secretion of IL-1. Chronic alcoholics have a significantly higher serum IFN concentration than controls.[55] The ability of PBMC from chronic alcoholics to produce IFNα in response to Sendai virus infection and IFNτ in response to LPS was suppressed, compared to controls.[55] Serum of chronic alcoholics contained eight times more IFNα inactivator than serum from controls. The activity of the IFNα inactivator was measured by adding known amounts of human IFNα to serum from alcoholics and controls, and then measuring the remaining IFN antiviral activity.[55] The high IFNα inactivator level could be the reason for the low amount of detected IFNα in PBMC supernatants as assessed with a bioassay. PBMC could have a normal IFNα secretion, but the high level of IFNα inactivator may have neutralized the antiviral activity of this cytokine. The increased serum IFNα level, together with the normal NK cell activity observed in these subjects, support this hypothesis. The *in vitro* culture of PBMC from healthy volunteers with various concentrations of alcohol suppressed the IFNτ secretion only at alcohol concentrations above 0.5% (v/v).[25] Alcohol *in vitro* is the simplest IFN inducer.[56] Primary chick embryo cells cultured *in vitro* with 5.5% (v/v) alcohol in the medium, produced a high amount of IFN. The authors speculate that alcohol may use a different molecular pathway for the induction of IFN than that used by viruses. The release of MIF which reportedly consists of several peptides, including IFNs,[1] is also affected by alcohol. MIF activity in rats administered alcohol by gavage was decreased in a dose-dependent manner.[57] These data are consistent with data generated from ferret model of oral alcohol ingestion.[58]

III. MECHANISMS OF ALCOHOL-INDUCED MODULATION OF CYTOKINE SECRETION

Several mechanisms for alcohol have been postulated to explain the alcohol-mediated changes in serum levels of cytokines. Alcohol and its metabolite, acetaldehyde, could directly interfere with cytokine-producing and secreting cells by altering signal transduction and membrane fluidity, affect synthesis of factors regulating cytokine production such as PGE_2, and cause tissue damage, and thereby indirectly induce cytokine release. The majority of the clinical studies showed increased plasma levels of cytokines, and increased cytokine release by PBMC from patients with alcoholic liver disease. The secretion of monokines such as IL-1 and TNFα and lymphokines such as IL-2 and IFNτ is under the control of PGE_2.[59-61] Therefore, alcohol could mediate its effect on cytokine secretion by modulating PGE_2 production. PBMC from alcoholics produced less PGE_2, and their PMN produced less LTB_4 than PBMC and PMN from controls.[62] The reduced PGE_2 production was corrected by the addition of exogenous arachidonic acid, despite a normal endogenous arachidonic acid and linoleate acid content in these cells. The authors concluded that chronic alcohol ingestion either inhibits membrane-bound phospholipase activity, or enhances the catabolism of eicosanoids. The acute addition of alcohol to murine peritoneal macrophages caused a dose-dependent release of both arachidonic acid and eicosanoids, indicating the activation of phospholipase A_2.[63] There was low metabolic turnover of the released arachidonic acid, and enzymes catalyzing prostaglandin synthesis were inhibited. Thus, alcohol appears to change the metabolic pathway involved in eicosanoid synthesis. Reduced synthesis of PGE_2 in alcoholic liver disease may predispose to cytokine-mediated hepatic inflammation and resultant fibrosis. PBMC from alcoholics further showed a significant reduction of both basal and stimulated cyclic adenosine monophosphate (cAMP) levels.[64] *In vitro* exposure of PBMC from healthy controls to alcohol resulted also in decreased cAMP levels.[65] Since cAMP is involved in signal transduction pathways leading to the production of cytokines, alcohol could interfere at the level of cAMP with cytokine production. Recently, it has been demonstrated that alcohol interacts with G_s, a member of the guanine nucleotide binding proteins (G proteins), that also play key roles in signal transduction.[66] Chronic alcoholics express low plasma concentrations of β-endorphin (β-end) compared with nonalcoholic controls, regardless of either alcoholic liver disease or of the time of abstinence studied.[67] β-end is known to stimulate *in vitro* the PGE_2 release by cultured human PBMC.[61] The low plasma β-end levels in chronic alcoholics may be related to the low PGE_2 levels observed in these patients.[62] *In vitro* studies observed stimulatory[68] as well as inhibitory effects[61] of β-end on IFNτ secretion by human PBMC. Alcohol could therefore mediate its immunomodulatory effect on IFNτ secretion by reducing β-end plasma levels.

Finally, alcohol could induce organ damage and, as a secondary effect, induce cytokine secretion in the damaged tissue. In the intestinal tract, alcohol damages intestinal walls[69] and induces mucosal IL-1 generation.[28] It increases intestinal permeability for macromolecules, including endotoxin,[69] which may result in chronic stimulation of endotoxin-clearing and cytokine secretion hepatic nonparenchymal cells. However, there is no relationship between cytokine concentrations and peripheral endotoxemia.[70] Nondrinking patients with alcoholic cirrhosis also have increased levels of circulating IL-1, and alcoholics without liver disease have normal plasma IL-1 levels,[20] which excludes alcohol as the primary cause of enhanced IL-1 secretion. Since patients with alcoholic hepatitis and cirrhosis have increased levels of circulating IL-1 and TNFα, but do not express activation markers on the cell surface,[20,31,32,70] it was suggested that hepatic nonparenchymal cells were the source of excess IL-1, IL-6 and TNFα. Animal studies revealed that Kupffer cells from chronically alcohol-fed rats release less TNFα than control Kupffer cells,[39] which leaves the question open regarding the source of the increased level of circulating cytokines. On the other hand, PBMC from chronically nonalcoholic cirrhosis patients showed a suppressed IL-2 secretion,[27] but binge drinking of alcohol also resulted in reduced IL-2 secretion by PBMC from healthy subjects.[46] At present, the existing clinical data allow no final conclusions whether alcohol-induced tissue damage is the causative factor for increased levels of circulating cytokines.

IV. SUMMARY

Cytokines regulate the immune response in narrow ranges by activating and suppressing immunocompetent cells. Alcohol ingestion is linked to an increased occurrence of bacterial infections, presumably by suppressing various immune responses. The exact mechanisms of alcoholic immunosuppression is not yet well-understood. Alcohol might interfere with the production and secretion of cytokines, and thereby initiate immunomodulation. Clinical studies with patients with alcoholic hepatitis and patients with alcoholic cirrhosis demonstrated increased plasma levels for IL-1, TNFα, IL-6, and IFNτ. *In vitro* studies suggest that chronic alcohol ingestion enhances IL-1, TNFα, and IL-6 secretion by cultured PBMC, but decreases the capacity of these cells to release IL-2, IFNτ, and IFNα. *In vitro* exposure to alcohol of PBMC from healthy subjects resulted generally in suppression of cytokine release, which indicates that acute, local alcohol effects differ markedly from chronic, systemic alcohol effects. Animal studies revealed also contradictory results between *in vivo* and *in vitro* exposure to alcohol. Data from chronic alcohol-feeding studies are in agreement with human studies, that the plasma monokine levels were increased, while *in vitro* exposure of spleen cells suppressed the cytokine release. IL-2 secretion by splenocytes was affected by alcohol exposure *in vivo* or *in vitro*. Alcohol could affect cytokine secretion by at least three different mechanisms:

1. It could have a direct effect on cytokine-secreting cells by affecting signal transduction and changing fatty acid composition in cell membranes.
2. It could affect synthesis of regulating factors of cytokine production such as PGE_2.
3. It could directly induce tissue damage with consecutive cytokine release.

ACKNOWLEDGMENT

This work was supported by Grant AA08037 from the National Institute on Alcohol Abuse and Alcoholism.

REFERENCES

1. **Oppenheim, J., Ruscetti, F., and Faltynek, C.,** Cytokines, in *Basic and Clinical Immunology,* Stites, D. P., Terr, A. I., Eds., Appleton and Lange, Norwalk, 1991, 78.
2. **MacGregor, R.,** Alcohol and immune defense, *JAMA,* 256, 1471, 1986.
3. **Cooper, B., and Maderazo, E.,** Alcohol abuse and impaired immunity, *Infections in Surg.,* 94, 101, 1989.
4. **Jerrells, T., Marietta, C., Bone, G., Weight, R., and Eckardt, M.,** Ethanol-associated immunosuppression, *Adv. Biochem. Psychopharmacol.,* 44, 173, 1988.
5. **Adams, G. and Jordan, C.,** Infections in the alcoholic, *Med. Clin. N. Am.,* 68, 179, 1984.
6. **Gluckman, S., Dvorak, V., and MacGregor, R.,** Host defenses during prolonged alcohol consumption in a controlled environment, *Arch. Intern. Med.,* 137, 1539, 1977.
7. **MacGregor, R., Gluckman, S., and Senior, J.,** Granulocyte function and levels of immunoglobulins and complement in patients admitted for withdrawal from alcohol, *J. Infect. Dis.,* 138, 747, 1978.
8. **MacGregor, R. and Gluckman, S.,** Effect of acute alcohol intoxication on granulocyte mobilization and kinetics, *Blood,* 52, 551, 1979.
9. **Imperia, P., Chikkappa, G., and Phillips, P.,** Mechanism of inhibition of granulopoiesis by ethanol, *Proc. Soc. Exp. Biol. Med.,* 175, 219, 1984.
10. **Liu, Y.,** Effects of alcohol on granulocytes and lymphocytes, *Semin. Hematol.,* 17, 130, 1980.
11. **Le, J. and Vilcek, J.,** Tumor necrosis factor and interleukin 1: cytokines with multiple overlapping biological activities, *Lab. Invest.,* 56, 234, 1987.
12. **Rimland, D.,** Mechanisms of ethanol-induced defects of alveolar macrophage function, *Alcoholism,* 8, 73, 1983.
13. **Mufti, S., Prabhala, R., Moriguchi, S., Sipes, I., and Watson, R.,** Functional and numerical alterations induced by ethanol in the cellular immune system, *Immunopharmacology,* 15, 85, 1988.
14. **Liu, Y.,** Phagocytic capacity of reticuloendothelial system in alcoholics, *J. Reticuloendoth. Soc.,* 25, 605, 1979.
15. **Tisman, G. and Herbert, V.,** *In vitro* myelosuppression and immunosuppression by ethanol, *J. Clin. Invest.,* 51, 1410, 1973.
16. **Glassman, A., Bennett, C., and Randall, C.,** Effects of ethyl alcohol on human peripheral lymphocytes, *Arch. Pathol. Lab. Med.,* 109, 540, 1985.
17. **Jerrells, T., Peritt, D., Marietta, C., and Eckardt, M.,** Mechanisms of suppression of cellular immunity induced by ethanol, *Alcohol.: Clin. Exp. Res.,* 13, 490, 1989.
18. **McClain, C., Cohen, D., Dinarello, C., Cannon, J., Shedlofsky, S., and Kaplan, A.,** Serum interleukin-1 (IL-1) activity in alcoholic hepatitis, *Life Sci.,* 39, 1479, 1986.
19. **Durum, S., Oppenheim, J., and Neta, R.,** Immunophysiologic role of interleukin 1, in *Immunophysiology,* Oppenheim, J. J. and Shevach, E. M., Eds., Oxford University Press, New York, 1990, 210.

20. **Allen, J. and Khoruts, A.,** Increased plasma tumor necrosis factor and interleukin-1 in patients with alcoholic liver disease, *Hepatology,* 10, 321, 1989.

21. **Felver, M., Mezey, E., McGuire, M., Mitchell, M., Herlong, H., Veech, G., and Veech, R.,** Plasma tumor necrosis factor α predicts decreased long-term survival in severe alcoholic hepatitis, *Alcohol.: Clin. Exp. Res.,* 14, 255, 1990.

22. **Yokota, M., Sakamoto, S., Koga, S., and Ibayashi, H.,** Decreased interleukin 1 activity in culture supernatant of lipopolysaccharide stimulated monocytes from patients with liver cirrhosis and hepatocellular carcinoma, *Clin. Exp. Immunol.,* 67, 335, 1987.

23. **Bird, G., Aria, K., Daniels, H., Alexander, G., and Williams, R.,** Contrasts in interleukin-1 and interleukin-2 activity in alcoholic hepatitis and cirrhosis, *Alcohol Alcoholism,* 24, 541, 1989.

24. **Rachmilewitz, D., Simon, P., Schwartz, L., Griswold, D., Fondacaro, J., and Wasserman, M.,** Inflammatory mediators of experimental colitis in rats, *Gastroenterology,* 97, 327, 1989.

25. **Watzl, B., Abdel-Fattah, G., Scuderi, P., and Watson, R.,** *In vitro* effect of ethanol (ETOH) on cytokine secretion in human mononuclear leukocytes, *Alcohol.: Clin. Exp. Res.,* 14, 351, 1990.

26. **Fox, E., Fenton, M., Broitman, S., and Thomas, P.,** Suppression of constitutive Kupffer cell interleukin 1 mRNA expression by ethanol, *Hepatology,* 13, 1991.

27. **Anastassakos, C., Alexander, G., Wolstencroft, R., Avery, J., Portmann, B., Panayi, G., Dumonde, D., Eddleston, W., and Williams, R.,** Interleukin-1 and interleukin-2 activity in chronic hepatitis B virus infection, *Gastroenterology,* 94, 999, 1988.

28. **Bingel, M., Lonnemann, G., Kock, K., Dinarello, C., and Shaldon, S.,** Enhancement of *in-vitro* human interleukin-1 production by sodium acetate, *The Lancet,* 1, 14, 1987.

29. **Nuutinen, H., Lindros, K., Hekali, P., and Salaspuro, M.,** Elevated blood acetate as indicator of fast ethanol elimination in chronic alcoholics, *Alcoholism,* 2, 623, 1985.

30. **Thiele, D.,** Tumor necrosis factor, the acute phase response and the pathogenesis of alcoholic liver disease, *Hepatology,* 9, 497, 1989.

31. **Stahnke, L., McClain, C., and Allen, J.,** Cytokine secretion by hepatic nonparenchymal cells in alcoholic liver disease, in *Cells of the Hepatic Sinusoid,* Vol. 3, Wisse, E., Knook, D., and McCuskey, R. S., Eds., Kupffer Cell Foundation, Rijswijk, The Netherlands, 1991, 472.

32. **Stahnke, L. and Allen, J.,** Plasma TNF concentrations correlate with peripheral blood monocyte TNF secretion and activation markers in alcoholic liver disease, *Hepatology,* 12, 926, 1990.

33. **McClain, C. and Cohen, D.,** Increased tumor necrosis factor production by monocytes in alcoholic hepatitis, *Hepatology,* 9, 349, 1989.

34. **Nelson, S., Bagby, G., Bainton, B., and Summer, W.,** The effects of acute and chronic alcoholism on tumor necrosis factor and the inflammatory response, *J. Infect. Dis.,* 160, 422, 1989.

35. **Nelson, S., Bagby, G., and Summer, W.,** Alcohol suppresses lipopolysaccharide-induced tumor necrosis factor activity in serum and lung, *Life Sci.,* 44, 673, 1989.

36. **D'Souza, N., Bagby, G., Nelson, S., Lang, C., and Spitzer, J.,** Acute alcohol infusion suppresses endotoxin-induced serum tumor necrosis factor, *Alcohol.: Clin. Exp. Res.,* 13, 295, 1989.

37. **Honchel, R., Marsano, L., Cohen, D., Shedlofsky, S., and McClain, C.,** A role for tumor necrosis factor in alcohol enhanced endotoxin liver injury, in *The Physiological and Pathological Effects of Cytokines,* Dinarello, C. A., Kluger, M. J., Powands, M. C., and Oppenheim, J. J., Eds., Wiley-Liss, New York, 1990, 171.

38. **Hansen, J., McClain, C., Cherwitz, D., Schlater, J., Stahnke, L., and Allen, J.,** Induction of tumor necrosis factor and interleukin-6 message in rats by ethanol administration and endotoxin, *Hepatology,* 12, 261, 1990.

39. **Watzl, B., Abril, E., Abbaszadegan, M., Scuderi, P., and Watson, R.,** Effects of ethanol *in vivo* on TNF secretion by cultured rat Kupffer cells, in *Cells of the Hepatic Sinusoid,* Vol. 3, Kirn, A., Knook, D., and Wisse, E., Eds., Kupffer Cell Foundation, Rijswijk, The Netherlands, 1991, 480.

40. **Datta, R., Sherman, M., and Kufe, D.,** Regulation of proto-oncogene and tumor necrosis factor gene expression by ethanol in HL-60 myeloid leukemia cells, *Blood,* 76, 298, 1990.

41. **Castell, J., Gomez-Lechon, M., David, M., Fabra, R., Trullenque, R., and Heinrich, P.,** Acute-phase response of human hepatocytes: regulation of acute-phase protein synthesis by interleukin-6, *Hepatology,* 12, 1179, 1990.

42. **Deviere, J., Content, J., Denys, C., Vandenbussche, P., Schandene, L., Wybran, J., and Dupont, E.,** High interleukin-6 serum levels and increased production by leucocytes in alcoholic liver cirrhosis. Correlation with IgA serum levels and lymphokines production, *Clin. Exp. Immunol.,* 77, 221, 1989.

43. **Mizel, S.,** The interleukins, *FASEB J.,* 3, 2379, 1989.

44. **Deviere, J., Dupont, E., Denys, C., Adler, M., Cremer, M., and Wybran, J.,** Mechanisms of defective lymphocyte activation in alcoholic liver cirrhosis, *J. Hepatol.,* 5, S119, 1987.

45. **Saxena, S., Nouri-Aria, K., Anderson, M., Eddleston, A., and Williams, R.,** Interleukin 2 activity in chronic liver disease and the effect of *in vitro* α-interferon, *Clin. Exp. Immunol.,* 63, 541, 1986.

46. **Bagasra, O., Kajdacsy-Balla, A., and Lischner, H.,** Effects of alcohol ingestion on *in vitro* susceptibility of peripheral blood mononuclear cells to infection with HIV and of selected T cell functions, *Alcohol.: Clin. Exp. Res.,* 13, 636, 1989.

47. **Kaplan, D.,** A novel mechanism of immunosuppression mediated by ethanol, *Cell. Immunol.,* 102, 1, 1986.

48. **Borgs, P., Witte, M., Way, D., and Watzl, B.,** Inter-well diffusion of ethanol in multiple well tissue culture plates: an important source of experimental error, *Clin. Res.,* 39, 426A, 1991.

49. **Tsukamoto, H., Gaal, K., and French, S.,** Insights into the pathogenesis of alcoholic liver necrosis and fibrosis: status report, *Hepatology,* 12, 599, 1990.

50. **Jerrells, T., Perritt, D., Eckardt, M., and Marietta, C.,** Alterations in interleukin-2 utilization by T cells from rats treated with an ethanol-containing diet, *Alcohol.: Clin. Exp. Res.,* 14, 245, 1990.

51. **Norman, D., Chang, M.-P., Castle, S., Van Zuylen, J., and Taylor, A.,** Diminished proliferative response of ConA-blast cells to interleukin-2 in adult rats exposed to ethanol *in utero, Alcohol.: Clin. Exp. Res.,* 15, 69, 1991.

52. **Chang, M.-P., Norman, D., and Castle, S.,** Impaired immune responses of T and B cells in young and old ethanol diet-fed mice, *FASEB J.,* 3, A6586, 1989.

53. **Chang, M.-P., Norman, D., and Makinodan, T.,** Immunotoxicity of alcohol in young and old mice. I. *In vitro* suppressive effects of ethanol on the activities of T and B immune cells of aging mice, *Alcohol.: Clin. Exp. Res.,* 14, 210, 1990.

54. **Levallois, C., Rouahi, N., Balmes, J.-L., and Mani, J.-C.,** Effects of ethanol *in vitro* on some parameters of the immune response, *Drug Alcohol Dependence,* 24, 239, 1989.

55. **Chadha, K., Whitney, R., Cummings, M., Norman, M., Windle, M., and Stadler, I.,** Evaluation of interferon system among chronic alcoholics, in *Alcohol, Immunomodulation, and AIDS,* Seminara, D., Watson, R., and Parolowski, A., Eds., New York, 1990, 123.

56. **Donnelly, M. and Sekellick, M.,** Alcohols induce interferon in primary chick embryo cells, *J. Interferon Res.,* 10, 25, 1990.

57. **Roselle, G., Mendenhall, C., and Grossman, C.,** Ethanol and soluble mediators of host response, *Alcohol.: Clin. Exp. Res.,* 13, 494, 1989.

58. **Roselle, G. and Mendenhall, C.,** Alteration of *in vitro* human lymphocyte function by ethanol, acetaldehyde, and acetate, *J. Clin. Lab. Immunol.,* 9, 33, 1982.

59. **Kunkel, S., Chenuse, S., and Phan, S.,** Prostaglandins as endogenous mediators of interleukin-1 production, *J. Immunol.,* 136, 219, 1988.

60. **Kunkel, S., Wiggins, R., and Larrick, J.,** Regulation of macrophage tumor necrosis factor production by prostaglandin E., *Biochem. Biophys. Res. Commun.,* 137, 404, 1986.

61. **Peterson, P., Sharp, B., Gekker, G., Brummitt, C., and Keane, W.,** Opioid-mediated suppression of interferon-τ production by cultured peripheral blood mononuclear cells, *J. Clin. Invest.,* 80, 824, 1987.

62. **Maxwell, W., Keating, J., Hogan, F., Kennedy, N., and Kelling, P.,** Prostaglandin E_2 and leukotriene B_4 synthesis by peripheral leucocytes in alcoholics, *Gut,* 30, 1270, 1989.

63. **Diez, E., Balsinde, J., Aracil, M., and Schiller, A.,** Ethanol induces release of arachidonic acid but not synthesis of eicosanoids in mouse peritoneal macrophages, *Biochem. Biophys. Acta,* 921, 82, 1987.

64. **Diamond, I., Wrubel, B., Estrain, W., and Gordon, A.,** Basal and adenosine receptor-stimulated levels of cAMP are reduced in lymphocytes from alcoholic patients, *Proc. Natl. Acad. Sci. U.S.A.,* 84, 1413, 1987.

65. **Nagy, L., Diamond, I., and Gordon, A.,** Effects of ethanol on cAMP levels in cultured lymphocytes from alcoholics. *FASEB J.,* 2, A6354, 1988.

66. **Hoffman, P. and Tabakoff, B.,** Ethanol and guanine nucleotide binding proteins: a selective interaction, *FASEB J.,* 4, 2612, 1990.

67. **Aguirre, J., Del Arbol, J., Raya, J., Ruiz-Requena, M., and Irles, J.,** Plasma β-endorphin levels in chronic alcoholics, *Alcohol,* 7, 409, 1989.

68. **Mandler, R., Biddison, D., Mandler, R., and Serrate, S.,** Beta-endorphin augments the cytolytic activity and interferon production of natural killer cells, *J. Immunol.,* 136, 934, 1986.

69. **Persson, J.,** Alcohol and the small intestine, *Scand. J. Gastroenterol.,* 26, 3, 1991.

70. **Khoruts, A., Stahnke, L., McClain, C. Y., Logan, G., Allen, Y. I.,** Circulating tumor necrosis factor, interleukin-1 and interleukin-6 concentrations in chronic alcoholic patients, *Hepatology,* 13, 267, 1991.

Chapter 6

THE ROLE OF TUMOR NECROSIS FACTOR IN HEALTH AND DISEASE

Steve Nelson, Carol Mason, Chester Nakamura, and Gregory Bagby

TABLE OF CONTENTS

103

I. INTRODUCTION

Cytokines are potent polypeptide mediators that modulate the host defense response to invasive disorders. Tumor necrosis factor-α (TNF) is one of these proinflammatory mediators derived primarily from mononuclear phagocytes that elicits a myriad of responses in the host. When TNF was first identified as a mediator during infection-like states, it was thought to be primarily responsible for many of the deleterious effects associated with overwhelming infections leading to shock and death. However, the protective effects of TNF and its role in normal immune mechanisms which have led to its preservation throughout mammalian evolution, remain to be clarified. Recent evidence indicates that, in fact, the TNF response is a critical component of the immune response to invading pathogens.

In addition to its central role in modulating inflammation, TNF is also cytotoxic to a number of human and murine tumor cell lines. Over one hundred years ago, it was observed that regression of cancer occurred in patients in association with bacterial infection. This observation, coupled with the isolation of bacterial products and their application to human cancer patients, was pioneered by William Coley in the early 1890s.[1] These bacterial products, known as Coley's toxins, proved effective in many patients. Shear later isolated lipopolysaccharide (LPS) from bacteria, and showed it to be a potent inhibitor of transplanted tumors in mice.[2] A characteristic of the endotoxic effect on a variety of tumors was the development of hemorrhagic necrosis followed by partial or complete tumor regression. Subsequently, it has been determined that this effect was mediated by TNF.[3]

Although alcohol use is commonly associated with an increased susceptibility to infections, clinicians frequently do not think of cancer when contemplating the medical consequences of alcohol abuse. However, in prospective studies of alcohol consumption, cancer is one of the major causes of increased morbidity and mortality. Invasive diseases, whether infectious or neoplastic, threaten the integrity of the host, and TNF may play an essential role in modulating host defenses against both of these pathological states.

II. TNF AND INFECTION

TNF is detectable in the systemic circulation of approximately one third of critically ill patients, and is frequently elevated in proportion to the severity of the underlying infection. Waage et al.[4] reported higher serum TNF activity in patients who subsequently succumbed to meningococcal meningitis than in those individuals who survived. Since then, other investigators have also found that high circulating levels of TNF appear to correlate with the severity of the underlying illness, but this has not been uniformly observed.[5-10]

To speculate that higher TNF levels are causally related to the lethal consequences of infections is tempting, but this conclusion cannot be firmly drawn from elevated TNF levels alone. A number of studies conducted in both patients and animals demonstrate that high TNF levels alone are not sufficient to produce the full complement of adverse symptoms seen during overwhelming infections. For example, in a study of Kiener et al.[11] both toxic and nontoxic forms of the lipid-A component of LPS produced similar increases in TNF. In preliminary studies in our laboratory, pretreatment of rats with the glucocorticoid antagonist RU 486 prior to endotoxin administration, converted a nonlethal challenge to a lethal one, while systemic TNF responses in these animals were similar. It is therefore likely that multiple factors, such as the duration of the TNF response, the presence of synergistic mediators, and/or endogenous modulators, and the site of infection are critical determinants of the host's response to both endogenous or exogenously administered TNF.

The site of infectious challenge has a substantial impact on the TNF response. Intravenous injections of bacterial endotoxins or live microorganisms yield large transient increases in circulating TNF levels that peak 1 to 2 h after challenge, and return to near nondetectable levels after 3 or 4 h.[12-14] Under these conditions, we reported that TNF remains nondetectable in fluid lavaged from the lungs throughout the study period.[13] Likewise, administering LPS directly into the lung results in a substantial increase of TNF in bronchoalveolar lavage fluid, while serum TNF remains nondetectable (Table 1).

The selective increase in TNF activity, after either intravenous or intrapulmonary lipopolysaccharide administration, may be an essential factor compartmentalizing the host's inflammatory response. This phenomenon may, under most conditions, serve to protect the host. Clearly, it would not be advantageous to either nonspecifically or systemically activate the inflammatory cascade during a localized infection, as this may inadvertently injure the host. Furthermore, this mechanism may serve to localize the inflammatory response at a specific site or within a selected compartment. In our laboratory, we have shown that administration of a lethal dose of TNF, if given intravenously, when administered directly into the lung, is not only noninjurious, but in fact, enhances the antibacterial defenses of the lung.[15]

Although TNF-alpha alone or in combination with other cytokines or bacterial products can produce symptoms seen during severe infections, other studies demonstrate that treatment of animals with this cytokine may potentiate the host defense response against bacterial infections. Nakano and associates[16] found that pretreating mice with TNF 6 to 12 h before intrapulmonary challenge with *Salmonella typhimurium* enhanced bactericidal activity within the peritoneal cavity. Moreover, the survival rate of infected mice was improved by pretreatment with TNF. Blanchard et al.[17] were able to protect mice from lethal *Legionella pneumophilia* pulmonary infections by locally instilling TNF, and demonstrated that such treatments enhanced bacterial clearance of the pathogen from the lungs of infected mice. Havell[18] and Desiderio et al.[19] were

TABLE 1
TNF Response in Serum and
Bronchoalveolar Lavage (BAL) Fluid is
Dependent on Route of LPS Administration

LPS	Peak serum TNF (1.5 h)	Peak bal fluid TNF (2.5 h)
None	ND	ND
Intravenous	High	ND
Intratracheal	ND	High

Note: ND, nondetectable.

able to protect mice from a lethal dose of *Listeria monocytogenes* by administering TNF to them 1 to 24 h before the bacterial challenge. Pretreatment with TNF has also been shown to afford protection against lethal endotoxemia and peritonitis produced by cecal ligation and puncture.[20] In the latter case, therapeutic benefit was demonstrated up to 6 h after initiating the insult. Hershman et al.[21] found TNF treatment of mice reduced mortality from *Klebsiella pneumoniae* wound infection when given for 5 d before bacterial challenge, or starting 1 h after initiating the infection, and continuing therapy for 7 d. Cross et al.[22] conducted interesting experiments in C3H/HeJ mice. This murine strain is resistant to endotoxin-induced shock and death, owing to the inability of its macrophages to produce TNF in direct response to LPS. However, these investigators found C3H/HeJ mice to be 100-fold more sensitive to *E. coli*-induced lethality. Furthermore, pretreatment of C3H/HeJ mice with a combination of recombinant murine TNF and interleukin-1 protected mice from intraperitoneal bacterial challenge. To further define the role of TNF in mediating pulmonary antibacterial defenses, we similarly challenged C3H/HeJ mice with intrapulmonary *Klebsiella pneumoniae*. These animals were unable to generate an inflammatory response, and the bacteria proliferated within their lungs (Figure 1). Interestingly, the C3H/HeJ macrophage is also defective in its tumoricidal capacity.[23] These studies show that TNF is essential in augmenting the host response to invasive disorders.

The consequences of passive immunization with antibodies directed against TNF offers the best means presently available for determining the role TNF plays during infections. Pretreatment of animals with these antibodies protects them from lethal doses of bacterial LPS and certain kinds of bacterial and parasitic insults. Beutler et al.[24] first demonstrated that passive immunization with anti-TNF serum rendered mice less sensitive to *E. coli* LPS. Other laboratories, including our own, have substantiated this finding.[12,25,26] Such data provide compelling evidence that TNF produced by endotoxin administration participates in its lethal consequences. The detrimental role of TNF has been extended to lethal bacteremia by studies in baboons. Tracey et al.[14]

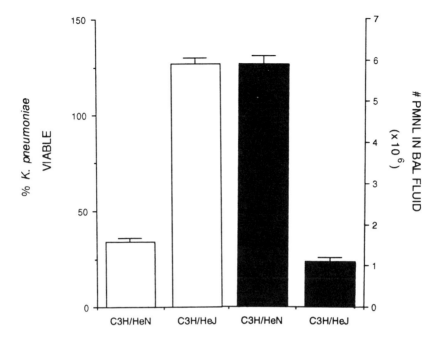

FIGURE 1. The percentage of *Klebsiella pneumoniae* remaining viable in the lung □, and the number of PMNL recovered by bronchoalveolar lavage ■ in C3H/HeJ and C3H/HeN (control) mice 4 h after bacterial challenge.

found that neutralizing monoclonal anti-TNF F(ab')₂ prevented death from a lethal intravenous challenge of live *E. coli* if administered 2 h before the bacterial challenge. An anti-TNF antibody used by Hinshaw et al.[27] was also effective when administered to baboons 30 min after initiating a 2-h infusion of bacteria.

However, lethality after other types of infections is not uniformly prevented by using antibodies against TNF. A lack of efficacy with anti-TNF antibodies has been reported in animals subjected to bacterial peritonitis. Evans et al.[25] were unable to prevent mortality from cecal ligation and puncture by pretreating mice with a monoclonal antibody directed against murine TNF. We have also attempted to reduce the mortality induced by bacterial peritonitis in an *E. coli* fecal inoculum model, without success.[26] In this case, low levels of TNF that are effectively neutralized by pretreatment with a goat anti-TNF immunoglobulin G are detected in both serum and the peritoneal cavity. Despite demonstrating that more than sufficient antibody was administered, mortality to Gram-negative bacterial peritonitis was not abrogated. Thus, significant differences exist between intravascular models of infection and bacterial peritonitis. Whereas TNF plays an important role in the lethal consequences of vascular models of infection, its role during severe peritoneal infections remains to be established.

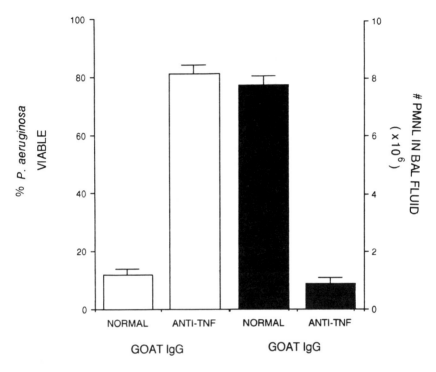

FIGURE 2.   Effect of anti-TNF IgG pretreatment on the percentage of *Pseudomonas aeruginosa* remaining viable in the lung ☐, and the number of PMNL recovered by bronchoalveolar lavage ■ 4 h after bacterial challenge.

These studies underscore the fact that anti-TNF therapy is not uniformly efficacious in mitigating the adverse consequences of severe infections. Furthermore, there is a growing body of literature demonstrating the fact that anti-TNF therapy may have a negative impact on host defense and increase host susceptibility to a variety of infectious insults.[18,19] In studies recently completed in our laboratory, we treated rats with anti-TNF IgG prior to an intrapulmonary challenge with *Pseudomonas aeruginosa*.[28] The antibody abolished the TNF response, and suppressed the recruitment of neutrophils from the vasculature into the alveoli by eightfold and significantly suppressed intrapulmonary bactericidal activity (Figure 2). Collectively, these studies suggest a central role of TNF in providing critical components of the host's response to invading pathogens, but also suggest that TNF may play a detrimental role when the inflammatory cascade is systemically activated.

III. CANCER AND TNF

TNF was originally described by Carswell et al.[3] as a transferable serum factor produced by mice primed with BCG or other immunostimulants, and subsequently exposed to endotoxin. This factor caused hemorrhagic necrosis and regression of a variety of murine tumors. Independent studies on the mechanisms involved in cachexia identified a serum factor from endotoxin primed macrophages which caused abnormal lipid metabolism in mice.[29] This factor was called cachectin. Amino acid sequencing and cloning of the cDNA genes encoding TNF and cachectin showed that the two molecules were identical.[30,31]

In vivo TNF causes regression of a wide range of murine tumors, and also has activity against human tumors heterotransplanted as xenografts in immune-suppressed mice.[3,32-36] Regression of tumors *in vivo* does not always reflect *in vitro* sensitivity, and some tumors which are resistant *in vitro* undergo regression in response to TNF *in vivo*.[37] Direct administration of TNF into the tumor appears to be the most effective route for achieving hemorrhagic necrosis and cure, possibly because of the high local TNF concentrations achieved while minimizing systemic toxicity. Toxicity is related to tissue damage to major organs, with metabolic changes similar to those seen in septic shock, namely fever, hypotension, and organ dysfunction.

As TNF is known to induce the release of other cytokines such as certain interleukins and colony-stimulating factors, there is experimental evidence to suggest that the antitumor activity of TNF *in vitro* and *in vivo* can be enhanced by other cytokines. For example, interferon-γ which induces the synthesis of TNF receptors and enhances TNF synthesis can augment the antitumor effects of TNF.[36,38] Furthermore, the cytotoxicity of TNF may also be increased by combination with chemotherapy drugs.[39,40]

Recently, it has been reported that macrophages can be directly stimulated by tumor cells to release TNF *in vitro*.[41] Further, monocytes and macrophages from tumor-bearing animals have an increased capacity for TNF release *in vitro*, and some patients with cancer demonstrate increased circulatory levels of TNF.[42,43] Whether this is a beneficial response or not, that is, the tumor-induced stimulation of TNF results in tumor cell death or leads to adverse consequences to the host, remains to be determined.

Although TNF has been used as an anticancer agent, its dual discovery as cachectin has implications for TNF as a mediator in cachexia seen in patients with cancer and severe infections. Oliff recently demonstrated that implantation of a xenograft constitutively producing human cachectin into nude mice led to tissue wasting and cachexia.[44] Furthermore, when mice bearing a transplantable sarcoma were passively immunized with an anti-TNF polyclonal antibody, the anorexia that normally develops was significantly attenuated.[45] Thus, neutralizing endogenous TNF production with antibodies significantly reduced tissue-wasting associated with experimental neoplastic disease. Balkwill and colleagues[43] first reported elevated cachectin levels in weight-losing patients with a variety of malignancies. However, this has not been consistently found in other series of patients, and may reflect the fact that tissue TNF production may be increased without increased levels in the circulation. In addition, patients and animals with tumors appear to be considerably more sensitive to the catabolic actions of TNF than are healthy hosts.[46]

IV. ALCOHOL AND TNF

Alcoholism is a major risk factor for severe bacterial pneumonia. Sir William Osler, in his *Principles and Practice of Medicine*,[47] stated that alcoholism was "perhaps the most potent predisposing factor" to lobar pneumonia. Numerous clinical investigations have reported evidence that alcoholics are at increased risk for pneumonia, and that mortality rates from bacterial pneumonia increase in proportion to the amount of alcohol consumed.[48-51] Despite technical advances and the development of potent antimicrobial agents, there has been little decline in the mortality associated with this disease in alcoholic patients.

The pathogenesis of bacterial pneumonia begins with colonization of the oropharynx.[52] Pneumonia follows the inability of pulmonary antibacterial defenses to kill aspirated challenges from the oropharynx. The alveolar macrophage is the only intraalveolar resident phagocyte, and is the first line of defense for the air spaces of the lower respiratory tract.[53] In addition, the polymorphonuclear leukocyte (PMNL), which is not a constituent of the normal alveolar cell population, can immigrate into the alveoli in response to bacterial challenges, and thus, provide auxiliary phagocytic defense capabilities to the lung.[54] Since the alveolar macrophage participates in directing the migration of PMNL from the intravascular compartment into the alveoli, a disorder of inflammatory signals may markedly impair normal host defenses against invasive bacteria.

Although numerous *in vitro* and *in vivo* studies have consistently reported ethanol-induced defects in PMNL adherence, mobilization, and delivery, the mechanisms by which ethanol alters these functions remain obscure.[55] The strong association between TNF production and LPS stimulation suggested to us that TNF may play a central role in mobilizing host defenses against pathogenic bacteria. Under certain conditions, TNF activates PMNL, stimulating their adhesion to endothelial cell surfaces, and enhancing their phagocytic and bactericidal activities.[56,57] Recently, TNF has been demonstrated to directly stimulate PMNL chemotaxis *in vitro* and *in vivo*.[58-60]

If TNF plays an important role in the inflammatory cascade supporting host defense, then factors modulating its production and release become critically important in understanding the pathophysiologic events leading to infection. Infection, particularly pneumonia, contributes substantially to the morbidity and mortality among individuals abusing alcohol, suggesting that alcohol is a potent immunosuppressive factor which undermines the normal host immune response. To investigate the effects of acute and chronic alcoholism on TNF activity, rats were systemically or intratracheally challenged

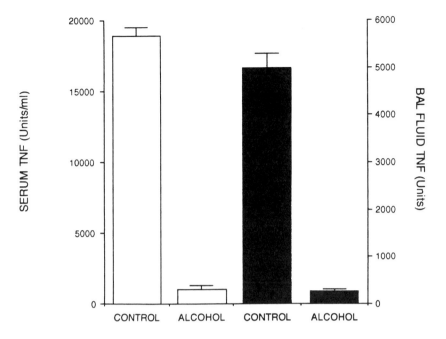

FIGURE 3. The effect of acute alcohol administration on lipopolysaccharide-induced TNF in serum ☐ and lung ◼.

with LPS. Four groups of animals were studied: normal, acute alcohol intoxication, chronic alcoholic, and acute alcohol intoxication of chronic alcoholic rats. TNF activity in serum and bronchoalveolar lavage fluid was determined over time. Total and differential cell counts in bronchoalveolar lavage fluid and serum were quantitated, and histopathology of the lung examined.

As observed in previous studies, intravenous administration of LPS produced large increases in serum TNF in normal animals. The response was transient, with peak levels occurring 90 min after LPS injection. By the third post-LPS hour, TNF levels had nearly returned to baseline levels. A similar time course was observed in chronic alcoholic rats, in which peak serum TNF levels did not differ from the levels seen in LPS-injected nonalcoholic rats. In contrast to these two groups, the LPS-induced increase in serum TNF levels was virtually abolished in nonalcoholic and chronic alcoholic rats given an acute injection of ethanol (Figure 3). In these animals, blood ethanol levels were in the range of 300 to 350 mg/dl during the 4-h observation period. In subsequent studies we showed that ethanol suppressed LPS-induced TNF in a dose-dependent fashion.[61]

A similar response was observed in rats challenged intratracheally with LPS. Nonalcoholic and chronic alcohol rats given an intratracheal challenge with LPS had substantial levels of TNF in fluid lavaged from their lungs at 1 and 4 h. In contrast, bronchoalveolar lavage fluid TNF levels remained near baseline when both groups were injected with ethanol 30 min before LPS challenge (Figure 3).

A different pattern emerged when TNF levels were assessed in alveolar macrophages lavaged from the lungs. Whereas TNF is barely detectable in association with alveolar macrophages obtained from rats not treated with LPS, cell-associated TNF was increased 1 and 4 h after intratracheal challenge with LPS. Unlike the attenuation observed in LPS-induced increases in bronchoalveolar lavage fluid TNF with acute alcohol administration, the response of cell-associated TNF to instilled LPS in normal rats was not dampened by acute ethanol intoxication. However, rats on the alcohol-containing diet did have significantly lower levels of TNF associated with bronchoalveolar lavage cells 1 and 4 h after LPS challenge. This was true in both groups of chronic alcoholic rats.

Acute ethanol intoxication, but not chronic alcohol consumption, had an adverse effect on migration of PMNL into the alveoli in response to intratracheal LPS instillation. At 1 and 4 h after LPS injection, bronchoalveolar lavage fluid macrophage cell number did not differ among the four groups. By 1 h after LPS, very few PMNLs were found in the bronchoalveolar lavage fluid. The PMNL count increased substantially ($35.5 \pm 5.1 \times 10^6$ cells) in normal rats by 4 h after LPS administration. A similar number of PMNLs was also found in bronchoalveolar lavage fluid of chronic alcoholic rats 4 h after LPS challenge. In contrast, acute ethanol administration substantially suppressed ($>90\%$) the number of PMNLs present in the bronchoalveolar lavage fluid. These data coincide with the pattern seen for bronchoalveolar lavage fluid TNF but not cell-associated TNF levels.

Numerous *in vitro* and *in vivo* studies have consistently reported ethanol-induced defects in PMNL adherence, mobilization, and delivery. In 1938, Pickrell[62] reported that acute intoxication in rabbits blocked the development of a local inflammatory infiltrate in response to the intracutaneous injection of bacteria; 30 years later, similar results were reported by using direct microscopic transillumination of injured tissue in a rabbit ear chamber.[63] Astry et al.[64] reported an ethanol-induced dose-dependent inhibition of PMNL migration into the alveoli in response to aerosolized Gram-negative bacterial challenges in mice. This failure of intoxicated subjects to mobilize a local PMNL response to inflammatory stimuli has been confirmed in humans using "skin window" abrasions.[65] The observation that PMNLs obtained from animals and humans after ethanol administration, maintain normal chemotaxis *in vitro*, suggests an impaired production of inflammatory mediators, rather than a direct toxic effect on PMNLs in subjects abusing alcohol.[66]

The mechanisms by which ethanol alters PMNL delivery to sites of inflammation remain obscure. Within the lung, the alveolar macrophage is the primary defender against invading microbes. In addition to its potent

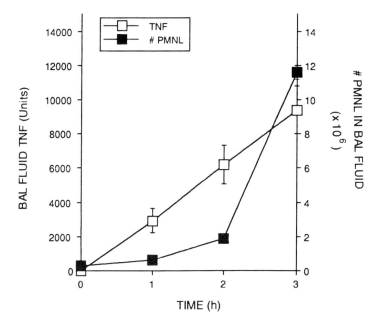

FIGURE 4. The temporal response of bronchoalveolar lavage TNF and PMNL number following an intratracheal challenge with lipopolysaccharide.

phagocytic capabilities, the alveolar macrophage is an active secretory cell, and can markedly influence the immune response of the host. The migration of PMNLs into the alveoli provides critical auxiliary phagocytic defenses. Expression of the antimicrobial functions of the PMNL is contingent on the ability of these cells to leave the circulation and enter infected sites. PMNL movement into the alveoli is an orderly reaction initiated from the alveolar site.

In our studies, the intrapulmonary TNF response to instilled LPS preceded PMNL recruitment into the alveolar compartment (Figure 4). TNF has been demonstrated to have diverse effects on phagocyte functions. TNF stimulates PMNL adhesion to endothelial cell surfaces, and enhances their phagocytic and bactericidal activity. Adherence of the PMNL to the vascular endothelium is an essential prelude to the effective migration of these cells to infected tissue sites *in vivo*. TNF has been demonstrated to directly stimulate PMNL chemotaxis *in vitro* and *in vivo*.[58,59] However, TNF has also been reported to inhibit *in vitro* PMNL chemotaxis under certain conditions.[67] These effects on chemotaxis appear to be dose-dependent. Recently, it was reported that low concentrations of TNF stimulate PMNL chemotaxis, while high concentrations inhibit this function.[60] Thus, TNF may possess the ability both to initiate the inflammatory process, and then subsequently to inhibit PMNL migration, which serves to localize the response. This would provide an effective mechanism of "stand and fight" by which these cells combat invading microorganisms. As the alveolar macrophage plays a pivotal role in host defense, the release of macrophage-derived TNF provides a possible mechanism for the initiation, amplification, and containment of inflammation during infection.

If TNF is an important factor in normal host defenses, then an impaired TNF response should be associated with an increased susceptibility to infections. These *in vivo* experiments demonstrate that acute alcohol intoxication markedly inhibits both the systemic and intrapulmonary TNF response to *E. coli* LPS. Within the lung, this suppression of LPS-induced TNF was associated with a markedly impaired inflammatory response. The additional phagocytic capacity afforded by the normal influx of PMNLs into the lung in response to bacteria is known to contribute essential defense capabilities against bacteria.[54] In subsequent studies, we showed that acute alcohol intoxication similarly suppresses lung TNF, elicited in response to intrapulmonary challenges with *Staphylococcus aureus* and *Klebsiella pneumoniae*.[68] In these studies, the suppressed TNF response was associated with proliferation of the bacteria within the lung. Thus, alcohol-induced suppression of TNF may be one mechanism underlying ethanol's reported deleterious effects on PMNL delivery and host defenses.

Recently, McClain et al.[69] reported that incubation of monocytes isolated from healthy individuals with ethanol suppressed LPS-stimulated TNF *in vitro*. Interestingly, monocytes from patients with alcoholic hepatitis had significantly increased spontaneous and LPS-stimulated TNF release, compared to monocytes from healthy volunteers. These findings suggest the occurrence of *in vivo* activation of these cells in patients with alcoholic hepatitis. In contrast, monocytes from patients with cirrhosis have a depressed LPS-induced TNF response.[70] These apparent discrepant findings may result from the underlying degree of endotoxemia in these patient groups. It is known that the majority of patients with cirrhosis have detectable endotoxemia which likely results from translocation of LPS from the gastrointestinal tract.[71] We have recently shown in an animal model that repeated doses of intravenous LPS leads to a failure of the animals to generate a subsequent systemic TNF response.[72] Perhaps these findings of altered TNF responses in patients relates to the development of "oral tolerance" which follows the progressive loss of intestinal barrier function, resulting in a state of acquired immune deficiency.

In our model, chronic alcoholism significantly decreased the amount of cell-associated TNF isolated from alveolar macrophages stimulated *in vivo* by LPS. *In vitro*, isolated macrophages have been demonstrated to contain detectable quantities of TNF messenger RNA, and little biologically active TNF is present before LPS administration.[73] After stimulation with LPS, transcriptional and post-transcriptional events lead to the rapid synthesis and

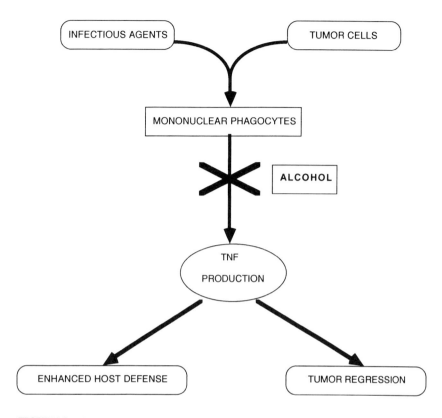

FIGURE 5. A proposed model for the deleterious effects of alcohol on the host response to both infection and cancer.

release of TNF. Recently, both membrane and cytoplasmic TNF have been demonstrated by immunohistochemical techniques in activated macrophages.[74] It is known that alcohol markedly affects membrane fluidity and disrupts membrane structure.[75] Perhaps these and other changes alter the distribution between membrane-associated and released TNF in cells from animals on a chronic alcoholic diet.

Our *in vivo* studies indicate that acute alcohol intoxication significantly inhibits the host's ability to produce and release TNF. The association of impaired inflammation with altered TNF activity in these studies strongly suggest an important relation of this cytokine to host defenses. Bacterial infections can usually be related to one or more deficiencies in regional and systemic defense capabilities. Alcohol markedly suppresses TNF and, thereby, seriously impairs the host's normal inflammatory response to invading pathogens. Further investigations may offer innovative approaches to the intervention of infections in these and other compromised hosts.

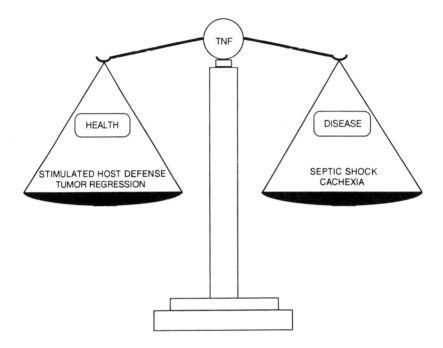

FIGURE 6.   A schematic diagram illustrating that the TNF response can elicit both beneficial and harmful effects in the host.

V. CONCLUSION

TNF, like most other inflammatory mediators, may be either beneficial or potentially harmful to the host (Figures 5 and 6). The ultimate outcome most likely relates to the specific stimulus, the location, magnitude, and duration of the response, and underlying host status. As both infectious agents and tumor cells directly stimulate the TNF response, this explains how apparently dissimilar stimuli can elicit similar systemic responses by activating a common pathway. As disease is the end clinical manifestation of multiple interactions involving immunologic defenses, metabolism, and nutrition, clearly, the diverse effects of alcohol on these factors renders the otherwise normal host more susceptible to infection and malignancy.

ACKNOWLEDGMENT

This work was supported by Grant AA 07710 from the National Institute on Alcohol Abuse and Alcoholism.

REFERENCES

1. **Coley, W. B.,** The treatment of malignant tumors by repeated inoculations of erysipelas: with a report of ten original cases, *Am. J. Med. Sci.,* 105, 487, 1893.

2. **Shear, W. J., Turner, F. C., Perrault, A., and Shovelton, T.,** Chemical treatment of tumors. V. Isolation of the hemorrhage-producing fraction forms *Serratia marcescens (Bacillus prodigiosus)* culture filtrate, *J. Natl. Cancer Inst.,* 4, 81, 1943.

3. **Carswell, E. A., Old, L. J., Kassel, R. L., et al.,** An endotoxin-induced serum factors that causes necrosis of tumors, *Proc. Natl. Acad. Sci. U.S.A.,* 72, 3666, 1975.

4. **Waage, A., Halstensen, A., and Espevik, T.,** Association between tumour necrosis factor in serum and fatal outcome in patients with meningococcal disease, *Lancet,* 1, 355, 1987.

5. **Cannon, J. G., Tompkins, R. G., Gelfand, J. A., et al.,** Circulating interleukin-1 and tumor necrosis factor in septic shock and experimental endotoxin fever, *J. Infect. Dis.,* 161, 79, 1990.

6. **Calandra, T., Baumgartner, J. D., Grau, G. E., et al.,** Prognostic values of tumor necrosis factor/cachectin, interleukin-1, interferon-alpha, and interferon-gamma in the serum of patients with septic shock, *J. Infect. Dis.,* 161, 982, 1990.

7. **Leroux-Roels, G. and Oftner, F.,** Tumor necrosis factor in sepsis, *JAMA,* 263, 1494, 1990.

8. **Marks, J. D., Marks, C. B., Luce, J. M., et al.,** Plasma tumor necrosis factor in patients with septic shock: mortality rate, incidence of adult respiratory distress syndrome, and effects of methylprednisolone administration, *Am. Rev. Respir. Dis.,* 141, 94, 1990.

9. **Damas, P., Reuter, A., Gysen, P., et al.,** Tumor necrosis factor and interleukin-1 serum levels during severe sepsis in humans, *Crit. Care. Med.,* 17, 975, 1989.

10. **DeGroote, M. A., Martin, M. A., Densen, P., et al.,** Plasma tumor necrosis factor levels in patients with presumed sepsis. Results in those treated with antilipid A antibody vs. placebo, *JAMA,* 262, 249, 1989.

11. **Kiener, P. A., Marek, F., Rodgers, G., et al.,** Induction of tumor necrosis factor, IFN-gamma, and acute lethality in mice by toxic and non-toxic forms of lipid A, *J. Immunol.,* 141, 870, 1988.

12. **Mathison, J. C., Wolfson, E., and Ulevitch, R. J.,** Participation of tumor necrosis factor in the mediation of gram negative bacterial lipopolysaccharide-induced injury in rabbits, *J. Clin. Invest.,* 81, 1925, 1988.

13. **Nelson, S., Bagby, G. J., Bainton, B. G., et al.,** Compartmentalization of intraalveolar and systemic lipopolysaccharide-induced tumor necrosis factor and the pulmonary inflammatory response, *J. Infect. Dis.,* 159, 189, 1989.

14. **Tracey, K. J., Fong, Y., Hesse, D. G., et al.,** Anti-cachectin/TNF monoclonal antibodies prevent septic shock during lethal bacteraemia, *Nature (London),* 330, 662, 1987.

15. **Nelson, S., Noel, P., Bokulic, R., et al.,** Murine recombinant tumor necrosis factor enhances host defenses against *Staphylococcus aureus, Am. Rev. Resp. Dis.,* (Abstr.), 139, A357, 1989.

16. **Nakano, Y., Onozuka, K., Terada, Y., et al.,** Protective effect of recombinant tumor necrosis factor-alpha in murine salmonellosis, *J. Immunol.,* 144, 1935, 1990.

17. **Blanchard, D. K., Djeu, J. Y., Klein, T. W., et al.,** Protective effects of tumor necrosis factor in experimental *Legionella pneumophilia* infections of mice via activation of PMN function, *J. Leukoc. Biol.,* 43, 429, 1988.

18. **Havell, E. A.,** Evidence that tumor necrosis factor has an important role in antibacterial resistance, *J. Immunol.,* 143, 2894, 1989.

19. **Desiderio, J. V., Kiener, P. A., Lin, P. F., et al.,** Protection of mice against *Listeria monocytogenes* infection by recombinant human tumor necrosis factor alpha, *Infect. Immun.,* 57, 1615, 1989.

20. **Sheppard, B. C., Fraker, D. L., and Norton, J. A.,** Prevention and treatment of endotoxin and sepsis lethality with recombinant human tumor necrosis factor, *Surgery,* 106, 156, 1989.

21. **Hershman, M. J., Pietsch, J. D., Trachtenberg, L., et al.,** Protective effects of recombinant human tumor necrosis factor-alpha and interferon-gamma against surgically simulated wound infection in mice, *Br. J. Surg.,* 76, 1282, 1989.

22. **Cross, A. S., Sadoff, J. C., Kelly, N., et al.,** Pretreatment with recombinant murine tumor necrosis factor-alpha/cachectin and murine interleukin-1 alpha protects mice from lethal bacterial infection, *J. Exp. Med.,* 169, 2021, 1989.

23. **Morrison, D. C.,** Bacterial endotoxins and pathogenesis, *Rev. Infect. Dis.,* 5, S733, 1983.

24. **Beutler, B., Milsark, I. W., and Cerami, A. C.,** Passive immunization against cachectin/tumor necrosis factor protects mice from lethal effect of endotoxin, *Science,* 229, 869, 1985.

25. **Evans, G. F., Snyder, Y. M., Butler, L. D., et al.,** Differential expression of interleukin-1 and tumor necrosis factor in murine septic shock models, *Circ. Shock,* 29, 279, 1989.

26. **Bagby, G. J., Plessala, K. J., Wilson, L. A., et al.,** Divergent efficacy of anti-TNF-alpha antibody in intravascular and peritonitis models of sepsis, *J. Infect. Dis.,* 163, 83, 1991.

27. **Hinshaw, L., Tekamp-Olson, P., Chang, A. C. K., et al.,** Survival of primates in LD100 septic shock following therapy with antibody to tumor necrosis factor (TNF-alpha), *Circ. Shock,* 30, 279, 1990.

28. **Nelson, S., Bagby, G., and Summer, W.,** Anti-tumor necrosis factor-alpha antibody suppresses pulmonary antibacterial defenses, *Am. Rev. Respir. Dis.,* 143S, 393, 1991.

29. **Beutler, B., Mahoney, J., Le Trang, N., Pekala, P., and Cerami, A.,** Purification of cachectin, a lipoprotein lipase-suppressing hormone secreted by endotoxin-induced RAW 264.7 cells, *J. Exp. Med.,* 161, 984, 1985.

30. **Pennica, D., Nedwin, G. E., Hayflick, J. S., et al.,** Human tumour necrosis factor; precursor structure, expression, and homology to lymphotoxin, *Nature (London),* 312, 724, 1984.

31. **Caput, D., Beutler, B., Hartog, K., Brown-Shimer, S., and Cerami, A.,** Identification of a common nucleotide sequence in the 3' untranslated region of mRNA molecules specifying inflammatory mediators, *Proc. Natl. Acad. Sci. U.S.A.,* 83, 1670, 1986.

32. **Haranaka, K., Satomi, N., and Sakaurai, A.,** Antitumor activity of murine tumor necrosis factor (TNF) against transplanted murine tumors and heterotransplanted human tumors in nude mice, *Int. J. Cancer,* 34, 263, 1984.

33. **Brouckaert, P. G. G., Leroux Roels, G. G., Guisez, Y., et al.,** In vivo antitumor activity of recombinant human and murine TNF, alone and in combination with murine IFN-gamma, on a syngeneic murine melanoma, *Int. J. Cancer,* 38, 763, 1986.

34. **Creasey, A., Reynolds, M. R., and Laird, W.,** Cures and partial regressions of murine and human tumors by recombinant human tumor necrosis factor, *Cancer Res.,* 46, 5687, 1986.

35. **Balkwill, F. R., Lee, A., Aldam, G., et al.,** Human tumor xenografts treated with recombinant human tumor necrosis factor alone or in combination with interferons, *Cancer Res.,* 46, 3990, 1986.

36. **Balkwill, F. R., Ward, B. G., Moodie, E., and Fiers, W.,** Therapeutic potential of tumor necrosis factor-alpha and alpha-interferon in experimental ovarian cancer, *Cancer Res.,* 47, 4755, 1987.

37. **Manda, T., Shimomura, K., Mukomoto, S., et al.,** Recombinant human tumor necrosis factor-alpha: evidence of an indirect mode of antitumor activity, *Cancer Res.,* 47, 3707, 1987.

38. **Aggarwal, B. B., Eessalu, T. E., and Hass, P. E.,** Characterisation of receptors for human tumour necrosis factor and their regulation by alpha-interferon, *Nature (London),* 318, 665, 1985.

39. **Alexander, R. B., Nelson, W. G., and Coffey, D. S.,** Synergistic enhancement by tumor necrosis factor of *in vitro* cytotoxicity from chemotherapeutic drugs targeted at DNA topoisomerase II, *Cancer Res.,* 47, 2403, 1987.

40. **Das, A. K., Walther, P. J., Buckley, N. J., and Poulton, S. H. M.,** Recombinant human tumor necrosis factor alone and in combination with chemotherapeutic agents, *Arch. Surg.,* 124, 107, 1989.

41. **Hasday, J. D., Shah, E. M., and Lieberman, A. P.,** Macrophage tumor necrosis factor-alpha release is induced by contact with some tumors, *J. Immunol.,* 145, 371, 1990.

42. **Yamazaki, M. and Okutomi, T.,** Augmentation of release of cytotoxin from murine bone marrow and peritoneal macrophages by tumor transplantation, *Cancer Res.,* 49, 352, 1989.

43. **Balkwill, F. F., Burke, D., Talbot, J., et al.,** Evidence for tumour necrosis factor/cachectin production in cancer, *Lancet,* 1, 1229, 1987.

44. **Oliff, A., Defeo-Jones, D., Boyer, M., et al.,** Tumors secreting human TNF/cachectin induce cachexia in mice, *Cell,* 50, 555, 1987.

45. **Moldawer, L. L., Sherry, B., Lowry, S. F., and Cerami, A.,** Endogenous cachectin/tumour necrosis factor-alpha production contributes to experimental cancer-associated cachexia, *Cancer Surv.,* 8, 853, 1989.

46. **Bartholeyns, J., Freudenberg, M., and Galanos, C.,** Growing tumors induce hypersensitivity to endotoxin and tumor necrosis factor, *Infect. Immun.,* 55, 2230, 1987.

47. **Osler, W.,** *The Principles and Practice of Medicine,* D. Appleton, New York, 1905.

48. **Nolan, J. P.,** Alcohol as a factor in the illness of university service patients, *Am. J. Med. Sci.,* 249, 135, 1965.

49. **Kolb, D. and Gunderson, E. K. E.,** Alcohol-related morbidity among older career navy men, *Drug Alcohol Depend.,* 9, 181, 1982.

50. **Tillotson, J. R. and Lerner, A. M.,** Pneumonias caused by gram-negative bacilli, *Medicine,* 45, 65, 1966.

51. **Capps, J. A. and Coleman, G. H.,** Influence of alcohol on prognosis of pneumonia in Cook County Hospital, *JAMA,* 80, 750, 1923.

52. **Johanson, W. G.,** Prevention of respiratory tract infection, *Am. J. Med.,* 76, 69, 1984.

53. **Green, G. M., Jakab, G. J., Low, R. B., and Davis, G. S.,** Defense mechanisms of the respiratory membrane, *Am. Rev. Resp. Dis.,* 115, 479, 1977.

54. **Toews, G. B.,** Determinants of bacterial clearance from the lower respiratory tract, *Semin. Respir. Infect.,* 1, 68, 1986.

55. **MacGregor, R. R., Safford, M., and Shalit, M.,** Effect of ethanol on functions required for the delivery of neutrophils to sites of inflammation, *J. Infect. Dis.,* 157, 682, 1988.

56. **Gamble, J. R., Harlan, J. M., Klebanoff, S. J., and Vadas, M. A.,** Stimulation of the adherence of neutrophils to umbilical vein endothelium by human recombinant tumor necrosis factor, *Proc. Natl. Acad. Sci. U.S.A.,* 82, 8667, 1985.

57. **Shalaby, M. R., Aggarwal, B. B., Rinderknecht, E., et al.,** Activation of human polymorphonuclear neutrophil functions by interferon and tumor necrosis factor, *J. Immunol.,* 135, 2069, 1985.

58. **Figari, I. S. and Palladino, M. A.,** Stimulation of neutrophil chemotaxis by recombinant tumor necrosis factors alpha and beta (Abst. 1431), *Fed. Proc.,* 46, 562, 1987.

59. **Averbook, B., Ulich, T., Jeffes, E., et al.,** Human alpha lymphotoxin and TNF induce different types of inflammatory responses in normal tissue *Fed. Proc.,* (Abstr. 1432), 46, 562, 1987.

60. **Yonemaru, M., Zheng, H., Stephens, K. E., et al.,** Biphasic effect of tumor necrosis factor on polymorphonuclear leukocyte chemotaxis (Abstr.), *Am. Rev. Resp. Dis.,* Suppl. 137, 42, 1988.

61. **D'Souza, N. B., Bagby, G. J., Nelson, S., et al.,** Acute alcohol infusion suppresses endotoxin-induced serum tumor necrosis factor, *Alcohol.: Clin. Exp. Res.,* 13, 295, 1989.

62. **Pickrell, K. L.,** The effect of alcoholic intoxication and ether anesthesia on resistance to pneumococcal infection, *Bull. Johns Hopkins Hosp.,* 63, 238, 1983.
63. **Moses, J. M., Geschickter, E. H., and Ebert, R. H.,** The relationship of enhanced permeability to leukocyte mobilization in delayed inflammation, *Br. J. Exp. Pathol.,* 49, 386, 1968.
64. **Astry, C. L., Warr, G. A., and Jakab, G. J.,** Impairment of polymorphonuclear leukocyte immigration as a mechanism of alcohol-induced suppression of pulmonary antibacterial defenses, *Am. Rev. Resp. Dis.,* 128, 113, 1983.
65. **MacGregor, R. R. and Gluckman, S. G.,** Effect of acute alcohol intoxication on granulocyte mobilization and kinetics, *Blood,* 52, 551, 1979.
66. **MacGregor, R. R.,** Alcohol and immune defense, *JAMA,* 256, 1474, 1986.
67. **Stephens, K., Ishizaka, A., Basilico, L., et al.,** Human tumor necrosis factor inhibits neutrophil chemotaxis (Abstr.), *Am. Rev. Respir. Dis.,* Suppl. 135, A338, 1987.
68. **Nelson, S., Bagby, G. J., and Summer, W. R.,** Alcohol-induced suppression of tumor necrosis factor: a potential risk factor for secondary infection in the acquired immuno-deficiency syndrome, *Prog. Clin. Biol. Res.,* 325, 211, 1990.
69. **McClain, C. J. and Cohen, D. A.,** Increased tumor necrosis factor production by monocytes in alcoholic hepatitis, *Hepatology,* 9, 349, 1989.
70. **Muzes, G., Deak, G., Lang, I., et al.,** Depressed monocyte production of interleukin-1 and tumor necrosis factor-alpha in patients with alcoholic liver cirrhosis, *Liver,* 9, 302, 1989.
71. **Bigatello, L. M., Broitman, S. A., Fattori, L., et al.,** Endotoxemia, encephalopathy, and mortality in cirrhotic patients, *Am. J. Gastroenterol.,* 82, 11, 1987.
72. **Nelson, S., Summer, W. R., and Bagby, G. J.,** LPS-induced inhibition of lung TNF and host defenses, *Prog. Leukocyte Biol.,* 10B, 141, 1990.
73. **Michie, H. R., Manogue, K. R., Spriggs, D. R., et al.,** Detection of circulating tumor necrosis factor after endotoxin administration, *N. Engl. J. Med.,* 318, 1481, 1988.
74. **Chensue, S. W., Remick, D. G., Shmyr-Forsch, C., et al.,** Immuno-histochemical demonstration of cytoplasmic and membrane-associated tumor necrosis factor in murine macrophages, *Am. J. Pathol.,* 133, 564, 1988.
75. **Rubin, E. and Rottenberg, H.,** Ethanol-induced injury and adaptation in biological membranes, *Fed. Proc.,* 41, 2465, 1982.

PART II
Fetal Alcohol Exposure, Immunity, and Neuroimmune Interactions

Chapter 7

FETAL ALCOHOL EXPOSURE AND IMMUNITY

Sandra J. Ewald

TABLE OF CONTENTS

I. INTRODUCTION

Exposure to ethanol in prenatal life has a detrimental effect on a number of organ systems. It would be surprising if the immune system of the developing organism were unaffected. A recent review[1] discusses the literature to 1988. Chapters 8 and 9 in this volume focus on the neuroimmune aspects of fetal alcohol exposure. There remains a scarcity of clinical data on the immune status of children diagnosed with fetal alcohol syndrome (FAS). Therefore, this chapter will deal, for the most part, with studies conducted in our laboratory examining the immune system of late-fetal and young adult mice that were prenatally exposed to ethanol, and recent studies using *in vitro* methods to determine direct effects of ethanol on the fetal thymus.

II. *IN VIVO* EFFECTS OF ETHANOL ON LYMPHOID ORGANS

A. ASSOCIATION BETWEEN FETAL ALCOHOL EXPOSURE AND DiGEORGE SYNDROME

Several authors have noted overlapping features of FAS and DiGeorge syndrome. Children with FAS frequently have heart defects, as well as the facial, neurological, and growth abnormalities that characterize the syndrome. Some of the heart defects and other anomalies in FAS resemble those seen in DiGeorge syndrome,[2] a complex of disorders that typically includes absence or reduction of thymus and parathyroid tissues, in addition to heart abnormalities. This pattern of overlapping features has led some clinicians[3,4] to suggest the two syndromes may be related. Furthermore, a study by Ammann et al.[3] noted a history of maternal alcoholism in four cases of DiGeorge syndrome, and suggested alcohol as the causative agent of DiGeorge syndrome in these children. Siebert's group[4] discussed the involvement of cephalic neural crest in formation of the tissues affected in DiGeorge and fetal alcohol syndrome, and proposed that abnormalities of neural crest could be involved in the pathogenesis of both.

In experimental animals, it is well known that acute exposure to ethanol in doses producing maternal blood alcohol levels (BAL) above 400 mg/100 ml, is teratogenic for the heart as well as other tissues.[5,6] In particular, Daft et al.[7] demonstrated that exposure to such high concentrations of ethanol at gestational day (g.d.) 8, 12 h and 16 h in mice, produced abnormalities of the heart and great vessels similar to the defects seen in children with DiGeorge syndrome. These authors suggest that the heart anomalies are due to an interference of neural crest cell migration by high doses of ethanol. Heart (as well as thymus[8]) has a contribution from neural crest tissue, and neural crest cells in the mouse migrate during gestational day eight.

We were interested in determining whether acute exposure of mouse embryos to teratogenic doses of ethanol (BAL >400 mg/100 ml) at a time when neural crest cells were migrating and the thymic anlage was forming, would lead to athymia. Pregnant C57Bl/6 mice were injected with two doses of ethanol given 4 h apart on one day of gestation (g.d. 7, 8, 9, 10, or 11), using a regimen that produced peak maternal BAL >400 mg/ml.[6] The fetuses from ethanol-injected and control saline-injected dams were examined on gestational day 18 for presence of a thymus, number of thymocytes, and expression of thymus differentiation antigens, as well as for gross external malformations. Eighteen-day fetuses injected on day 9 of gestation demonstrated a very high incidence of forelimb malformations, as previously described by Webster et al.[6] None of the 18-day fetuses exposed to ethanol on any of the days tested demonstrated athymia, and fetuses exposed on days 7, 8, or 9 did not have altered subpopulation ratios.[9]

The possibility remains that *in utero* ethanol exposure can cause athymia, but requires more prolonged exposure to alcohol or a genetic predisposition lacking in C57Bl/6 mice. Genetic differences in susceptibility to ethanol-induced limb defects have been demonstrated.[10] It should also be noted that in our experiments, the smallest fetuses from dams injected on gestational day 8 had a reduced thymus/body weight ratio compared to controls, suggesting that those fetuses most affected by ethanol (with evidence of intrauterine growth retardation) may have also suffered a partial loss of thymic tissue. Because exposure to ethanol occurred well before colonization of the anlage by lymphoid cells, the effect of ethanol must have been on development of thymic epithelium or stem cells.

B. LYMPHOCYTE POPULATIONS AND RESPONSES IN LATE-TERM FETUSES AND NEONATES FOLLOWING CHRONIC EXPOSURE TO ETHANOL *IN UTERO*

A previous review[1] discussed data from our laboratory relating to changes in the thymus of 18-day fetuses exposed throughout gestation to ethanol. In brief, C57Bl/6 dams were fed a complete liquid diet containing ethanol in a concentration of 25% ethanol-derived calories (25% EDC) from gestational day 1 to 18. Thymocytes from their 18-day fetuses were greatly reduced in number, and proliferative responses to mitogens were reduced compared to thymocytes from fetuses whose mothers were fed a control liquid diet.[11] Thymuses from ethanol-exposed fetuses also appeared to be immature, as assessed by histology and expression of the T cell differentiation antigens CD4(L3T4) and CD8(Lyt-2).[12] When C57Bl/6 mice were exposed to ethanol *in utero* from g.d. 1 to 13 (by feeding the pregnant dam 25% EDC diet), their thymuses were still hypocellular, and the thymocytes less differentiated than controls at g.d. 18.[13] By 6 days after birth, however, neonates exposed to ethanol through g.d. 13 had normal numbers and subpopulations of both thymocytes and splenocytes.

C. EFFECT OF ETHANOL ON MATERNAL TRANSFER OF IMMUNITY TO THE FETUS AND NEONATE

Data from Seelig and co-workers[14] demonstrate that chronic ethanol consumption by rats alters the structure of mammary glands. Specifically, female rats fed a liquid diet containing 36% ethanol-derived calories before mating, throughout pregnancy, and during lactation, demonstrated reduced alveolar epithelium and increased connective tissue at day 2 of lactation but not at day 10 of lactation. This group also reports that there are alterations in numbers of T-lymphocytes (particularly T-helper lymphocytes) and of IgA$^+$ B cells in connective tissue surrounding alveoli of lactating rats fed an 18% protein diet, but not a high (25%) protein diet.[15] Such studies illustrate the interaction of alcohol and nutrition in effects on the immune response. The observed changes in mammary structure and immune cells within mammary tissue following ethanol consumption may indicate altered lactational transfer of immunity.

The same group provides evidence that chronic alcohol consumption by the pregnant dam impairs lactational transfer of anti-parasite immunity to her offspring, if the dam is fed the ethanol diet before primary infection with *Trichinella spiralis*.[16]

Jollie[17] performed a study to examine effects of ethanol on trans-placental transfer of IgG in a rat model. He reports alterations in the Golgi elements of yolk-sac epithelial cells from dams chronically fed a 36% EDC diet during pregnancy. An *in vitro* culture method also indicates reduced sorting and translocation of IgG across the epithelium in cells from ethanol-exposed dams.

D. FETAL ALCOHOL EXPOSURE AND POSTNATAL IMMUNITY

Much of the work dealing with immune responses in young or adult animals (and humans) prenatally exposed to ethanol has been reviewed previously,[1] and therefore will be briefly summarized here. In humans, two reports[18,19] indicated that children diagnosed with fetal alcohol syndrome had increased incidence of infection and reduced T and B cell numbers, as well as reduced T cell mitogen responses. More recently, a study focusing on hearing disorders in children with FAS, reported a high incidence of serous otitis media in these children, as well as a history of recurrent respiratory infections;[20] the authors attribute the susceptibility to otitis media, at least in part, to Eustachian tube malformations that are part of the constellation of craniofacial anomalies characteristic of FAS. Although the authors speculate that immunodeficiency also contributes to the increased susceptibility to infections in these children, they did not examine the children immunologically. As with most studies dealing with humans, the interpretation of alcohol as etiologic for the increased susceptibility to infection is complicated by the fact that many of the mothers abused other drugs in addition to alcohol, or were undernourished. To summarize the data with respect to humans, surprisingly little information has been published concerning the immune status of children with fetal alcohol syndrome or fetal alcohol exposure.

In animals, experiments have been performed with mice and rats fed an ethanol-containing liquid diet during pregnancy. Somewhat conflicting reports have resulted as to whether such prenatal ethanol exposure leads to immune alterations in offspring examined as adults. The data from rats are largely in agreement that *in utero* alcohol exposure leads to reduced responses of splenocytes to T cell mitogens,[21-24] although one of these groups found the impairment restricted to only males.[24] In mice there are two published reports, one of which shows no effect of prenatal ethanol exposure on delayed type hypersensitivity, T-dependent antibody responses, or mitogen responses,[25] and the other reporting a reduction in contact sensitivity responses of mice in the ethanol-exposed group.[26] Our own work[44] examined adult offspring of C57Bl/6 dams fed a 23% EDC diet during pregnancy. This diet regimen produced blood alcohol levels >100 mg/100 ml in the dams, and 18-day fetuses from the ethanol-exposed dams had thymuses that were smaller and less mature than those of controls. Nonetheless, when offspring were studied immunologically at the age of 5 to 8 weeks after birth, no significant differences were seen in immune responses of ethanol-exposed and control animals, as assessed by T-dependent antibody production, delayed-type hypersensitivity, contact sensitivity, or mitogen proliferative responses. We also found no difference between the two experimental groups in numbers of CD4$^+$, CD8$^+$, Thy-1$^+$, or immunoglobulin-positive (B–) spleen cells.

Possible reasons for somewhat conflicting results from different groups may relate to variations in ethanol dose, special differences, transience of immune deficits in postnatal life, and in the rat model, interaction of nutritional deficiency and ethanol. It has been suggested that rats fed a 36% EDC diet (the standard Lieber-DeCarli diet used in most rat studies) are undernourished because they limit their food intake rather significantly[27,28] due to aversion to high alcohol levels; the same absolute amount of daily alcohol intake by a dam will have a much more dramatic effect on her pups (weight, mortality) if the alcohol represents a high percent of total calories (36%) than if it represents a lower percent of calories in the diet (e.g., 30%). One advantage of the mouse model is that C57Bl/6 mice fed a 23 or 25% EDC diet consume almost as much of the alcohol-containing diet as mice administered a control diet *ad libitum,* and yet these alcohol-containing diets produce high maternal BAL in our hands (peak BAL >100 mg/100 ml).

III. POSSIBLE MECHANISMS OF ETHANOL EFFECTS ON THE DEVELOPING IMMUNE SYSTEM

Two clear aspects of ethanol exposure in fetal life emerge:

1. Immediate effects of ethanol on development of lymphoid organs such as the thymus or bone marrow, or on transfer of maternal immunity
2. Protracted effects of *in utero* alcohol exposure that persist for at least some time after birth (and cessation of alcohol exposure)

The former issue is relatively straightforward, as it is easy to appreciate that the lymphoid organs are likely to suffer damage as long as ethanol is in the system. Because the lymphoid compartment of tissues, such as the thymus, have vigorous regenerative capacity, long-term effects of prenatal alcohol exposure on the immune system would have to be mediated through damage to the stroma (such as occurs in DiGeorge syndrome, and more subtly, following total lymphoid irradiation),[29] alterations of the neuroendocrine system that interact with the immune system, persistent damage to the lymphoid stem cell compartment, or long-lived lymphocytes[30] that underwent aberrant maturation during the period of ethanol exposure. Indirect effects of prenatal ethanol on the immune system after birth could result from neuroendocrine changes that alter feeding behavior in the offspring,[31,32] leading to nutritional deficiency that could secondarily produce immune impairment.

Possible mechanisms by which ethanol could affect development of lymphoid tissues include:

1. Direct effects of ethanol on lymphoid cells or the stromal elements that induce their differentiation
2. Toxic effects of metabolites of ethanol (such as acetaldehyde)
3. Increased levels of hormones such as glucocorticoids, which are known to be elevated in ethanol-consuming animals,[33] and are lytic for immature thymocyte subpopulations[34]
4. Undernourishment of the dam due to reduced food consumption[27,28]
5. Reduced absorption or transport of nutrients such as amino acids[35] or zinc[36] across the placenta
6. Fetal hypoxia,[37,38] damage to the placenta, or other mechanisms

We have addressed the question of whether ethanol or its immediate metabolite acetaldehyde directly affect fetal thymus development by using fetal thymus organ cultures. These cultures have the advantage of maintaining the normal architecture and cellular make-up of the thymus, while allowing for controlled addition of ethanol in the absence of maternal effects. When 14-day fetal thymus lobes are grown *in vitro,* both proliferation of thymocytes and differentiation occur. Lymphocytes in the thymus at g.d. 14 are immature — devoid of T cell antigens such as CD3, T cell receptor, CD4 and CD8 antigens. After a number of days in culture, however, thymocytes differentiate, such that all the normal phenotypically defined subpopulations are present.[39]

In recent unpublished studies,[45] we have shown that inclusion of ethanol at either 0.2 or 0.4% (w/v) does not inhibit thymocyte differentiation. After 5 days' culture, in fact, thymuses incubated in 0.2 or 0.4% ethanol, had 50% more $CD4^+CD8^-$ cells than did control cultures. Because these cells represent a mature and functional subset of thymocytes (the T-helper population), the data indicate that ethanol at physiological concentrations enhances thymocyte differentiation. This interpretation is reinforced by data demonstrating that thymuses cultured in the presence of ethanol also contain proportionately lower numbers of cells expressing the receptor for interleukin 2, a marker of immature thymocytes.[40] Total cell numbers were reduced by about 25% in cultures to which 0.4% ethanol had been added at the start of culture. These data contrast with results of thymus development in 18-day fetuses exposed to ethanol *in vivo,* in which thymocyte numbers were reduced about 75% relative to controls, and the percentages of cells expressing CD4 and CD8 antigens were greatly reduced.

The *in vivo* effects of ethanol on thymus development we have noted in the late-term mouse fetus undoubtedly represent complex effects of ethanol, both direct and indirect. At least part of the impaired maturation is probably due to indirect effects of ethanol, such as reduced absorption of nutrients by the dam or elevated glucocorticoids. In fact, thymus growth retardation subsequent to *in utero* alcohol exposure could simply be a developmental delay that reflects the over-all growth retardation seen in the fetuses.

In rodents, the thymus normally reaches maturity (in terms of subpopulations identified by antigenic phenotype and T cell receptor expression) coincident with parturition. Analysis of thymus populations in pups exposed to ethanol both pre- and postnatally would provide a more "steady-state" picture that could provide insights as to other effects of ethanol (i.e., direct effects, glucocorticoids) acting on thymus development. Postnatal exposure of the pup through alcohol delivery to the dam, however, introduces additional variables such as effects of ethanol (both pre- and postnatally) on nursing behavior of the offspring.

IV. CONCLUSIONS

Clearly, it is impossible to control all the variables (such as nutritional status) that relate to ethanol exposure in the intact organism. It is likely that direct effects of ethanol contribute to the ultimate picture of thymus development in animals and humans exposed *in utero.* As ethanol has been demonstrated to affect intracellular signal transduction through interaction with biological membranes in other tissues (most notably neuronal),[41] it is probable that developing lymphoid tissue is similarly affected. Thymocyte development is sensitive to changes in intracellular mediators: increased levels of intracellular cyclic adenosine monophosphate (cAMP), for example, enhance rearrangement of antigen receptor genes,[42] and activate apoptotic processes related to negative selective of immature thymocytes.[43] If ethanol affects processes of positive and negative selection by altering signal transduction through the T cell receptor in immature thymocytes, it could thereby alter the antigenic repertoire of mature T cells.

ACKNOWLEDGMENTS

This work was supported by Research Grant AA07010 and Research Scientist Development Award AA00105, both from the Alcohol, Drug Abuse, and Mental Health Administration awarding unit National Institute on Alcohol Abuse and Alcoholism.

REFERENCES

1. **Ewald, S. J.**, Effects of prenatal drugs of abuse on development of lymphoid organs, in *Drugs of Abuse and Immune Function,* Watson, R. R., Ed., CRC Press, Boca Raton, FL, 1990, 49.
2. **Conley, M. E., Beckwith, J. B., Mancer, J. F. K., and Tenckhoff, L.,** The spectrum of the DiGeorge syndrome, *J. Pediatr.,* 94, 883, 1979.
3. **Ammann, A. J., Wara, D. W., Cowan, M. J., Barrett, D. J., and Stiehm, R.,** The DiGeorge syndrome and the fetal alcohol syndrome, *Am. J. Dis. Child.,* 136, 906, 1982.
4. **Siebert, J. R., Graham, J. M., and MacDonald, C.,** Pathologic features of the CHARGE association: support for involvement of the neural crest, *Teratology,* 31, 331, 1985.
5. **Webster, W. S., Germain, M.-A., Lipson, A., and Walsh, D.,** Alcohol and congenital heart defects: an experimental study in mice, *Cardiovasc. Res.,* 18, 335, 1984.
6. **Webster, W. S., Walsh, D. A., McEwen, S. E., and Lipson, A. H.,** Some teratogenic properties of ethanol and acetaldehyde in C57BL/6J mice: implications for the study of the fetal alcohol syndrome, *Teratology,* 27, 231, 1983.
7. **Daft, P. A., Johnston, M. C., and Sulik, K. K.,** Abnormal heart and great vessel development following acute ethanol exposure in mice, *Teratology,* 33, 93, 1986.
8. **Bockman, D. E. and Kirby, M. L.,** Dependence of thymus development on derivatives of the neural crest, *Science,* 223, 498, 1984.
9. **Ewald, S. J. and Huang, C.,** Lymphocyte populations and immune responses in mice prenatally exposed to ethanol, in *Alcohol, Immunomodulation, and AIDS,* Seminara, D., Watson, R. R., and Pawlowski, A., Eds., Alan R. Liss, New York, 1990, 191.
10. **Gilliam, D. M., Kotch, L. E., Dudek, B. C., and Riley, E. P.,** Ethanol teratogenesis in selectively bred long-sleep and short-sleep mice: a comparison to inbred C57BL/6J mice, *Alcohol.: Clin. Exp. Res.,* 13, 667, 1989.
11. **Ewald, S. J. and Frost, W. W.,** Effect of prenatal exposure to ethanol on development of the thymus, *Thymus,* 9, 211, 1987.
12. **Ewald, S. J. and Walden, S. M.,** Flow cytometric and histological analysis of mouse thymus in fetal alcohol syndrome, *J. Leuk. Biol.,* 44, 434, 1988.
13. **Ewald, S. J.,** T-lymphocyte populations in fetal alcohol syndrome, *Alcohol.: Clin. Exp. Res.,* 13, 485, 1989.
14. **Steven, W. M., Bulloch, B., and Seelig, L. L.,** A morphometric study of the effects of ethanol consumption on lactating mammary glands of rats, *Alcohol.: Clin. Exp. Res.,* 13, 209, 1989.
15. **Steven, W. M., Barron, R. A., Stewart, G. L., and Seelig, L. L.,** The effects of maternal ethanol consumption on the distribution of leukocyte subsets in the lactating mammary gland of rats, *Alcohol and Alcoholism,* 26, 615, 1991.
16. **Seelig, L. L., Steven, W. M., and Stewart, G. L.,** Maternal alcohol consumption and lactational transfer of anti-parasitic immunity in rats, *Alcohol.: Clin. Exp. Res.,* 14 (Abstr.), 336, 1990.

17. **Jollie, W. P. and Aly, H. M.,** Effects of chronic alcohol intake on placental transport of IgG, in *Alcohol, Immunomodulation, and AIDS,* Seminara, D., Watson, R. R. and Pawlowski, A., Eds., Alan R. Liss, New York, 1990, 201.

18. **Johnson, S., Knight, R., Marmier, D. J., and Steele, R. W.,** Immune deficiency in fetal alcohol syndrome, *Pediatr. Res.,* 15, 908, 1981.

19. **Calvani, M., Ghirelli, D., and Fortuna, C.,** Fetal alcohol syndrome: clinical, metabolic and immunologic follow-up in 14 cases, *Minerva Pediatr.,* 37, 77, 1985.

20. **Church, M. W. and Gerkin, K. P.,** Hearing disorders in children with fetal alcohol syndrome: findings from case reports, *Pediatrics,* 82, 147, 1988.

21. **Monjan, A. A. and Mandell, W.,** Fetal alcohol and immunity: depression of mitogen-induced lymphocyte blastogenesis, *Neurobehav. Toxicol.,* 2, 213, 1980.

22. **Norman, D. C., Chang, M.-P., Castle, S. C., Van Zuylen, J. E., and Taylor, A. N.,** Diminished proliferative response of ConA-blast cells to interleukin 2 in rats exposed to ethanol *in utero, Alcohol.: Clin. Exp. Res.,* 13, 69, 1989.

23. **Redei, E., Clark, W. R., and McGivern, R. F.,** Alcohol exposure *in utero* results in diminished T cell function and alterations in brain corticotropin-releasing factor and ACTH content, *Alcohol.: Clin. Exp. Res.,* 13, 439, 1989.

24. **Jerrells, T. and Weinberg, J.,** Suppression of immune responsiveness following prenatal ethanol exposure, *Alcohol.: Clin. Exp. Res.,* 13 (Abstr.), 320, 1989.

25. **Zidell, R. H., Hatoum, N. S., and Thomas, P. T.,** Fetal alcohol effects: evidence of developmental impairment in the absence of immunotoxicity, *Fund. Appl. Toxicol.,* 10, 189, 1988.

26. **Gottesfeld, Z., Christie, R., Felten, D. L., and LeGrue, S. J.,** Prenatal ethanol exposure alters immune capacity and noradrenergic synaptic transmission in lymphoid organs of the adult mouse, *Neuroscience,* 35, 185, 1990.

27. **Rao, G. A., Larkin, E. C., and Derr, R. F.,** Chronic alcohol consumption during pregnancy: alleviation of untoward effects by adequate nutrition, *Nutr. Res.,* 8, 421, 1988.

28. **Rao, G. A., Larkin, E. C., and Derr, R. F.,** Nutritional adequacy versus ethanol toxicity in chronic alcoholic rats: is the 36% ethanol liquid diet model nutritionally adequate?, *Biochem. Arch.,* 6, 1, 1990.

29. **Adkins, B., Gandour, D., Strober, S., and Weissman, I. L.,** Total lymphoid irradiation leads to transient depletion of the mouse thymic medulla and persistent abnormalities among medullary stromal cells, *J. Immunol.,* 140, 3373, 1988.

30. **Freitas, A. A., Rocha, B., and Coutinho, A. A.,** Lymphocyte population kinetics in the mouse, *Immunol. Rev.,* 91, 5, 1986.

31. **Middaugh, L. D., Randall, C. L., and Favara, J. P.,** Prenatal ethanol exposure in C57 mice: effects on pregnancy and offspring development, *Neurotoxicol. Teratol.,* 10, 175, 1988.

32. **Rockwood, G. A. and Riley, E. P.,** Alterations in suckling behavior in preweanling rats exposed to alcohol prenatally, *Teratology,* 33, 145, 1986.

33. **Tabakoff, B., Jaffe, R. C., and Ritzmann, R. F.,** Corticosterone concentrations in mice during ethanol drinking and withdrawal, *J. Pharm. Pharmacol.,* 30, 371, 1978.

34. **Screpanti, I., Morrone, S., Meco, D., Santoni, A., Gulino, A., Paolini, R., Crisanti, A., Mathieson, B. J., and Frati, L.,** Steroid sensitivity of thymocyte subpopulations during intrathymic differentiation. Effects of 17 beta-estradiol and dexamethasone on subsets expressing T cell antigen receptor or IL-2 receptor, *J. Immunol.,* 142, 3378, 1989.

35. **Snyder, A. K., Singh, S. P., Pullen, G. L., and Eman, S.,** Effects of maternal ethanol ingestion on the uptake of alpha-aminoisobutyric acid by fetal rat liver, lung and brain, *Biol. Neonate,* 56, 277, 1989.

36. **Ghishan, F. K., Patwardhan, R., and Greene, H. L.,** Fetal Alcohol Syndrome: inhibition of placental zinc transport as a potential mechanism for fetal growth retardation in the rat, *J. Clin. Lab. Med.,* 100, 45, 1982.

37. **Altura, B. M., Altura, B. T., Carella, A., Chatterjee, M., Halevy, S., and Tejani, N.,** Alcohol produces spasms of human umbilical blood vessels: relationship to fetal alcohol syndrome (FAS), *Eur. J. Pharmacol.,* 86, 311, 1982.

38. **Mukherjee, A. B. and Hodgen, G. D.,** Maternal ethanol exposure induces transient impairment of umbilical circulation and fetal hypoxia in monkeys, *Science,* 218, 700, 1982.

39. **Ceredig, R.,** Differentiation potential of 14-day fetal mouse thymocytes in organ culture. Analysis of CD4/CD8-defined single-positive and double-negative cells, *J. Immunol.,* 141, 355, 1988.

40. **Ceredig, R., Lowenthal, J. W., Nabholz, M., and MacDonald, H. R.,** Expression of interleukin-2 receptors as a differentiation marker on intrathymic stem cells, *Nature (London),* 314, 98, 1985.

41. **Hoffman, P. L. and Tabakoff, B.,** Ethanol and guanine nucleotide binding proteins: a selective interaction, *FASEB J.,* 4, 2612, 1990.

42. **Menetski, J. P. and Gellert, M.,** V(D)J recombination activity in lymphoid cell lines is increased by agents that elevate cAMP, *Proc. Natl. Acad. Sci. U.S.A.,* 87, 9324, 1990.

43. **McConkey, D. J., Orrenius, S., and Jondal, M.,** Agents that elevate cAMP stimulate DNA fragmentation in thymocytes, *J. Immunol.,* 145, 1227, 1990.

44. **Ewald, S. J., Huang, C., and Bray, L.,** Effect of prenatal alcohol exposure on lymphocyte populations in mice, in *Drugs of Abuse, Immunity and Immunodeficiency,* Friedman, H., Ed., Plenum Press, New York, 1991, 237.

45. **Bray, and Ewald, S. J.,** Effect of ethanol on development of fetal mouse thymocytes in organ culture, submitted.

Chapter 8

NEUROIMMUNE EFFECTS OF PRENATAL AND EARLY POSTNATAL ALCOHOL EXPOSURE

Zehava Gottesfeld

TABLE OF CONTENTS

I. INTRODUCTION

Clinical and experimental studies indicate that exposure to alcohol *in utero* is associated with long-lasting immune deficits. This may account for the increased susceptibility to bacterial and parasitic infection, as well as high frequency of carcinogenesis (reviewed in Reference 1). Mechanisms which underlie the immune anomalies are not clearly understood. Most investigators studying prenatal alcohol effects have focused on various immune parameters, but much of the research is phenomenological, and the site of alcohol action is far from clear.

There is no single mechanism which can account for such a complex biological phenomenon as immune regulation. The immune system is traditionally considered autonomous, but increasing evidence indicates that the immune response is also modulated by the central nervous system (CNS).[2] Accordingly, antigenic challenges prompt activated lymphocytes to secrete cytokines which mediate immunologic signals to other lymphocytes, as well as to the CNS. The brain, in turn, modulates the immune response via two pathways: (1) humoral channels involving the hypothalamo-pituitary-endocrine axis, and (2) neural projections from the autonomic nervous system (Figure 1). This suggests that reciprocal communications between the immune and nervous system are essential for maintaining the wellness of the host. Consequently, integrated studies of the neuro-immune-endocrine networks are necessary for a better understanding of mechanisms by which alcohol effects immune competency.

The role of the nervous system in mediating prenatal or early postnatal alcohol effects on the immune system has not been studied heretofore. Our hypothesis was that prenatal alcohol exposure alters neural regulation of immunity.[3,4] We focused attention, therefore, on the sympathetic innervation of lymphoid organs ("sympatho-lymphoid axis"), the final common pathway between the brain and the immune system that plays an important role in immune modulation.[5] The purpose of this chapter is to present our observations on the immune capacity, as well as activity of the sympatho-lymphoid axis, displayed by rodents exposed to either prenatal or lactational alcohol.[3,4,16]

II. EFFECTS OF PRENATAL ALCOHOL EXPOSURE ON IMMUNE COMPETENCE

A. CELLULAR IMMUNE RESPONSES

Young adult C57Bl/6J mice exposed to prenatal alcohol, or the pair-fed cohorts, were assigned to one of two immunologic tests: (1) contact hypersensitivity (CHS), or (2) the local graft vs. host (LGvH) response. The CHS response of alcohol-exposed mice to the contact-sensitizing hapten trinitrochlorobenzene (TNCB) was reduced significantly ($p < 0.001$) when compared with that of the pair-fed controls.[3] The depressed responsiveness persisted for

BRAIN

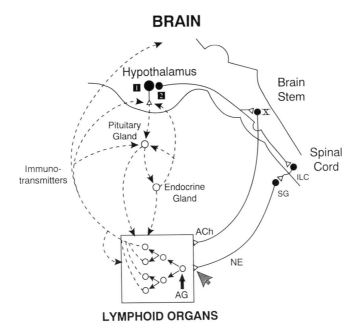

LYMPHOID ORGANS

FIGURE 1. Schematic illustration of reciprocal communications between the immune and the central nervous system. In response to an antigenic (AG) challenge, activated lymphocytes (LYMPHOID ORGANS) undergo proliferation and secrete cytokines (Immunotransmitters).[6] The secretory products carry signals to various lymphocytes as well as to the BRAIN. The latter, in turn, utilizes peripheral neural networks, as well as hormones, from the pituitary and endocrine glands to modulate the immune response. As indicated in the diagram, cells (1) in the hypothalamus secrete releasing or release-inhibiting hormones which trigger/inhibit the release of pituitary hormones, and, consequently, of endocrine hormones which act as immune modulators. Other cells (2) in the hypothalamus regulate the autonomic neural outflow, including the parasympathetic dorsal motor nucleus of the vagus (×) in the brainstem, and the preganglionic sympathetic neurons in the spinal intermediolateral cell column (ILC), innervating spinal ganglia (SG). The parasympathetic neural projections secrete acetylcholine (ACh), and the sympathetic neural axons release norepinephrine (NE) to interact with adrenoceptors on lymphocytes. (Adapted from Shepherd, G. M., *Neurobiology*, Oxford University Press, New York, 1988, 495.) The gray arrowhead indicates the focal point of our studies, i.e., the sympatho-lymphoid synapse, the final link of communication between the brain and the immune system.

at least as long as eight to nine weeks of age. It is noteworthy, however, that during the suckling on control dams, the prenatal alcohol-exposed pups did not display the suppressed CHS response. The immune anomalies were expressed only after weaning (Figure 2). These observations are consistent with the suggestion that breast-feeding facilitates the transmission of passive immunity from the nursing mother to the infant during the critical period of the nascent immune system.[8-10]

The LGvH response was determined using the popliteal lymph node weight-gain assay.[3] A significant ($p < 0.001$) reduction was observed in the

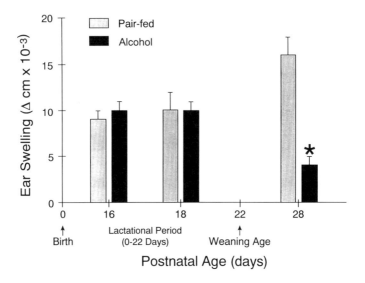

FIGURE 2.   Effects of prenatal alcohol exposure on cellular immune responses in infant mice suckling on untreated control dams, as well as in young weanlings. Contact hypersensitivity responses to TNCB were determined by measuring differences in swelling (Δcm $\times$ 10^{-3} $\pm$ SEM) between the TNCB-treated and vehicle-treated ears (n = 6/group). *Significant (p <0.001) decrease in ear swelling of the prenatal alcohol-exposed mouse after weaning, but not during lactation, as compared to the pair-fed cohorts.

weight of the draining popliteal lymph nodes of adult F1 mice challenged in the footpad with splenocytes from ethanol-exposed mice.[3]

B. IMMUNE RESPONSE TO PARASITIC INFECTION

Previous studies demonstrated that maternal alcohol consumption during nursing can have adverse effects on the lactational transfer of immunity.[11] This was expressed by a higher intestinal worm count as compared to pair-fed controls. There were no reports, however, as to whether exposure to alcohol *in utero* alters immune responsiveness to the parasitic challenge. We addressed the question in the following experiment.[26] Young-adult male Sprague-Dawley rats exposed to prenatal alcohol, or their pair-fed and control cohorts, were administered a primary infection by oral inoculation with 1.5×10^3 *Trichinella spiralis* larvae. The latter were recovered from infected mouse skeletal muscle by pepsin digestion.[12] Some of the rats (eight per group) were killed by decapitation two weeks following the primary infection, and intestinal worms were recovered and counted, as previously described.[13] The remaining rats (eight per group) received a secondary inoculation of 1000 *T. spiralis* larvae 35 days post-primary infection. Twenty-four hours later, worms were recovered from the intestine and counted.

The results indicated that there were no significant differences in the immune response to the parasitic infection between prenatal alcohol-exposed rats and their pair-fed controls. This is consistent with previous studies showing that prenatal alcohol exposure is associated with differential sensitivity to various antigenic challenges, as reflected by a variety of immunologic tests.[1] Alternately, the increased sensitivity to parasitic infection displayed by animals suckling on alcohol-consuming dams,[11] may reflect increased vulnerability during the critical period of early postnatal development.[16]

III. EFFECTS OF PRENATAL ALCOHOL EXPOSURE ON THE SYMPATHO-LYMPHOID AXIS

Previous studies demonstrated that the autonomic nervous system, especially the sympathetic noradrenergic pathways, plays an important role in immune modulation.[5] We examined effects of prenatal alcohol exposure on activity of the sympathetic neural projections to lymphoid organs by studying the turnover of tissue norepinephrine (NE), reflecting release of the amine. In addition, we examined the affinity and density of β-adrenoceptors on splenocyte and thymocyte membranes, that may indicate altered NE release.

A. TISSUE CONCENTRATION AND TURNOVER OF NOREPINEPHRINE

Mice exposed to alcohol *in utero* displayed a significant increase in NE turnover in the thymus ($p < 0.001$) and spleen ($p < 0.01$), but not the heart as compared to the pair-fed cohorts.[3] The increase in amine release may have been attributed, at least partly, to the observed decreased NE concentration selectively in lymphoid organs.[3] The amine deficit in the spleen and thymus of animals exposed to prenatal alcohol was observed as early as postnatal day one.[4] The magnitude of the deficit became progressively larger as the animal grew older, because thymic and splenic weight-gain became more restricted in the alcohol group.[4] Cardiac noradrenergic neural development and activity were not influenced by prenatal alcohol exposure.[3,4]

B. β-ADRENOCEPTORS IN LYMPHOID TISSUES

Mice exposed to prenatal alcohol displayed a significant ($p < 0.001$) and selective reduction in the apparent number (B_{max}), but not affinity (Kd) of β-adrenoceptors on splenocyte and thymocyte membranes.[3,4] The differences between the alcohol-exposed and pair-fed cohorts were apparent as early as postnatal day one, but became more pronounced at progressive stages of the development.[4] The decrease in β-adrenoceptor density is consistent with the enhanced turnover, i.e., increased release of NE. This is in agreement with the report that sympathectomy elicited an upregulation of lymphocytic β-adrenoceptors.[24]

IV. EFFECTS OF LACTATIONAL ALCOHOL ON IMMUNITY

Clinical and experimental studies suggest that chronic heavy alcohol use by adult subjects is associated with severe immune deficits.[14,15] We studied the consequences of alcohol consumption on the suckling mouse during early postnatal life.[16] This period in rodent development is characterized by rapid brain growth spurt that is comparable to the human third trimester,[17] as well as by the development and maturation of the immune system.[18,19] Thus, alcohol in maternal breast milk may render the suckling rodent vulnerable to immunologic challenges during the critical period of immune development. Indeed, we observed that young adult mice which suckled on alcohol-consuming dams displayed diminished cellular immune capacity, including suppressed contact hypersensitivity, as well as local graft vs. host responses.[16] In addition, this is reminiscent of previous studies demonstrating increased susceptibility to parasitic infection during early postnatal life.[11]

V. EFFECTS OF LACTATIONAL ALCOHOL EXPOSURE ON THE SYMPATHO-LYMPHOID AXIS

Development of the noradrenergic innervation of lymphoid organs in rodents occurs predominantly during early postnatal life,[4,20,21] coincident with the development and maturation of the immune competence.[16,17] This is consistent with the suggestion that sympathetic innervation of lymphoid organs plays an important role in regulating the development of lymphoid compartmentalization,[21] as well as of lymphocyte proliferation and differentiation.[25] We observed that young adult mice which were nursed by alcohol-consuming dams, displayed a significant ($p < 0.01$) reduction in both content and concentration of NE in the thymus and spleen, but not the heart.[16] The decrease in amine levels may have been attributable to the increased utilization rate, i.e., the ratio between the major metabolite MHPG and the parent amine NE (MHPG:NE),[22] selectively in lymphoid organs of the alcohol-suckling mice, as compared to the pair-fed controls.[16] The increased release of NE from the sympatho-lymphoid axis may have accounted for the observed immune deficits of the alcohol-exposed subjects. This is in agreement with the general consensus that NE facilitates the dampening of the immune response.[5] Alternatively, the enhanced turnover of NE in lymphoid organs may reflect a compensatory response to altered local activity,[23] and, thus, partly explain the selectivity of the observed effects.

Changes in the release of NE may influence the expression of noradrenergic receptors. Indeed, we observed a significant ($p < 0.001$) decrease in the apparent number, not affinity, of β-adrenoceptor in thymocyte and splenocyte plasma membranes isolated from young adult mice exposed to lactational alcohol.[16]

VI. CONCLUSIONS

Our studies demonstrate that exposure to alcohol *in utero* or during early postnatal life is associated with lasting cell-mediated immune deficits and an increased activity of the sympatho-lymphoid axis. The data demonstrate that the changes in noradrenergic synaptic transmission occur selectively in lymphoid organs. Furthermore, we suggest that the neurochemical changes are metabolic in nature, since no anatomical changes nor shifts in noradrenergic compartmentation were revealed by histofluorescent studies.[3]

The magnitude of the immune deficits and sympatho-lymphoid axis activity displayed by animals exposed to lactational alcohol was similar to that associated with prenatal alcohol exposure. It is noteworthy, however, that blood alcohol concentrations occurring in suckling pups were considerably lower.[16] This suggests that the nascent immune and nervous system are not only vulnerable to alcohol exposure during the critical period of early postnatal development, but may also be more sensitive to perturbation than at other times. It remains to be determined whether the same mechanisms underlie immune deficits associated with adult alcohol consumption and perinatal alcohol exposure.

Multiple factors are considered to play a role in regulating the immune response. Disruption of any of the functional components, whether neural, humoral, or immune-derived factors, can be translated into immune anomalies. Our studies demonstrate that exposure to alcohol during critical developmental periods is associated with altered neural-immune communication at the level of the sympatho-lymphoid synapse, the final site of communication between the brain and the immune system. It remains to be determined whether the effects of alcohol are directly aimed at the sympatho-lymphoid axis, or occur indirectly, by altering brain responsiveness to immunologic signals.

ACKNOWLEDGMENTS

Studies in the author's laboratory were supported by National Institute on Alcohol Abuse and Alcoholism Grants AA06158 and AA08667, as well as National Institutes of Health Biomedical Research Support Grant (UTMSH). Dr. Stephen J. LeGrue, Department of Immunology, M. D. Anderson Cancer Center, Houston, contributed to the immunologic studies. A note of gratitude to Peggy Gibbons for her excellent secretarial assistance, and to Keith Patricio for the illustrations.

REFERENCES

1. **Gottesfeld, Z. and Abel, E. L.,** Maternal and paternal alcohol use: effects on the immune system of the offspring, *Life Sci.,* 48, 1, 1991.
2. **Besedovsky, H. O., del Rey, A. G., and Sorkin, E.,** What does the immune system and the brain know about each other? *Immunol. Today,* 4, 342, 1983.
3. **Gottesfeld, Z., Christie, R., Felten, D. L., and LeGrue, S. J.,** Prenatal ethanol exposure alters immune capacity and noradrenergic synaptic transmission in lymphoid organs of the adult mouse, *Neuroscience,* 35, 185, 1990.
4. **Gottesfeld, Z., Morgan, B., and Perez-Polo, J. R.,** Prenatal alcohol exposure alters the development of sympathetic synaptic components and of nerve growth factor receptor expression selectively in lymphoid organs, *J. Neurosci. Res.,* 26, 308, 1990.
5. **Felten, D. L., Felten, S. Y., Bellinger, D. L., Carlson, S. L., Ackerman, K. D., Madden, K. L., Olschowska, J. A., and Livnat, S.,** Noradrenergic sympathetic neural interactions with the immune system: structure and function, *Immunol. Rev.,* 100, 225, 1987.
6. **Hall, N. R., McGillis, J. P., Spangello, B. L., and Goldstein, A. L.,** Evidence that thymosins and their biologic response modifiers can function as neuroactive immuno-transmitters, *J. Immunol.,* 135, 806s, 1985.
7. **Shepherd, G. M.,** *Neurobiology,* Oxford University Press, New York, 1988, 495.
8. **Faden, H. and Ogra, P. L.,** Breast milk as an immunologic vehicle for transport of immunocompetence, in *Textbook of Gastroenterology and Nutrition in Infancy,* Lebenthal, E., Eds., Raven Press, New York, 1981, 355.
9. **Migliore-Samour, D. and Jolles, P.,** Casein, a prohormone with an immunomodulating role for the newborn?, *Experientia,* 44, 188, 1988.
10. **Pitt, J., Barlow, D., Heird, W. C., and Snatuli, T. V.,** Macrophages and the protective action of breast milk on necrotizing enterocolitis, *Pediatr. Res.,* 8, 384, 1974.
11. **Seelig, L. L., Jr., Steven, W. M., and Stewart, G. L.,** Maternal alcohol consumption and lactational transfer of anti-parasitic immunity in rats, *Alcohol.: Clin. Exp. Res.,* 14, 33, 1990.
12. **Castro, G. A. and Fairbarn, D.,** Carbohydrates and lipids of *Trichinella spiralis* larvae and their utilization *in vitro, J. Parasitol.,* 55, 51, 1969.
13. **Russell, D. A. and Castro, G. A.,** Physiological characteristics of a biphasic immune response to *Trichinella spiralis* in the rat, *J. Inf. Dis.,* 139, 304, 1979.
14. **MacGregor, R. R.,** Alcohol and immune defense, *JAMA,* 256, 1474, 1986.
15. **Watson, R. R., Eskelson, C., and Hartmann, B. R.,** Severe alcohol abuse and cellular immune functions, *Arizona Med.,* 41, 665, 1984.
16. **Gottesfeld, Z. and LeGrue, S. J.,** Lactational alcohol exposure elicits long-term immune deficits and increased noradrenergic synaptic transmission in lymphoid organs, *Life Sci.,* 47, 457, 1990.
17. **Dobbing, J. and Sands, J.,** Comparative aspects of brain growth spurt, *Early Hum. Devl.,* 3, 79, 1979.
18. **Kimura, S., Eldridge, J. H., Michalek, S. M., Morisaka, I., Hamada, S., and McGhee, J. R.,** Immunoregulation in the rat: ontogeny of B cell responses to types 1, 2, and T-dependent antigens, *J. Immunol.,* 134, 2839, 1985.
19. **Veerman, A. J. P.,** The postnatal development of the white pulp in the rat spleen and the onset of immunocompetence against a thymus-independent and a thymus-dependent antigen, *Z. Immun. Forsch.,* 150, 45, 1975.
20. **Ackerman, K., Felten, S. Y., Bellinger, D. L., and Felten, D. L.,** Noradrenergic sympathetic innervation of the spleen. III. Development of innervation in the rat spleen, *Exp. Neurol.,* 103, 239, 1987.

21. **Ackerman, K., Felten, S. Y., Dijkstra, C. D., Livnat, S., and Felten, D. L.,** Parallel development of noradrenergic innervation and cellular compartmentation in the rat spleen, *Exp. Neurol.,* 103, 239, 1989.

22. **Lavielle, S., Tassin, J.-P., Thierry, A.-M., Blanc, H., Herve, D., Barthelemy, C., and Glowinski, J.,** Blockade by benzodiazepines of the selective high increase in dopamine turnover induced by stress in mesocortical dopaminergic neurons of the rat, *Brain Res.,* 168, 585, 1978.

23. **Del Rey, A. and Besedovsky, H. O.,** in *Hormones and Immunity,* Berczi, I. and Kovacs, I., Eds., Kluvier Academic Publishers Group, Boston, 1987, 215.

24. **Fuchs, B. A., Campbell, K. S., and Munson, A. E.,** Norepinephrine and serotonin content of the murine spleen: its relationship to lymphocyte β-adrenergic receptor density and the humoral immune response *in vivo* and *in vitro, Cell. Immun.,* 117, 339, 1988.

25. **Ackerman, K. D., Madden, K. S., Livnat, S., Felten, S. Y., and Felten, D. L.,** Neonatal sympathetic denervation alters the development of *in vitro* spleen cell proliferation and differentiation, *Brain. Behav. and Immunity,* 5, 235, 1991.

26. **Harai, Y., Castro, G. A., and Gottesfeld, Z.,** unpublished observations.

Chapter 9

FETAL ALCOHOL EXPOSURE AND NEUROIMMUNE SURVEILLANCE

Francesco Chiappelli, Carol Wong, Raz Yirmiya, Dean Norman, Mei-Ping Chang, and Anna N. Taylor

TABLE OF CONTENTS

5761-6/93/$0.00 + $.50

143

I. INTRODUCTION

The breadth of central and peripheral dysfunctions seen in children exposed prenatally to alcohol has been described as far back as the earliest reports on the teratogenic effects of ethanol in 1968.[1] Today, the pathogenesis of the fetal alcohol syndrome remains still largely undefined.[2] Among the most promising lines of investigation are the several animal models developed for characterizing the development and maturation of the brain, of behavioral and cognitive patterns, of neuroendocrine processes, and of immune responses, following prenatal exposure to alcohol. This chapter describes rodent models as reliable systems for research of the developmental and teratological outcomes of fetal alcohol exposure (FAE) on immune competence and surveillance. Emphasis is given specifically to the outcome of FAE on the development of the interaction between the hormones produced by the hypothalamic-pituitary-adrenal (HPA) axis and cell-mediated immunity (CMI), the immune-hypothalamic-pituitary-adrenal axis.[3]

II. THE HPA AXIS IN FETAL ALCOHOL EXPOSURE

In the past decade, we[4] and others[5] have examined developmental and long-term effects of maternal ethanol consumption (5% w/v ethanol-containing liquid diet [35% ethanol-derived calories]) in Sprague Dawley rats during the last two to three weeks of gestation on the function and regulation of the HPA axis. These studies have established that FAE animals manifest significant alterations in adrenocortical development and function.

We found that FAE pups have neonatal plasma corticosterone levels that are close to twofold higher than those of matched control animals. When we fostered all the pups to normal lactating females at birth, and recorded the characteristic drops in corticosterone levels in all animals by day 3, we noted that FAE rats retained corticosterone levels much higher than controls. Similar trends were also seen with whole brain corticosterone levels.[6,7]

The data of Shoemaker and collaborators[8] support the findings that prenatal alcohol exposure is associated with activation of the HPA axis during perinatal development. These investigators demonstrated that certain brain regions (e.g., midbrain, hindbrain) were significantly richer in the pro-opiomelanocortin (POMC) gene product, β-endorphin (bE), in FAE rats, compared to controls. By contrast, pituitary bE levels were higher in FAE, compared to control rats at postnatal day 4, but lower than control at days 8, 14, and 22 postnatally.[9] The ontogeny of the bE response to stress was also reported to be altered in FAE rats[10] (bE is generally believed to be released simultaneously with the major POMC gene product adrenocorticotropic hormone, ACTH).

Several additional endogenously produced opiate-like peptides have now been described which, together with bE, compose the endogenous opioid system (EOS). Taken together, the data to date suggest that FAE may be associated with significant alterations in EOS ontogeny,[8-10] which may contribute to the altered immune competence and surveillance seen in FAE rats and described in this chapter.

To study the regulation of the HPA axis in FAE rats, we administered various doses of dexamethasone (3.1 to 50 µg/kg) to adult (150 to 210 days) female Sprague-Dawley rats. Corticosterone was measured 4 h later, immediately before the onset of the activity cycle (lights off). FAE rats suppressed corticosterone levels as effectively as control animals at higher dexamethasone concentrations. At lower dexamethasone concentrations, FAE animals showed an early escape from dexamethasone suppression, and hypersecretion of adrenal steroids after dexamethasone.[11] These results suggest that FAE may lead to altered regulation of the HPA axis, which may be reflected as well in HPA/CMI dysregulation, as described below.

The HPA axis plays a central role in the neuroendocrine response to a variety of stressful stimuli, and drugs such as morphine and ethanol. We tested whether or not prenatal alcohol exposure may be associated with significant alterations of HPA responses. Experiments have measured the levels of plasma corticosterone 60 min following injection of morphine (30 mg/kg) or ethanol (1.5 g/kg). FAE pups (7 days old) showed an adrenocorticoid response to these drugs that was significantly lower than that obtained in control pups treated in parallel. Within 5 days, however, this anomalous adrenal response was overcome, and all groups responded equally to ethanol and morphine stimuli by day 12 to 18.[12] Older FAE rats (75 to 90 days), by contrast, manifested a significantly higher secretion of corticosterone in response to the ethanol[13] and the morphine stimulus,[14] compared to control rats. Some stressful stimuli (e.g., noise/shaking), but not others, (e.g., cold) also elicited elevated adrenocortical responses in adult (75 to 100 days) FAE animals.[15] Similar findings on HPA responsiveness of neonatal and adult FAE rats were obtained by Weinberg.[5,16] In summary, FAE results in significant long-lasting alterations in the neuroendocrine regulation of the HPA axis under stressful conditions. These lines of research, taken together with the recent body of literature describing the neuroimmune system, suggest that FAE may impair neuroendocrine-immune interactions as well. FAE-mediated alterations in immune surveillance mechanisms are described below.

III. IMMUNE SURVEILLANCE IN FAE

Alcohol consumption[17,18] and prenatal exposure to alcohol lead to many alterations in immune competence (for review, see Chapters 7 and 8 of this volume). The focus on the effects of FAE on the development and function of thymocytes is relevant to the present discussion, because it is in the thymus that T cells develop their functional ability (i.e., acquisition of the T cell receptor), their specificity (i.e., helper T cells vs. suppressor T cells), and their discriminative ability (i.e., self vs. nonself recognition via the major histocompatibility complex [MHC]).[19]

A. THYMIC ONTOGENY

The thymus is central to the development of immune competence. Its ontogenesis is determined by a series of precisely timed events during which the pharyngeal pouch endoderm interacts with embryonic connective tissue and migrating blood-borne lymphoid stem cells. The portion of the neural crest associated with the developing hindbrain migrates ventrolaterally through the bronchial arches. It will become the mesenchyme that will form the layers around the epithelial primordia of the thymus. Experimental alterations of this sequence of events or ablation of the cranial neural crest before its migration to the nascent thymus results in delayed, aborted, or abnormal thymic ontogenesis, and in aberrant development of immune competence.[20] The HPA-thymus interaction[21,22] and the deleterious effects of FAE on HPA ontogenesis predict that substantial damaging effects of FAE on thymic ontogenesis should be expected.

Some of the effects of fetal exposure to alcohol upon thymic ontogeny have been characterized in a murine FAE model (C57BL/6, 4.8% w/v ethanol, up to two weeks before and throughout pregnancy)[23] (see also Chapter 7 of this volume). Histologically, the cortico-medullary junction, which normally appears at 17 to 19 days of fetal life in the mouse as the thymus becomes functionally mature, was not apparent in FAE mice. The absence of this landmark of thymic development suggests that FAE may lead to a retardation of thymic ontogeny. Three lines of evidence support this hypothesis:[23]

1. A positive linear relationship was obtained between fetal weight and thymocyte number in 18-day old fetal mice. FAE animals were clustered in the lower left quadrant, but control animals were found in the upper ranges of thymocyte number and fetal weight.
2. Immature thymocytes are generally enlarged, and reduce their size as they traverse the thymus and acquire signs of thymocyte maturity. By flow cytometric forward scatter analysis, thymocytes from FAE fetuses appeared generally enlarged, compared to thymocytes from control cohorts.
3. The murine pan-thymocyte and pan-T lymphocyte marker, Thy-1, is acquired early during thymic ontogeny and thymocyte maturation. This membrane antigen, a 18 to 25 kDa glycoprotein of the immunoglobulin superfamily, is associated with the phosphatidylinositol transmembrane signaling system, and is expressed in cerebellar and brain stem neurons, as well as in thymocytes and T lymphocytes.[24]

Committed T cell precursors from the murine hematopoietic fetal liver — where toxic alcohol metabolites may be produced in FAE animals — initially migrate to the thymic primordia by day 10 to 11 of gestation. These enlarged basophilic cells engage in active differentiation and maturation within the thymus, and express Thy-1 by day 15.[25] By day 16 of gestation, thymocytes acquire Lyt-2. The appearance of L3T4 generally does not occur before day 17. By day 18 to 19 of fetal life, the time point examined by Ewald and Walden,[23] murine fetal thymocytes generally express the Lyt-2 and L3T4 antigens in a proportion similar to that found in adult mice. Helper T cell activity is conferred to the L3T4$^+$/Lyt-2$^-$ subpopulation, and cytotoxic/suppressor T cell activity resides in the L3T4-/Lyt-2$^+$ thymocyte subpopulation in mature normal mice. Double negative populations are immature, and remain in the thymus. By single color fluorescence-flow cytometry measurements, the proportion of Thy-1$^+$ fetal murine thymocytes was not different in FAE vs. control animals, but the proportions of L3T4$^+$ and Lyt-2$^+$ thymocytes were two to threefold reduced in FAE animals compared to controls.[23]

The generation of functionally competent T cells from thymocyte precursors involves several finely regulated processes modulated in part by the interaction between thymocytes and the thymic epithelium,[26] as well as the intrathymic environment, determined in part by secreted cytokines.[27-29] In addition, different subpopulations of thymocytes are characterized biochemically by the expression of distinct isozymes of protein kinase C, and maturation of thymocytes seems linked to the sequential expression and de-expression of these isozymes.[30,31]

Recent data reveal that several of the patterns of intrathymic T cell development identified thus far are common across many species, including rodents and humans.[32] The extent to which FAE alters any of these patterns of thymic development, however, is still unknown.

B. THYMIC INNERVATION

Both myelinated and nonmyelinated fibers of the autonomic nervous system innervate the thymus. Acetylcholinesterase-positive fibers innervate the murine thymic cortex and the cortico-medullary junction as early as embryonic day 18. This pattern of innervation is similar to that seen in fully developed mature murine thymus. Perivascular catecholaminergic innervation of the thymus is also evident at gestational day 18. In mature thymus, catecholaminergic innervation is both perivascular and nonperivascular within the cortical area particularly. This pattern of innervation is apparent only within the third week of postnatal life in the mouse.[33] The hypothesis that catecholaminergic innervation of the thymus modulates the regulation of the influx/efflux of lymphocytes from the blood stream through the thymic tissue, while innervation by cholinergic fibers is critical to the maturation and differentiation of the thymus, has been proposed by Bulloch and colleagues[33] and requires testing, particularly within the context of FAE.

Biochemical evidence confirms the existence of adrenergic receptors early in thymic development. At gestational day 18, the level of β-adrenergic receptors in fetal thymus is comparable to that found in adult thymus, as determined by binding studies with the potent β-adrenergic antagonist, dihydroalprenolol.[34] The immunofunctional relevance of lymphocytic adrenergic receptors is suggested by studies, such as those demonstrating an enhancement of expression of the activation marker, Tac (low molecular weight subunit of the interleukin-2 [IL-2] receptor), by human lymphocytes after treatment with the β-adrenoreceptor antagonist, propanolol $(10^{-6} M)$.[35]

C. THYMIC FUNCTION IN FAE

From the functional standpoint, the proliferative response to mitogen stimulation is generally lower in FAE animals, compared to control cohorts. Studies have used the male offspring of Sprague Dawley rats intubated daily with 6 g/kg ethanol from two weeks before mating until delivery, to measure the response of splenocytes at 7, 11, and 18 months of postnatal life. No differences in proliferation were obtained between FAE and control animals when the B cell mitogen, lipopolysaccharide (LPS), was used. The T cell mitogen, concanavalin A (ConA) showed a suppression in proliferative response that was greatest at 7 months (5% of control), less pronounced at 11 months (40% of control), and all but abolished at 18 months (90 to 100% of control).[36]

The proliferative response to ConA was also examined in splenocytes and thymocytes of 21-day-old offspring from Sprague Dawley rats treated with ethanol (35% ethanol-derived calories) during the last week of gestation. Neuroendocrine assessments indicated similar HPA dysfunctions in FAE animals (elevated hypothalamic ACTH, but decreased hypothalamic CRF and pituitary ACTH compared to control animals at day 1, postnatally). The ConA response was suppressed eightfold in splenocytes and twofold in thymocytes, compared to control three weeks after birth.[37]

Our laboratory demonstrated that maximal suppression of the proliferative response of splenocytes to ConA could be obtained at 3 to 5 months in male adult Sprague Dawley FAE rats exposed to alcohol (5% w/v) during the last two weeks of gestation (Figure 1).[38] Splenocytes obtained from these adult FAE animals preactivated with ConA were also much less responsive to further stimulation with crude ConA supernatant or with recombinant IL-2, compared to controls. This loss of responsiveness was age-dependent (Figure 2).[38,39] Preliminary flow cytometric analyses of splenocyte populations suggested that FAE alters the proportion of T cell subsets that home to the spleen, and that these alterations may be sustained into adulthood.[40]

In a parallel series of studies, we demonstrated an age-dependent increase (over eightfold, $p < 0.01$) in response to ConA by thymocytes by postnatal day 44 in male FAE rats, as opposed to the twofold decrease in response by splenocytes noted above (Figure 1). Stimulated thymocytes from FAE rats were less responsive to further stimulation with crude ConA supernatant compared to normal rats at day 44, as were stimulated splenocytes. Contrary

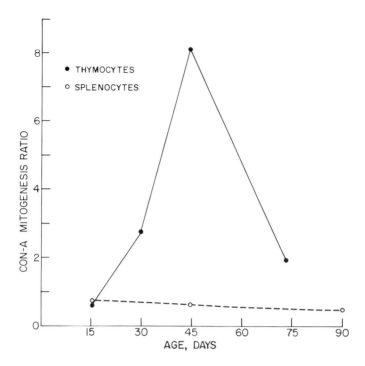

FIGURE 1. Effect of fetal alcohol exposure on ConA mitogenesis in thymocytes and splenocytes between postnatal days 16 and 90. Date expressed as the ratio of the mitogenic response obtained with cells from FAE rats to the response of cells from normal rats.

to splenocytes,[38] the response of stimulated thymocytes tended to normalize by young adulthood (day 72) (Figure 2).[41] We do not yet fully understand the striking differences in response between FAE thymocytes and FAE splenocytes, compared to cell populations obtained from normal rats. We are now engaged in testing working hypotheses to test this effect by immunofunctional and immunophenotypic approaches, based upon our current knowledge of the intrathymic events leading to T cell generation briefly outlined above.

Studies to date have used the male progeny primarily to avoid the complexities associated with the possible neuroimmune outcomes derived from the neuroendocrine fluctuations of the estrous cycle. However, and based upon putative neuroimmune sexual dimorphic characteristics,[42] studies designed to characterize the outcome of FAE on immune surveillance mechanisms in females must now be conceived. One such study has recently contrasted the effects of FAE in 60- to 70-day-old male and female Sprague Dawley rats. The results showed that alterations in T cell responsiveness were primarily evident in males.[43]

Different outcomes of prenatal alcohol exposure may be attributed at least in part to different schedules of fetal exposure to ethanol. Critical periods in

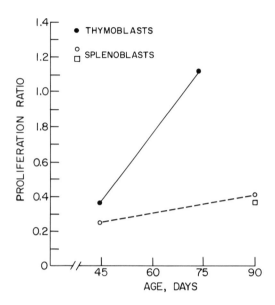

FIGURE 2.   Effect of fetal alcohol exposure on the mitogenic response of ConA-thymoblasts and ConA-splenoblasts (open squares, crude ConA supernatant; open circles, recombinant IL-2) to further stimulation between postnatal days 16 and 90. Data expressed as the ratio of the proliferation response obtained with cells from FAE rats to the response of cells from normal rats.

the development of the CNS have been described,[44] and in all likelihood exist for the immune system as well. FAE has several distinct outcomes during CNS development,[45-47] and several outcomes are similarly likely to occur during the development of CMI and of immune surveillance.[23,48] A simple test of this hypothesis will entail subjecting animals to different schedules of prenatal alcohol exposure, and assessing HPA and cell-mediated immunity responses peri- and postnatally.

Immediate future studies should be designed to test whether or not FAE retards:

1. The appearance of mature and functional T cell receptors (i.e., interference with the rearrangement and expression of the T cell receptor chain genes by fetal ethanol exposure [as determined, for instance, by *in situ* hybridization techniques[25]])

2. The development of the self vs. nonself discriminative ability of mature thymocytes (i.e., interference of the "positive" [thymocytes whose T cell receptor recognizes and binds to the MHC on the thymic epithelium are preserved] vs. "negative" [thymocytes with excessive affinity for self-antigens are eliminated] selection process of thymocyte development[49,50])

Furthermore, and because of the role of neuroendocrine products in the regulation of the expression of lymphocyte adhesion and homing molecules,[51] it is not inconceivable — considering the substantial degree of neuroendocrine abnormalities in FAE — that the expression of these membrane molecules may be significantly altered in FAE thymocytes and splenocytes, compared to normal animals.

In summary, structural, morphologic, and phenotypic lines of evidence support the hypothesis that FAE delays the development of the thymus, and impairs CMI ontogeny and immune surveillance. Studies should systematically characterize the effects of FAE on the development of immune, neuroendocrine, and neuroimmune processes. Clearly, these studies also must consider the possibility that the effects of FAE on thymic cell maturation may be indirect, in that FAE may impair prothymocyte seeding of the thymus,[52] or result from the serious aberration in hepatic biology and metabolism induced by FAE, among which are the depletion in retinoid levels and the reduction in retinoic acid synthesis.[53] These latter observations appear particularly relevant to the general focus of this work when one considers the role of retinoids in the control and regulation of cancer progression.[54]

IV. FAE AND NEUROIMMUNOLOGY

Few studies have investigated the outcome of FAE specifically on the neuroimmune system. As noted above, research has usually characterized the adverse effects of FAE, either on the neuroendocrine, or the immune system. A notably exception is the recent report by Gottesfeld and co-workers[55] (see also Chapter 8 of this volume). These investigators showed that the young adult (5 to 10 weeks) progeny of C57BL/6J mice born from dams exposed to ethanol (4.8% w/v) throughout gestation exhibited:

1. Decreased *in vivo* measures of cell-mediated immunity (e.g., contact hypersensitivity, local graft-vs.-host response)
2. Altered synaptic transmission of noradrenergic fibers in the spleen — that is, a rise in splenic (and thymic, but not cardiac) norepinephrine turnover, a drop in norepinephrine content, and a drop in beta-adrenergic receptor number, but a retention of "sympatolymphoid" noradrenergic system of innervation to the spleen

As discussed in the preceding sections, FAE animals have profound disturbances in the HPA axis and the EOS. Therefore, and since melatonin effectively counteracts stress-induced immune suppression consequential to EOS activation,[56] it will be interesting to test the effects of melatonin on immune surveillance in stressed FAE rats. In fact, and in further support of this research direction, it is possible that FAE animals may exhibit disturbances in melatonin metabolism and pineal ontogeny and functioning, a hypothesis that is now being tested in our laboratory.

As indicated above, bE has complex immunomodulatory effects on cytotoxic and proliferative responses of immune effector cells. It is now clear that bE has multiple modulatory effects on transmembrane signaling events, crucial in immune surveillance. We have shown that bE inhibits phosphoinositol phosphate metabolism, and that bE also enhances, or inhibits the phosphorylation of the gamma chain of CD3 in a dose-dependent manner.[57] Thus, bE, and perhaps other EOS products, can modulate several membrane transduction processes simultaneously, and some of these outcomes may counter others. The immunomodulatory effects of bE in FAE now remain to be explored.

In a slightly different context, and based on previous studies of social confrontation in fish where social submissiveness results in profound suppression of proliferative response to mitogen and cytotoxicity, data show that this suppression in immune competence can be blocked in part by naltrexone,[58] implicating EOS. Social confrontation in rodents has also been shown to induce EOS responses.[59,60] Therefore, it can be expected that social confrontation paradigms in FAE rats should be associated with an enhanced adrenocortical response and a more pronounced suppression of *in vitro* CMI measures. Thus, social confrontation paradigms may contribute to the elucidation of the physiological mechanisms responsible for impaired immune surveillance following prenatal exposure to alcohol.

V. CONCLUSION

Cross-disciplinary investigations are now necessary to characterize the interaction between brain, behavior, and immunity, and to elucidate the effects of prenatal alcohol exposure upon these interactive processes, in general, and upon neuroimmune surveillance mechanisms, in particular. Animal models are practical systems to address developmental and teratological issues of FAE. These models are likely to remain systems of choice in the investigation of developmental neuroimmunology of FAE, and of its consequences on immune surveillance.

ACKNOWLEDGMENTS

During portions of this study, Francesco Chiappelli was a post-doctoral fellow in the Psychoneuroimmunology Program at UCLA, and warmly thanks the late Mr. Norman Cousins and the UCLA Task Force on Psychoneuroimmunology for their guidance and support; Dr. Chiappelli also held a post-doctoral fellowship in Clinical and Fundamental Immunology (NIAID AI 07126).

The authors warmly thank Ms. B. J. Branch for her most valuable contributions throughout these studies.

This study was supported in part by funds obtained from the UCLA Psychoneuroimmunology Program (Kettering Foundation, Grant CO-6642-01) (Francesco Chiappelli); and Veteran's Administration Medical Research Service (Anna N. Taylor).

REFERENCES

1. **Lemoine, P., Harousseau, H., Borteryu, J. P., and Menuet, J. C.,** Les enfants de parents alcooliques. Anomalies observées à propos de 127 cas., *Ouest Médical,* 21, 476, 1968.
2. **Schenker, S., Becker, H. C., Randall, C. L., Phillips, D. K., Baskins, G. S., and Henderson, G. I.,** Fetal alcohol syndrome: current status of pathogenesis, *Alcohol.: Clin. Exper. Res.,* 14, 635, 1990.
3. **Bateman, A., Singh, A., Kral, T., and Solomon, S.,** The immune-hypothalamic-pituitary-adrenal axis, *Endocrine Rev.,* 10, 92, 1989.
4. **Nelson, L. R. and Taylor, A. N.,** Long-term behavioral and neuroendocrine effects of prenatal alcohol exposure, in *Genetic and Perinatal Effects of Abused Substances,* Braude, M. C. and Zimmerman, A. M., Eds., Academic Press, Orlando, 1987, 177.
5. **Weinberg, J.,** Prenatal alcohol exposure alters adrenocortical development of the offspring, *Alcohol.: Clin. Exper. Res.,* 13, 73, 1989.
6. **Taylor, A. N., Branch, B. J., Kokka, N., and Poland, R. E.,** Neonatal and long-term neuroendocrine effects of fetal alcohol exposure, *Monographs in Neural Sci.,* 9, 140, 1983.
7. **Taylor, A. N., Branch, B. J., Cooley-Mathews, B., and Poland, R. E.,** Effects of maternal ethanol consumption on basal and rhythmic pituitary-adrenal function in neonatal offspring, *Psychoneuroendocrinology,* 7, 49, 1982.
8. **Shoemaker, W. J., Baetge, G., Azad, R., Sapin, V., and Bloom, F. E.,** Effect of prenatal alcohol exposure on amine and peptide neurotransmitter systems, *Monographs in Neural Sci.,* 9, 130, 1983.
9. **Gianoulakis, C.,** Effect of prenatal exposure to ethanol on body growth and the pituitary beta-endorphin, *Alcohol.: Clin. Exp. Res.,* 11, 567, 1987.
10. **Angelogianni, P. and Gianoulakis, C.,** Prenatal exposure to ethanol alters the ontogeny of the beta-endorphin response to stress, *Alcohol.: Clin. Exp. Res.,* 13, 564, 1987.
11. **Nelson, L. R., Redei, E., Branch, B. J., Liebeskind, J. C., and Taylor, A. N.,** Corticosterone response to dexamethasone in fetal ethanol-exposed rats, *Proc. Pharmacol. Soc.,* 28, 299, 1985.
12. **Taylor, A. N., Branch, B. J., Nelson, L. R., Lane, L. A., and Poland, R. E.,** Prenatal ethanol and ontogeny of pituitary-adrenal responses to ethanol and morphine, *Alcohol,* 3, 255, 1986.
13. **Taylor, A. N., Branch, B. J., Liu, S., Weichman, A. F., Hill, M. A., and Kokka, N.,** Fetal exposure to ethanol enhances pituitary-adrenal and temperature responses to ethanol in adult rats, *Alcohol.: Clin. Exp. Res.,* 5, 237, 1981.
14. **Nelson, L. R., Taylor, A. N., Lewis, J. E., Poland, R. E., Redei, E., and Branch, B. J.,** Pituitary-adrenal responses to morphine and footshock stress are enhanced following prenatal alcohol exposure, *Alcohol.: Clin. Exp. Res.,* 10, 397, 1986.
15. **Taylor, A. N., Branch, B. J., Liu, S. H., and Kokka, N.,** Long-term effects of fetal alcohol exposure on pituitary-adrenal response to stress, *Pharmacol. Biochem. Behav.,* 16, 585, 1982.

16. **Weinberg, J.,** Hyperresponsiveness to stress: differential effect of prenatal ethanol in male and female, *Alcohol.: Clin. Exp. Res.,* 12, 647, 1989.

17. **MacGregor, R. R.,** Alcohol and immune defense, *JAMA,* 256, 1474, 1986.

18. **Seminara, D., Ed.,** Recent advances in alcohol and immunology, *Alcohol.: Clin. Exp. Res.,* 13, 467, 1989.

19. **Roitt, I., Brostoff, J., and Male, D.,** *Immunology,* 2nd ed., Gower Medical Publishing, London, 1989.

20. **Bockman, D. E. and Kirby, M. L.,** Neural crest interactions in the development of the immune system, *J. Immunol.,* 135, 766s, 1985.

21. **Hall, N. R. S., O'Grady, M. P., and Farah, J. M.,** Thymic hormones and immune function: mediation via neuroendocrine circuits, in *Psychoneuroimmunology II,* Ader, R., Felten, D. L., and Cohen, N., Eds., Academic Press, San Diego, CA, 1990, 515.

22. **Chiappelli, F., Wong, C. M. K., and Taylor, A. N.,** Endocrine-immune developmental patterns in rat thymocytes, in *Proc. 1st Int. Congr. Biomarkers Aging,* Licastro, F. and Caldarera, C. M., Eds., Editrice CLUEB, Bologna, 309, 1992.

23. **Ewald, S. J. and Walden, S. M.,** Flow cytometric and histological analysis of mouse thymus in fetal alcohol syndrome, *J. Leukocyte Biol.,* 44, 434, 1988.

24. **Greene, M. I., Kokai, Y., Gaulton, G. N., Powell, M. B., Geller, H., and Cohen, J. A.,** Receptor systems in tissues of the nervous system, *Immunol. Rev.,* 100, 153, 1987.

25. **Pardoll, D. M., Fowlkes, B. J., Lechler, R. I., Germain, R. N., and Schwartz, R. H.,** Early genetic events in T cell development analyzed by *in situ* hybridization, *J. Exp. Med.,* 165, 1624, 1987.

26. **Singer, K. H.,** Interactions between epithelial cells and T lymphocytes: role of adhesion molecules, *J. Leukocyte Biol.,* 48, 367, 1990.

27. **Cardioz, S. R., Hayday, A. C., and Bottomly, K.,** Cytokines in T cell development, *Immunol. Today,* 12, 239, 1991.

28. **Montgomery, R. A. and Dallman, M. J.,** Analysis of cytokine gene expression during fetal thymic ontogeny using the polymerase chain reaction, *J. Immunol.,* 147, 554, 1991.

29. **Street, N. E. and Mosman, T. R.,** Functional diversity of T lymphocytes due to secretion of different cytokine patterns, *FASEB J.,* 5, 171, 1991.

30. **Freire-Moar, J., Cherwinski, H., Hwang, F., Ranson, J., and Webb, D.,** Expression of protein kinase C isozymes in thymocyte subpopulations and their different regulation, *J. Immunol.,* 147, 405, 1991.

31. **Helman Finkel, T., Kubo, R. T., and Cambier, J. C.,** T cell development and transmembrane signaling: changing biological responses through an unchanging receptor, *Immunol. Today,* 12, 79, 1991.

32. **Aspinall, R., Kampinga, J., and van den Bogaerde, J.,** T cell development in the fetus and the invariant series hypothesis, *Immunol. Today,* 12, 7, 1991.

33. **Bulloch, K., Cullen, M. R., Schwartz, R. H., and Longo, D. L.,** Development of innervation within syngeneic thymus tissue transplanted under the kidney capsule of the nude mouse: a light and ultrastructural microscope study, *J. Neurosci. Res.,* 18, 16, 1987.

34. **Singh, U., Millson, D. S., Smith, P. A., and Owen, J. J. T.,** Identification of beta-adrenoreceptors during thymocyte ontogeny in mice, *Eur. J. Immunol.,* 9, 31, 1979.

35. **Malec, P. and Nowak, Z.,** Propanolol enhances *in vitro* interleukin-2 receptor expression on human lymphocytes, *Immunol. Lett.,* 17, 319, 1988.

36. **Monjan, A. A. and Mandell, W.,** Fetal alcohol and immunity: depression of mitogen-induced lymphocyte blastogenesis, *Neurobehav. Toxicol.,* 2, 213, 1980.

37. **Redei, E., Clark, W., and McGivern, R. F.,** Alterations in immune responsiveness, ACTH, and CRF content of brains in animals exposed to alcohol during the last week of gestation, *Alcohol.: Clin. Exp. Res.,* 13, 439, 1989.

38. **Norman, D. C., Chang, M.-P., Wong, C. M. K., Branch, B. J., Castle, S., and Taylor, A. N.,** Changes with age in the proliferative response of splenic T cells from rats exposed to ethanol *in utero, Alcohol.: Clin. Exp. Res.,* 15, 428, 1991.

39. **Norman, D. C., Chang, M.-P., Castle, S. C., van Zuylen, J. E., and Taylor, A. N.,** Diminished proliferative response of ConA blast cells to interleukin-2 in adult rats exposed to ethanol *in utero, Alcohol.: Clin. Exp. Res.,* 13, 69, 1989.

40. **Norman, D. C., Chang, M.-P., and Taylor, A. N.,** Diminished T cell proliferative response of fetal alcohol exposed (FAE) rats is not due to excessive suppressor cell activity, *Alcohol.: Clin. Exp. Res.,* 15, 342, 1991.

41. **Wong, C., Chiappelli, F., Chang, M.-P., Norman, D. C., Cooper, E. L., Branch, B. J., and Taylor, A. N.,** Prenatal exposure to alcohol enhances thymocyte mitogenic responses postnatally, *Int. J. Immunopharmacol.,* 14, 303, 1992.

42. **Grossman, C. S.,** Are the underlying immune-neuroendocrine interactions responsible for immunological sexual dimorphism?, *Prog. NeuroEndocrine Immunol.,* 3, 75, 1990.

43. **Weinberg, J. and Jerrells, T. R.,** Suppression of immune responsiveness: sex differences in prenatal ethanol effects, *Alcohol.: Clin. Exp. Res.,* 15, 525, 1991.

44. **Erzurumlu, R. S. and Killackey, H. P.,** Critical and sensitive periods in neurobiology, in *Current Topics in Developmental Biology,* Vol. 17, 1982, 207.

45. **West, J. R., Ed.,** *Alcohol and Brain Development,* Oxford University Press, New York 1986.

46. **West, J. R. and Hamre, K. M.,** Effects of alcohol exposure during different periods of development: changes in hippocampal mossy fibers, *Dev. Brain Res.,* 17, 280, 1985.

47. **Chiappelli, F., Taylor, A. N., Espinosa de los Monteros, A., and de Vellis, J.,** Fetal alcohol delays the expression of myelin basic protein and transferrin in rat cultured primary oligodendrocyte cultures, *Int. J. Dev. Neurosci.,* 9, 67, 1990.

48. **Ewald, S.,** T lymphocyte populations in the fetal alcohol syndrome, *Alcohol.: Clin. Exp. Res.,* 13, 485, 1989.

49. **Ezine, S.,** The thymus: colonization and ontogeny, *Bull. l'Institut Pasteur,* 87, 171, 1989.

50. **von Boehmer, H.,** The developmental biology of T lymphocytes, *Annu. Rev. Immunol.,* 6, 309, 1988.

51. **Chiappelli, F.,** Neuroimmunological perspectives on lymphocyte homing and adhesion, *Int. J. Immunopathol. Pharmacol.,* 4, 115, 1991.

52. **O'Neil, H. C.,** Prothymocyte seeding in the thymus, *Immunol. Lett.,* 27, 1, 1991.

53. **Pullarkat, R. R.,** Hypothesis: prenatal ethanol-induced birth defect and retinoic acid, *Alcohol.: Clin. Exp. Res.,* 15, 565, 1991.

54. **Virma, A. K.,** Modulation of carcinogenesis by vitamin A and its analogs (retinoids), in *Vitamins and Cancer Prevention,* Laidlaw, S. and Swendseid, M. E., Eds., Wiley Liss, New York, 1991, 25.

55. **Gottesfeld, Z., Christie, R., Felten, D. L., and LeGrue, S. J.,** Prenatal ethanol exposure alters immune capacity and noradrenergic synaptic transmission in lymphoid organs of the adult mouse, *Neuroscience,* 35, 185, 1990.

56. **Maestroni, G. J. M. and Conti, A.,** Role of the pineal neurohormone melatonin in the psycho-neuroendocrine network, in *Psychoneuroimmunology II,* Ader, R., Felten, D. L., and Cohen, N., Eds. Academic Press, San Diego, 1990, 495.

57. **Chiappelli, F., Kavelaars, A., and Heijnen, C. J.,** Beta-endorphin effects on membrane transduction in human lymphocytes, *Annals of the New York Academy of Sciences,* 650, 211, 1991.

58. **Faisal, M., Chiappelli, F., Ahmed, I. I., Cooper, E. L., and Weiner, H.,** Social confrontation "stress" in aggressive fish is associated with an endogenous opioid-mediated suppression of proliferative response to mitogens and nonspecific cytotoxicity, *Brain. Behav. Immunity,* 3, 223, 1989.

59. **Miczek, K. A. and Thompson, M. L.,** Analgesia resulting from defeat in social confrontation: the role of endogenous opioids in brain, in *Modulation of Sensorimotor Activity during Alterations in Behavioral States,* Alan R. Liss, New York, 1984, 431.
60. **Smelik, P. G.,** Differential control of ACTH-related peptides and the importance of the behavioral situation, in *Neurobiological Approaches to Human Diseases,* Hellhammer, D., Florin, D. and Weiner, H., Eds., Hans Huber, Toronto, 1987, 286.

PART III
Alcohol and Cancer

Chapter 10

ALCOHOL AND CANCERS OF THE ESOPHAGUS AND LIVER

Siraj I. Mufti

TABLE OF CONTENTS

5761-6/93/$0.00 + $.50

159

I. INTRODUCTION

An association between long-term chronic alcohol consumption and increased risk of cancers in humans has long been suspected. This association was first demonstrated for cancers of the oropharynx, larynx, and esophagus in a large number of epidemiological studies relating national or regional per capita alcohol consumption to age-adjusted cancer mortality.[1-5] The observations were then confirmed by prospective cohort studies of groups of people who consume great quantities of alcoholic beverages; for example, brewery workers who get drinks free of charge, have shown an increased cancer risk.[6-9] The conclusions were also supported by case-control studies where patients with malignant disease are examined for the relative risk of cancer.[10-16] Additional evidence for association has been provided by studies among traditional abstainers, such as Seventh Day Adventists and Mormons.[17,18] In addition to upper gastrointestinal tract cancer, these studies also indicated an association with liver cancers. Other sites associated with alcohol abuse are the pancreas,[19] breast,[20] stomach,[21-24] and colon, but the evidence for these associations is not as strong.[15,25-29] The subject of association of alcohol with cancers has been reviewed by several investigators,[30-34] including recent reviews by us.[35-37] This article outlines some of the evidence for association with cancers of the esophagus and liver, indicating that environment, including alcohol consumption, plays an important role in cancer causation. Despite the abundance of epidemiologic evidence, however, the experimental evidence does not associate alcohol by itself as a cause for cancer. Most cancers are of multifactorial origin, and alcohol may play a role, along with a multiplicity of other factors. Therefore, discussion of the major etiological factors that may underlie alcohol-associated cancers is also included. Finally, based on results of our recent studies, mechanisms are postulated that could explain occurrence of alcohol-related cancers.

II. EPIDEMIOLOGICAL EVIDENCE

A. ASSOCIATION WITH ESOPHAGEAL (AND ORAL CAVITY) CANCERS

Clinicians were first to discover that there was a high occurrence of laryngeal and esophageal cancers in males who drank excessively. Schwartz et al.[1] questioned the cancer patients, and found that drinkers had the highest incidence of cancers of the buccal cavity, tongue, oropharynx, hypopharynx, larynx, and esophagus. The best evidence for an association of excessive chronic alcohol consumption and cancer comes from case-control studies in which the contribution of alcohol is separated from smoking, a frequently associated risk factor.[39-45] This is supported by evidence from cohort studies in alcoholics demonstrating that excessive drinkers have an increased risk of cancers. Rothman and Keller[41] observed that the risk of developing oral cancer was two to six times greater in heavy drinkers, compared with abstainers. Similar results were obtained for head and neck cancer by Feldman et al.[43] Alcohol and tobacco apparently interact synergistically to enhance cancer risk. For example, the above-noted two studies found that individuals who combined the use of alcohol and tobacco had an oral cancer risk that was more than 15 times greater than for those who neither smoke nor drink. Other studies found that the relative cancer risk also depended on, and increased with, the amount of tobacco smoked. For example, McCoy and Wynder[46] observed that heavy smoking alone resulted in no more than a two- to threefold increase in oral cancer. However, the relative risk of developing oral cavity and larynx cancers among individuals who consumed seven or more ounces of alcohol a day and smoked more than one pack of cigarettes a day, increased 20- to 27-fold compared with nondrinkers and nonsmokers.[46] Studies have indicated a dose-response relationship and a gradient in risk according to the ethanol concentration of the drinks and the amount of ethanol consumed. (See, for example, Reference 47).

A number of other studies have shown a high degree of association between esophageal cancer and alcohol consumption in different geographical areas, such as China,[48] France,[49] the U.S.,[50] Puerto Rico,[40] and South Africa.[51] About 75% of the cancers of the esophagus in men and women in the U.S. are attributable to the consumption of alcohol.[31] A high rate of esophageal carcinoma among Blacks in the U.S. was related to a high consumption of alcoholic beverages.[52]

Especially remarkable is the geographical variation in worldwide occurrence of esophageal cancers. In low-risk areas, including the U.S., the incidence is less than 10 per 100,000, while in high-risk areas of Northwestern China, around Caspian Littoral in Russia and Iran, and Transkei in South Africa, the incidence is about 50 per 100,000, with rates reaching 100 to 200 per 100,000 in areas within these regions, and being as high as 800 per 100,000 within the high-risk age group.[53-58] Also, in the Kazakhstan Province of Russia, where esophageal carcinoma is the most commonly diagnosed cancer, consumption of alcohol is high.[59] On the other hand, near the Caspian Sea in Iran, another high-risk area, there is little or no consumption of alcohol. Even more remarkable is the observation that along Caspian Littoral, a 30-fold gradient in the incidence of disease is reported along a strip of several hundred kilometers.[60] However, the incidence falls to low levels in areas of close proximity, indicating that there are strong factors present in local environment that play a major role in causation.

That the environment has a major etiological role in causing cancer is borne out by a number of studies. For example, in China, when immigrants move from the high-incidence province of Honan, to Hubei, a low-incidence province, they also transfer with them their high-incidence of esophageal carcinoma. Since the incidence of cancers among fowl in high- and low-incidence areas (reared on remnant household foods) also paralleled the incidence among immigrant populations,[61-63] the observation suggests that dietary factors play important roles in the carcinogenetic process. Another noteworthy example comes from Transkei in South Africa, where an association of esophageal cancer has been found with a particular soil strata that are low in content of trace elements and high in silica.[64,65] In these areas, marked differences in the amounts of trace elements, particularly molybdenum, zinc, copper, iron, and magnesium, were found in plants grown in gardens of cancer sufferers, vs. areas where no esophageal cancers were reported.[66] Furthermore, food grown in an experimental plot in the high-risk area produced degenerative changes in basal cell nuclei of the rat esophagus.[67] These epidemiologic observations suggest the predominant role of environmental factors in the etiology of esophageal cancers.

B. ASSOCIATION WITH LIVER CANCERS

Worldwide, liver cancer is one of the most common forms of cancers. Although, in the U.S. and most Western countries, liver cancer is relatively uncommon and has an incidence rate of about 4 per 100,000[68] (accounting for about 1% of total cancer deaths), in sub-Saharan Africa and Southeast Asia, the incidence of liver cancer is high. The incidence of primary liver cancer is about 50 or more per 100,000 in Africa and the Far East; in Hong Kong and Taiwan, it is the second most common malignant tumor.[69-71] Despite low incidence, about 36% of liver cancers in the U.S. are attributable to alcohol consumption.[31]

Several case control studies in the U.S.[72,73] and Japan[74,75] have suggested a positive association of drinking with liver cancer, especially hepatocellular carcinoma (HCC). This observation is supported by cohort studies that have mostly shown a weak or moderately positive correlation with drinking.[76-80] A study in Japan has shown a considerably high risk with Shochu or strong Japanese spirits.[81] Yu and Henderson[72,82] and Austin et al.,[73] in case-control studies in Los Angeles and Hong Kong, found that drinkers of more than 65 cumulative drinks per year exhibited twofold increased risk of primary HCC, compared to nondrinkers. Drinkers of 80 + g ethanol per day had a relative risk of 3.3 after adjusting for cigarette smoking. Kono and his colleagues,[80] in a study that started in 1965 and was followed for 19 years, observed mortalities among 5130 male Japanese physicians, and found that liver cancer was significantly related to alcohol consumption. Yu et al.[83] have reviewed case control and prospective studies on the relationship of chronic alcohol abuse and alcoholic cirrhosis as factors in pathogenesis of primary liver cancer, and observed that the relative risk estimates varied from 2.0 to 8.0 for various studies in the U.S. and Japan. In one study, Tanaka et al.[84] found a relatively low risk of two with heavy drinking, but argued that, although the relative risk does not appear to be great, it may present a substantial proportion of HCC, because drinking is very common among Japanese males. The positive correlation between alcohol consumption and HCC is particularly significant among hepatitis B surface antigen (HBsAg)-negative subjects with no history of blood transfusion, but who had been drinking heavily in their younger years. The current upward trend of HCC among Japanese males, despite a reduction in hepatitis B virus (HBV) infection, could be explained as due to increasing alcohol consumption. Additional support for association with alcohol is provided in studies by Ohnishi and co-workers,[85,86] indicating that the average age of HCC patients who drank moderately or heavily was significantly younger than those who did not drink, regardless of the state of HBV seromarkers. The observation is justified, since most of the patients died within two years, with only a small fraction surviving more than five years.

Similar observations have been reported in other parts of the world. For example, in Scandinavian countries, including Finland and Sweden, the incidence of HBV infection is low,[87] and alcohol consumption is considered the most important predisposing factor for HCC.[88] Similarly, in Italy, the incidence of HBV infection varies, but there is in general high daily alcohol intake.[89] Karhunen and Penttila[90] studied consecutive autopsy series of 95 males, age 35 to 69 years, in Helsinki, Finland and found that parenchymal hyperplastic nodules of clear cells were significantly associated with liver cirrhosis, liver enlargement, and heavy alcohol consumption.

As discussed above, incidence of primary HCC varies a great deal in different areas of the world. This suggests that environmental factors are involved in the etiology of this disease. Much research has gone into identifying these factors, just as for esophageal cancer discussed in Section II.A. Among many chemicals studied as possible etiologic agents, aflatoxins are of special interest because of their widespread occurrence (for a discussion see Section III.A.2). Increasingly, also the importance of viral infection, particularly by hepatitis viruses B and C, has been realized (also discussed in Section III.B). Prospective epidemiological studies have shown a high incidence of primary liver cancer among HBV carriers in HBV-endemic areas. These epidemiologic studies are supported by clinical examinations, showing that most primary liver cancer patients are carriers of the hepatitis B surface antigen, and suffer from chronic active hepatitis. The existing evidence implicates HBV as a major etiologic factor for primary liver cancer in populations of such areas as Taiwan and the People's Republic of China. On the other hand, epidemiologic studies from Africa indicate that liver cancer is associated more strongly with aflatoxin than with viral infection (see, for example, References 91 to 94).

III. UNDERLYING ETIOLOGICAL FACTORS

A. CHEMICAL CARCINOGENS
1. Nitrosamines

A variety of carcinogenic congeners, such as nitrosamines,[95] polycyclic hydrocarbons,[96] and asbestos fibers,[97] have been shown to be present in various alcoholic beverages. Among these, nitrosamines are the prime suspect carcinogens. They are particularly interesting because they exhibit site specificity, and could induce tumors in the upper GI (gastrointestinal) tract, liver, and other sites in experimental animals.[98,99] In the Western countries, low levels of nitrosamines are present in nitrite-cured and preserved meats, and in fish in the West.[100-104] Similarly, small amounts have been identified in various alcoholic beverages.[105] In general, the levels of food or beverage contamination with nitrosamines in the Western World are low and sporadic, and, therefore, they are not considered imminent hazards. However, tobacco-specific nitrosamines are important contributors, and their contribution to alcohol-tobacco related synergism discussed above need be clearly understood. In other parts of the world, nitrosamines may contribute a great deal, even as contaminants. For example, in areas of Africa, the high rate of esophageal and liver tumors may be attributable to drinking of locally brewed maize beer that is highly contaminated with nitrosamines.[106,107] Studies indicate that in China and the Far East, nitrosamines may be important contributors to cancer incidence. For example, in Hong Kong, a high incidence of nasopharyngeal and esophageal cancer might be related to the diet that frequently includes salted fish and dried shrimp that contain dimethylnitrosamine and nitrosopyrrolidine.[108,109] High incidence of liver cancer in Taiwan and The Peoples Republic of China may be similarly explained. Fong et al.[110,111] observed that the urine of rats fed salted fish showed increased mutagenic activity, while the activity returned to normal when the rats were returned to regular chow diet. In a study of foods from the high-incidence area of Linxian (China), nitrosamines were present in 23% of the samples, compared to 1.2% from the low incidence Fanxian area.[112]

Nitrosamines could be readily formed from precursor nitrites and secondary or tertiary amines under the acidic conditions of the mammalian stomach, and, to some extent, on interaction with saliva.[113-115] Residues of nitrates, common plant fertilizers, are carried in food materials, and can be reduced to nitrites by endogenous bacterial flora, and by reaction with saliva, while amines are breakdown products of various proteins. The average concentration of nitrates and nitrites in drinking water showed a positive correlation with the rates of incidence of esophageal carcinoma in high-incidence areas in China. A marked epithelial hyperplasia was also correlated with nitrite content of saliva in these areas.[116,117] Fong et al.[118] showed that treating experimental rats with methylbenzylamine and sodium nitrite, the precursors of methylbenzylnitrosamine, produced esophageal tumors. In China, contaminations with nitrososarcosine are common, and its precursors fed to the fowls of Linxian County induced pathological changes in the pharynx, esophagus, and glandular stomach.[61,62] Li et al.[119,120] and Lu et al.,[121] found that some common fungus species (mostly belonging to the genera, *Fusarium, Geotrichum, Aspergillus*), not only reduce nitrates to nitrites, but also decompose proteins into nitrites and amines.

The carcinogenicity of nitrosamines has been attributed to their capability to alkylate DNA and produce O-alkylated purines.[122,123] Such O-alkylated bases mispair and cause transition mutations. In fact, the mutagenic/carcinogenic potential of compounds has been related to their capacity to produce O-alkylated bases, and the susceptibility of tissues to the extent and persistence of these bases.[124-133] That metabolic activation of nitrosamines may involve mutations in oncogenes has recently been shown by Hirani-Hojatti et al.[134] *In vitro* reaction of an N-nitroso compound, N-nitrosomethyl(acetoxymethyl)-amine with a plasmid containing the human C-Ha-ras-1 gene, generated a transforming oncogene, when the methylated DNA was transfected into NIH3T3 cells.

2. Aflatoxins

A number of studies indicate that aflatoxin intake is an important contributor to the incidence of liver cancer. Extensive studies have been made of the carcinogenic properties of aflatoxins, various aspects of the mechanisms of their action, and evidence for their occurrence as common food contaminants (for a review, see Reference 91). Following is the summary of more salient features of aflatoxins. Aflatoxins, and especially aflatoxin B (AFB_1), are encountered so frequently in human food, as to constitute a virtually unavoidable contaminant. This is particularly so in parts of Africa. An extensive amount of data has accumulated associating elevated exposures to aflatoxins with elevated incidence of liver cancer. For example, Van Rensburg et al.[92] have provided listings of liver cancer incidence from a low of 1.2 in a locality situated at a high altitude of Kenya, to 17.7 in parts of Mozambique per 100,000 cases per year. The data, in general, show a strong parallel incidence of liver cancer with increasing aflatoxin intake values. Intakes of aflatoxins in these studies were measured by analyzing food samples collected from homes in relation to the quantities of food eaten by family members. Recently, methods that monitor individual exposure to aflatoxin and the genetic damage caused by these agents, have been applied in the design of epidemiological studies.[93,135] These analyses also quantitate levels of carcinogen adducts formed with DNA and blood proteins, and, therefore, would provide more precise estimates of the exposure.

Much research has gone into elucidating the mechanisms of action of aflatoxins in inducing carcinogenesis. Studies of the metabolism of aflatoxin AFB_1 have shown that the compound is converted into its active electrophilic DNA-binding form through an epoxidation pathway.[135] The pathway of aflatoxin metabolism is similar in human cells and in animal experimental systems. There is evidence that the reactive intermediates can covalently modify human DNA under conditions of natural exposure. Furthermore, both in experimental animals and in humans, the DNA adducts show identical profiles with the N^7-position of guanine representing the only site of adduct formation. AFB_1 is a potent mutagen in human cell cultures and a potent hepatic carcinogen for several diverse animal species, ranging from trout fish to subhuman primates. Recent studies have implicated oncogene activation in the mechanisms underlying aflatoxin-induced hepatocarcinogenesis.[94,136,137] Taken together, the evidence strongly suggests that humans consuming diets contaminated with aflatoxins are at elevated risk of developing liver cancer.

B. VIRAL INFECTIONS

Available evidence incriminates a number of viruses in the etiology of cancer. It is felt that the viral genome abnormally activates host protooncogenes, and the products of these genes have a role in cellular transformation.[138] The relationship of syphilis to oral cancer, particularly to cancer of the tongue, has long been established.[139-141] Both herpes simplex viruses (HSV) type 1 and type 2 can cause malignant cell transformation *in vitro,* and the transformed cells continue to express HSV antigens.[142] It has been suggested that there is an interaction between HSV type 1 and tobacco smoke in the development of oral tumors.[143] Human papilloma virus (HPV) is involved in a number of infections, and is implicated in the etiology of oral squamous cell carcinoma,[144] and carcinomas of the genital tract, bronchi, larynx, and esophagus.[145-148] Biopsies of some oral squamous cell carcinomas show histological features of HPV,[149,150] and a case of nodular leukoplakia exhibiting HPV viral antigens has been reported to progress to squamous cell carcinoma.[151]

The role of infections by hepatitis B virus in the development of HCC is well recognized. For example, Geer et al.[152] found that 90% of their primary liver cancer (PLC) patients in a referral hospital in Hawaii tested positive for hepatitis antigen reaction. Gibson et al.,[153] in a post-mortem study in Hong Kong, found that 55% of 196 hepatitis B surface antigen-positive (HBsAg⁺) cirrhotics had HCC, but only 27% of 121 HBsAg had a liver tumor. Furthermore, it appears that there are racial and genetic differences in incidence of HBV infections, which could explain the differences in incidence of HCC. For example, Peters et al.,[154] in an autopsy study in Los Angeles, found that 46% of the Oriental patients with HBsAg⁺ cirrhosis had liver cancers, while only 10 to 25% of patients from other races that were exposed to HBsAg had such cancers. In areas of South Africa, non-Caucasians developing some form of cirrhosis have a 40 to 50% risk of developing liver cancer,[155] while for comparable incidence of cirrhosis in Chicago, the risk of liver cancer is only 5%.[156] Lam et al.,[157] in Hong Kong, observed that 18% of Chinese patients without liver cancer and 82% of patients with liver cancer had HBsAg⁺ reactions. Additional support for association of HBV and HCC is provided by the observation that liver cancer patients with hepatitis-positive reactions in these studies, were younger than those without positive reactions for hepatitis.

There is a large amount of evidence indicating involvement of HBV in worldwide occurrence of HCC. The areas in Asia and Africa with a high incidence of primary liver cancer also have a high incidence of HBV infection.

Several case-control and cohort studies from various geographic areas of the world have indicated an association between HCC and chronic HBV infection[158-176] as shown by the presence of HBsAg. The most notable of these studies is a prospective study of 22,707 Chinese men in Taiwan, showing that the relative risk of HCC in carriers of HBsAg was 223.[177] However, the best estimates of relative risks in most other studies are in the range of 20 or so. In general, it has been estimated that as much as 80% of HCC patients have HBsAg in their serum, while others have antibodies to HBV antigens.[177] There is evidence that HCC could occur in the absence of HBV or hepatitis A virus (HAV) infections. For example, in Japan, Tanaka et al.[84] noted that, whereas about 40% of HCC patients in 1968 to 1977 were HBsAg$^+$, only 21% were so in their current study, suggesting that factors other than chronic HBV infection are playing an increasingly important role in causation. Patients with a history of blood transfusion showed a significantly elevated relative risk of 3 to 4.9, and most of these were noncarriers of HBV, as determined by HBsAg and antibody to hepatitis B core antigen (anti-HBc) titers. These studies have shown that infections by nonA, nonB hepatitis (NANBH), or hepatitis C virus (HCV), the major agent associated with NANBH, contribute to the prevalence of HCC. In Japan, an upward trend in HCC, despite a reduction in prevalence of HBV, could be explained as due to NANBH, particularly in individuals with a history of blood transfusions.[178-180] Recently, the cloned genome of HCV has been used to assay for the prevalence of antibodies to HCV (anti-HCV), and the assay has shown positivity at a number of geographic localities.[181-191] Studies indicate that, in the U.S., NANBH and HCV account for a substantial proportion of liver malignancy.[187,192] More recently, tests for anti-HCV have been found positive in 30 to 60% of patients with alcoholic cirrhosis, and even higher frequencies have been observed in alcoholics with HCC suggesting a causal relationship.[193-196] However, the relative contribution of these and other unknown viruses, and the exact mechanism of viral pathogenesis of HCC still remains to be clarified.

HBV genome has been detected, both in the hepatic DNA of carriers, and of patients with HCC,[197,198] further supporting the role of virus in the etiology of neoplasm. The child of a mother who is a chronic carrier carries an especially high risk of developing HCC, and the risk is even higher if the father is negative for surface antibodies to the virus, indicating that he is immunologically defective.[109]

C. NUTRITIONAL FACTORS

Malnutrition is commonly associated with alcohol abuse. An excess or deficiency of several dietary factors can modify the process of carcinogenesis. Generally, cancers are more prevalent in individuals of low socioeconomic status who have a diet that is frequently nutritionally deficient. High cancer frequency is associated with low intake of fresh vegetables, fruits, animal proteins, and deficiencies of vitamins A, B, C, pyridoxine, folic acid, riboflavin, and of trace elements, such as iron, zinc, molybdenum, and co-balt.[200-208] For a review of nutrient deficiencies in relation to cancer, see References 208 and 209. Among the mechanisms suggested are that these deficiencies can alter the susceptibility of the target tissue to carcinogens, or can affect the endogenous production, activation, or inactivation of carcinogens, either directly or indirectly, for example, by their effect on intestinal flora.[205,209-211] Nutrients and trace elements also act as co-factors in essential body reactions, and a deficiency would produce adverse effects. They are needed for healthy tissues and maintenance of immune surveillance. A few of the important dietary nutrients with special reference to esophageal cancer are discussed below; for a more detailed discussion, see a recent review by Leonard et al.[208]

Vitamin A is important for maintaining the normal integrity of epithelia.[212] In malignancy occurring with vitamin A deficiency, normal differentiation of epithelia is altered, and abnormal epithelium is formed instead.[213] Vitamin A and its analogs have a protective effect against the action of various carcinogens.[214,215] The inverse relationship observed between intake of green and yellow vegetables and cancer incidence may be due to the presence of carotene or provitamin A. In addition, other micro- or macronutrients may also be involved. Studies have indicated a significant association between high intake of vegetables containing carotenoids and low cancer mortality.[216] There is a correlation between incidence of upper aerodigestive tract cancer and deficiency of vitamin A, beta-carotene, and retinol. Such a correlation has been observed in the high-incidence areas for esophageal carcinoma in Iran and China.[204,207] In high oral cancer incidence areas of India and Pakistan, lower levels of vitamin A and beta-carotene were observed in patients with oral and oropharyngeal carcinoma than in controls.[217,218] A decrease in plasma levels of vitamin A has been noted in human squamous cancers of the oral cavity, pharynx, and esophagus.[219,220] Esophageal mucosa become dysplastic and keratinized in the absence of vitamin A; the keratinization can be prevented by supplementation with retinoids.[221,222] In animal models, vitamin A and other retinoids have been shown to inhibit carcinogenesis at various sites.[219,222-224]

Another micronutrient studied a good deal in relation to cancer, particularly gastrointestinal tumors, is zinc. Zinc is intimately involved in the metabolism of vitamin A.[225] It appears that body distribution of zinc is regulated, and that its redistribution is affected by malignancy.[226] In experimental animals, a deficiency of zinc reduced the induction period and increased the incidence of chemically-induced esophageal tumors.[227,228] In humans, a decrease in plasma zinc has been associated with squamous cancers of the head and neck, and with lung cancers.[229,230] In China, a decrease of plasma zinc has been found to occur with esophageal squamous cancer.[231] In the U.S., Mellow et al.[220] found, that in patients with esophageal carcinoma, plasma zinc and vitamin A were both significantly less than in age-matched healthy controls.

Plummer-Vinson (Paterson-Kelly) syndrome, a complex symptom of chronic dysphagia and atrophy of the upper GI mucosa, has been described in middle-aged women as an important syndrome in the development of carcinoma of the meso- and hypopharynx, buccal mucosa, tongue, and esophagus.[233-236] A report of the committee on Diet, Nutrition, and Cancer[237] and Shamberger[238] notes that improved nutrition, particularly that of iron and vitamins, has almost eliminated Plummer-Vinson in formerly endemic areas of Sweden. Siassi[239] observed that, in high incidence areas of Northern Iran, children from families of esophageal cancer patients had significantly lower serum iron and transferrin saturation levels, compared to the children from control households in these areas. The differences among children from low-risk areas were not significant. Siassi[239] suggests that iron deficiency may be an important etiological factor for esophageal cancers, in early growth and development. Iron supplementation starting in early childhood may alleviate cancer incidence in high-risk areas but this has not been tried as yet.

Areas of low selenium have increased mortality from cancers of the esophagus, stomach, urinary bladder, and rectum, and small increases in cancers of the pharynx, large intestine, liver, and kidney.[240] Mortality from cancers is low in high- and intermediate selenium areas.[241] A study in 27 countries indicated that selenium in diet correlated inversely with cancer mortality.[242] Many studies have attempted to correlate blood selenium levels with the incidence of cancer.[241,243,244] However, blood selenium levels may not indicate cancer risk, since they may change with dietary changes, or may alter with the onset of disease and subsequent treatment.[238,245]

Other potential vitamin deficiencies in the upper GI tract and liver that are also associated with alcohol abuse are those of pyridoxine,[246] folic acid,[247,248] and vitamin B_{12}.[249] Alcoholic and cirrhotic patients with chronic folate deficiency have increased incidence of esophageal cancers.[250] Ascorbic acid (vitamin C) inhibits formation of nitrosamines from precursor amines and nitrites; it has no protective effect against preformed nitrosamines, the effect being exerted largely on reaction with nitrite and nitrous acid.[251] A 100% protection by vitamin C supplementation on esophageal carcinoma induced by nitrite and methylbenzylamine was observed in experimental rats.[252] Riboflavin (vitamin B_2) functions in biological oxidations, where it is provided as an active site of the prosthetic group of flavoproteins. Deficiency of riboflavin is associated with angular stomatitis (a preneoplastic lesion). Riboflavin deficiency produced hyperkeratosis and hyperplasia in the skin and esophagus in mice.[200,253] Thurnham et al.[254] observed that dietary riboflavin supplementation in the esophageal cancer high-risk area in Henan Province (China), resulted in significantly fewer lesions, compared to control placebos. Molybdenum is a constituent of several oxidation-reduction enzymes, and a deficiency results in accumulation of harmful nitrates in plants. A deficiency of molybdenum was found to occur in samples of serum, hair, and urine from Linxian County, compared to low-risk areas.[117]

IV. MECHANISMS OF ALCOHOL-RELATED CARCINOGENESIS

Since ethanol by itself is generally not considered carcinogenic, ethanol may affect in association with other carcinogens/oncogens.

Experimental evidence indicates that ethanol interferes with first-pass clearance, and influences the pharmacokinetics of carcinogens by affecting their distribution in extrahepatic tissues.[255-257] Thus, carcinogens may appear in other organs which are more susceptible to carcinogens and get exposed to their damaging effects. In general, the results obtained depend on the carcinogen used, its dose and time of exposure, and on the amount of ethanol fed and its schedule of administration.

A. EFFECTS OF ETHANOL ON INITIATION OF CARCINOGENESIS

Most studies of the concurrent feeding of ethanol with carcinogen administration did not indicate an increase that could be attributed to ethanol. But the results are by no means in agreement. For example, Schmahl and his colleagues[258,259] did not observe an increase in hepatic tumors when rats were fed commercial brandy with administration of nitrosodiethylamine (NDEA) or with methylphenylintrosamine. Further, Habs and Schmahl[260] found that simultaneous administration of ethanol with a low dose of NDEA significantly reduced the incidence of liver tumors, but not of esophageal tumors. Teschke et al.[261] did not observe an increase in the number of tumors, or a change in target organ, when rats were fed an ethanol diet in four cycles of three weeks, followed by two weeks of regular chow diet, with doses of dimethylnitrosamine given in the latter period. In contrast to the above, Schwarz et al.[262] found an increase in preneoplastic lesions indicated by gamma glutamyltransferase-altered foci when NDEA was administered at the same time as 10% ethanol in drinking water.

Similarly, the carcinogenicity of substances other than nitrosamines may be affected variously by ethanol. For example, Radlike et al.[263] found that hepatocarcinogenicity of vinyl chloride is increased by concurrent ethanol administration. Yamamoto et al.[264] did not find any increase in tumors induced by 2-fluorenyl-acetamide. Similarly, Yanagi et al.[265] did not find any significant difference in rat hepatic lesions initiated with 3-methyl-4-dimethylaminoazobenzene that could be ascribed to 5, 10, or 15% of ethanol in drinking water. In our recent studies, we found that ethanol fed before and during treatment with methylbenzylnitrosamine (NMB_zA) inhibited incidence of esophageal tumors.[266] It appears that ethanol competes with nitrosamines for the active site on the dimethylase enzyme,[267,268] and the extent of inhibition depends on the relative lipophilicity of the specific nitrosamine. On the other hand, under conditions when ethanol enhances the effect of carcinogen, it may lead to increased tumor incidence.

B. EFFECT OF ETHANOL ON PROMOTION OF CARCINOGENESIS

Similar are the results on effect of ethanol on tumor promotion when ethanol is fed following treatment by a carcinogen. Takada et al.[269] observed that 20% ethanol in drinking water used as a promoter increased the number of gamma-glutamyl transpeptidase (GGT)-altered foci induced by NDEA. However, Schwarz et al.[262] found no effect of 10% ethanol in drinking water on the promotion of GGT-altered foci. On the other hand, in studies by Driver and McLean,[270] even 5% ethanol in drinking water starting a week after a single dose of 30 mg/kg NDEA, significantly increased hepatocellular carcinoma, equal in effect to 1000 μg/ml sodium phenobarbitone given for 15 months.

In recently completed studies where ethanol constituting 36% of total caloric intake was administered for 12 months after treatment with a NDEA regimen, we observed an increase neither in liver tumors nor in GGT-altered foci that could be attributed to tumor-promoting effects of ethanol.[271] These studies were prompted by our earlier studies[266] that indicated an increase in esophageal tumors occurring only when ethanol was administered post-initiation by NMB_zA. Following these studies,[271-274] we observed that, whereas an increase in generation of lipid peroxidation products as measured by ethane exhalation, hepatic diene conjugates, and fluorescent lipid products, which was observed with administration of ethanol, was unaffected by NMB_zA treatment, such an increase was obliterated with a NDEA treatment regimen. Also with the NDEA treatment, there was a corresponding increase in hepatic glutathione, the peroxidation scavenger. Similarly, there was a drastic reduction in cytochrome P-450 levels, and a significant decrease in concentration of cytochrome c reductase in the NDEA-treated ethanol-fed rats, indicating an absence of reactive oxygen intermediates that are normally generated by ethanol in microsomal ethanol-oxidizing system. Our other studies[275,276] showed that intraperitoneal (i.p.) injections or concurrent feeding of vitamin E decreased lipid peroxidation due to ethanol. These studies implicate free radicals generated by ethanol in its tumor promoting effects, a finding that is in line with tumor-promoting effects of a variety of tumor promoters.[277]

From the above discussion it appears that ethanol acts as a tumor promoter to enhance carcinogenesis. Further, it appears that this tumor promotion effect is exerted through the effect of ethanol on generation of free radicals and their products. Ethanol would thus promote carcinogenesis under conditions where free radicals are generated unobtrusively during its metabolism, and it would not have an effect on carcinogenesis where such free radical generation is inhibited. If this hypothesis is correct, then it could hold promise for controlling ethanol-related carcinogenesis, in that we could resort to supplemental feeding of antioxidants, such as vitamin E, to inhibit generation of free radicals.

V. CONCLUSIONS

It is now generally recognized that alcohol is a major contributor to human cancers. The risk is particularly great when combined with tobacco. Less clear, however, is how alcohol may contribute to development of cancers, since ethanol by itself in generally not considered a carcinogen. Among etiological factors that may underlie alcohol-related carcinogenesis in the esophagus and liver are chemical carcinogens such as nitrosamines and aflatoxins, infections by viruses such as HBV and HCV, and a deficiency of a variety of nutritional elements. Chemical carcinogens are defined by their initiating activity; oncogenic viruses also possess some tumorigenic potential. Nutritional deficiencies affect the target tissue or metabolism of endogenous and exogenous carcinogens. Moreover, it is increasingly evident that most human cancers are the result of synergistic interactions between these various factors. The carcinogenic process by its very nature is a long-term process, often encompassing several decades in humans, and involves distinct multiple stages of initiation, promotion, and progression, and that makes it likely that a variety of factors interact to produce cancer.[278] Other host factors such as genetic background, hormonal, and immunological systems are also involved. Alcohol may play an indirect role through these factors in enhancing cancer incidence. That free radicals and their products are generated during ethanol metabolism offers one possibility through which ethanol may directly exert its deleterious effects.

ACKNOWLEDGMENT

The research described in this paper that was carried out in the laboratory of the author was supported by a Grant No. CA51088 from the National Institutes of Health.

REFERENCES

1. **Schwartz, D., Lellouch, J., Flamant, R., and Denoix, P. F.,** Alcohol et cancer-resultats d'une enquete retrospective. Revue Fr. Etud., *Clin. Biol.,* 7, 590, 1962.
2. Finnish Foundation for Alcohol Studies and World Health Organization (Europe), *International Statistics on Alcoholic Beverages, Production, Trade, and Consumption,* Vol. 27, Finnish Foundation for Alcohol Studies, Helsinki, 1977.
3. **Tuyns, A. J.,** Incidence trends of laryngeal cancer in relation to national alcohol and tobacco consumption, in *Trends in Cancer Incidence, Causes and Practical Implications,* Magnus, K. Ed., Hemisphere, Washington, D.C., 1982, 199.
4. **Breslow, N. E. and Enstrom, J. E.,** Geographic correlations between cancer mortality rates and alcohol-tobacco consumption in the United States, *J. Natl. Cancer Inst.,* 53, 631, 1974.

5. **Tuyns, A. J.,** Cancer of the oesophagus, further evidence of the relation to drinking habits in France, *Int. J. Cancer,* 5, 152, 1970.

6. **Hakulinen, T., Lehtimaki, L., Lehtonen, M., and Teppo, L.,** Cancer morbidity among two male cohorts with increased alcohol consumption in Finland, *J. Natl. Cancer Inst.,* 52, 1711, 1974.

7. **Monson, R. R. and Lyons, J. L.,** Proportional mortality among alcoholics, *Cancer,* 36, 1077, 1975.

8. **Jensen, O. M.,** Cancer morbidity and causes of death among Danish brewery workers, *Int. J. Cancer,* 23, 454, 1979.

9. **Prior, P.,** Long term cancer risk in alcoholics, *Alcohol Alcohol,* 23, 163, 1988.

10. **Vincent, R. G. and Marchetta, F.,** The relationship of the use of tobacco and alcohol to cancer of the oral cavity, pharynx, and larynx, *Am. J. Surg.,* 106, 501, 1963.

11. **Martinez, I.,** Factors associated with cancer of the esophagus, mouth, and pharynx in Puerto Rico, *J. Natl. Cancer Inst.,* 42, 1069, 1969.

12. **Rothman, K. J. and Keller, A. Z.,** The effect of joint exposure to alcohol and tobacco on risk of cancer of the mouth and pharynx, *J. Chronic Dis.,* 25, 711, 1972.

13. **Tuyns, A. J., Pequignot, G., Jensen, O. M., and Pomeau, Y.,** La consommation individuelle de bossons alcoolisees et de tabac dans un echantilon de la population en We-et-Vitaine, *Rev. Alcohol.,* 21, 105, 1975.

14. **Feldman, J. G., Hazan, M., Nagarajen, M., and Kissin, B.,** A case-control investigation of alcohol, tobacco and diet in head and neck cancer, *Prev. Med.,* 4, 444, 1975.

15. **Williams, R. R. and Horm, J. W.,** Association of cancer sites with tobacco and alcohol consumption and socio-economic status of patients: interview study for the Third National Cancer Survey, *J. Natl. Cancer Inst.,* 58, 525, 1977.

16. **Wynder, E. L.,** The dietary environment and cancer, *J. Am. Diet. Assoc.,* 71, 385, 1977.

17. **Lemon, F. R., Walden, R. T., and Woods, R. W.,** Cancer of the lung and mouth in Seventh-Day Adventists. Preliminary report on a population study, *Cancer,* 17, 486, 1964.

18. **Lyon, J. L., Gardner, J. W., Klauber, M. R., and Smart, C. R.,** Low cancer incidence and mortality in Utah, *Cancer,* 39, 2608, 1977.

19. **Burch, C. E. and Ansari, A.,** Chronic alcoholism and carcinoma of the pancreas: a correlative hypothesis, *Arch. Intern. Med.,* 122, 273, 1968.

20. **Rosenberg, L., Shapiro, S., Slone, D., Kaufman, D. W., Helmrich, S. P., Miettinen, D. S., Stolley, P. D., Levy, M., Rosenshein, N. B., Schottenfeld, D., and Engle, R. L.,** Breast cancer and alcoholic beverage consumption, *Lancet,* 1, 267, 1982.

21. **MacDonald, W. C.,** Clinical and pathological features of adenocarcinoma of the gastric cardia, *Cancer,* 29, 724, 1972.

22. **Haenszel, W., Kurihara, M., Segi, M., and Lee, R. K. C.,** Stomach cancer among Japanese in Hawaii, *J. Natl. Cancer Inst.,* 49, 969, 1972.

23. **Hoey, J., Montvernay, C., and Lambert, R.,** Wine and tobacco: risk factors for gastric cancer in France, *Am. J. Epidemiol.,* 113, 668, 1981.

24. **Trichopoulos, D., Ouranos, G., Day, N. E., Tzonou, A., Manousos, O., Papadimitriou, C., and Trichopoulos, A.,** Diet and cancer of the stomach: a case-control study in Greece, *Int. J. Cancer,* 36, 291, 1985.

25. **Potter, J. D., McMichael, A. J., and Hartshorne, J. M.,** Alcohol and beer consumption in relation to cancers of bowel and lung: an extended correlation analysis, *J. Chronic Dis.,* 35, 833, 1982.

26. **Bgelke, E.,** Frequency of use of alcoholic beverages and incidence of cancer of the large bowel and other sites. Prospective study of 12,000 Norwegian men, paper presented at the Meeting on Alcohol and Cancer, IARC, Lyon, France, 1974.

27. **Hinds, M. W., Kolonel, L. N., Lee, J., and Hirohata, T.,** Associations between cancer incidence and alcohol/cigarette consumption among five ethnic groups in Hawaii, *Br. J. Cancer,* 41, 929, 1980.

28. **Kozarevic, D., Vojvodic, N., Gordon, T., Kaelber, C. T., McGee, D., and Zukel, W.,** Drinking habits and death: the Yugoslavia cardiovascular disease study, *Int. J. Epidemiol.,* 12, 145, 1983.

29. **Potter, J. D. and McMichael, A. J.,** Diet and cancer of the colon and rectum: a case control study, *J. Natl. Cancer Inst.,* 76, 557, 1986.

30. **Tuyns, A. J.,** Epidemiology of alcohol and cancer, *Cancer Res.,* 39, 2840, 1979.

31. **Rothman, K., Garfinkel, L., Keller, A. Z., Muir, C. S., and Schottenfeld, D.,** The proportion of cancer attributable to alcohol consumption, *Prev. Med.,* 9, 174, 1980.

32. National Research Council, *Diet, Nutrition and Cancer,* The Committee on Diet, Nutrition and Cancer, Assembly of Life Sciences. National Academy Press, Washington, D.C., 1982.

33. **Doll, R. and Peto, R.,** The causes of cancer: quantitative estimates of avoidable risks of cancer in the United States today, *J. Natl. Cancer Inst.,* 66, 1191, 1981.

34. **Lieber, C. S., Garro, A. J., Leo, M. A., Mak, K. M., and Worner, T.,** Alcohol and cancer, *Hepatology,* 6, 1005, 1986.

35. **Mufti, S. I., Darban, H. R., and Watson, R. R.,** Alcohol, cancer, and immunomodulation, *CRC Crit. Rev. Oncol. Hematol.,* 9, 243, 1989.

36. **Mufti, S. I., Garewal, H. S., and Watson, R. R.,** Role of environment, drugs of abuse, and nutritional factors in the etiology and prevention of the cancers of oral cavity and esophagus, in *Biochemistry and Physiology of Substance Abuse,* Vol. II, Watson, R. R., Ed., CRC Press, Boca Raton, FL, 1990, 1.

37. **Mufti, S. I.,** Liver cancer: role of alcohol and other factors, in *Liver Pathology and Alcohol,* Watson, R. R., Ed., Humana Press, Totowa, NJ, 1991, 195.

38. **Schwartz, D., Lellouch, J., Flamant, R., and Denoix, P. F.,** Alcool et cancer — resultats d'une enquete retrospective, *Revue Fr. Etud. Clin. Biol.,* 7, 590, 1962.

39. **Vincent, R. G. and Marchetta, F.,** The relationship of the use of tobacco and alcohol to cancer of the oral cavity, pharynx, and larynx, *Am. J. Surg.,* 106, 501, 1963.

40. **Martinez, I.,** Factors associated with cancer of the esophagus, mouth, and pharynx in Puerto Rico, *J. Natl. Cancer Inst.,* 42, 1069, 1969.

41. **Rothman, K. J. and Keller, A. Z.,** The effect of joint exposure to alcohol and tobacco on risk of cancer of the mouth and pharynx, *J. Chronic Dis.,* 25, 711, 1972.

42. **Tuyns, A. J., Pequignot, G., Jensen, O. M., and Pomeau, Y.,** La Consommation individuelle de boissons alcoolisees et de tabac dans un echantillon de la population en We-et-Vitaine, *Rev. Alcool,* 21, 105, 1975.

43. **Feldman, J. G., Hazan, M., Nagarajen, M., and Kissin, B.,** A case-control investigation of alcohol, tobacco, and diet in head and neck cancer, *Prev. Med.,* 4, 444, 1975.

44. **Williams, R. R. and Horm, J. W.,** Association of cancer sites with tobacco and alcohol consumption and socioeconomic status of patients: interview study from the Third National Cancer Survey, *J. Natl. Cancer Inst.,* 58, 525, 1977.

45. **Wynder, E. L.,** The dietary environment and cancer, *J. Am. Diet. Assoc.,* 71, 385, 1977.

46. **McCoy, G. D. and Wynder, E. L.,** Etiological and preventive implications in alcohol carcinogenesis, *Cancer Res.,* 39, 2844, 1979.

47. **Tuyns, A. J., Pequignot, G., and Abatucci, J. S.,** Oesophageal cancer and alcohol consumption: importance of type of beverage, *Int. J. Cancer,* 23, 443, 1979.

48. **Wu, Y. K. and Loucks, H. H.,** Carcinoma of the esophagus or cardia of the stomach, *Ann. Surg.,* 134, 946, 1951.

49. **Tuyns, A. J., Pequignot, G., Gignoux, M., and Valla, A.,** Cancers of the digestive tract, alcohol and tobacco, *Int. J. Cancer,* 39, 9, 1982.

50. **Schoenberg, B. S., Bailar, J. C., and Fraumeni, J. F.,** Certain mortality patterns of esophageal cancer in the United States, 1930–1967, *J. Natl. Cancer Inst.,* 46, 63, 1971.

51. **McGlashan, N. D., Bradshaw, E., and Harington, J. S.,** Cancer of the oesophagus and the use of tobacco and alcoholic beverages in Transkei, 1975–6, *Int. J. Cancer,* 29, 249, 1982.

52. **Pottern, L. M., Morris, L. E., Blot, W. J., Ziegler, R. G., and Fraumeni, J. F.,** Esophageal cancer among Black men in Washington, D.C. I, Alcohol, tobacco, and other risk factors, *J. Natl. Cancer Inst.,* 67, 777, 1981.

53. **Warwick, G. P. and Harrington, J. S.,** Some aspects of the epidemiology and etiology of esophageal cancer with particular emphasis on the Transkei, South Africa, *Adv. Cancer Res.,* 17, 81, 1973.

54. The Coordinating Group for Research on Etioloty of Esophageal Cancer in North China. The epidemiology and etiology of esophageal cancer in North China, *Chin. Med. J.,* 1, 167, 1975.

55. **Mahboubi, E.,** The epidemiology of oral cavity, pharyngeal, and esophageal cancer outside of North America and Western Europe, *Cancer,* 40, 1879, 1977.

56. **Miller, R. W.,** Cancer epidemics in the People's Republic of China, *J. Natl. Cancer Inst.,* 60, 1195, 1978.

57. **Yang, C. S.,** Research on esophageal cancer in China: a review, *Cancer Res.,* 40, 2633, 1980.

58. **Rose, E. F.,** Esophageal cancer in Transkei — The pattern and associated risk factors, in *Cancer of the Esophagus,* Vol. 1, Pfeiffer, C. J., Ed., CRC Press, Boca Raton, FL, 1982, 19.

59. **Doll, R.,** The geographical distribution of cancer, *Br. J. Cancer,* 23, 1, 1969.

60. **Mahboubi, E., Kmet, J., Cook, P. J., Day, N. E., Ghadirian, P., and Salmasizadeh, S.,** Oesophageal cancer study in the Caspian Littoral of Iran: the Caspian center registry, *Br. J. Cancer,* 28, 197, 1973.

61. Cancer Institute, Chinese Academy of Medical Sciences, Epidemiology and pathological morphology of pharyngeal and esophageal cancers in domestic fowls, *Acta Zool. Sin.,* 19, 309, 1973.

62. Cancer Institute, Chinese Academy of Medical Sciences, Epidemiology and pathology of pharyngoesophageal cancers in domestic fowls from Honan migrant communities and native inhabitants in Zhongxian County, Hubei Province, *Acta Zool. Sin.,* 22, 319, 1976.

63. Cancer Institute, Chinese Academy of Medical Sciences and Cancer Hospital, Hubei Province Report, *Acta Zool. Sin.,* 22, 314, 1976.

64. **Marais, J. A. H. and Drewes, E. F. R.,** The relationship between solid geology and esophageal cancer distribution in Transkei, *Ann. Geol. Surv. S. Afr.,* 1, 105, 1962.

65. **Rose, E. F.,** The role of demographic risk factors in carcinogenesis, in *Prevention and Detection of Cancer,* Part II, Vol. 1, Neiburgs, H. W., Ed., Marcel Dekker, New York, 1978, 25.

66. **Burrell, R. J. W., Roach, W. A., and Shadwell, A.,** Esophageal cancer in Bantu of Transkei associated with mineral deficiency in garden plants, *J. Natl. Cancer Inst.,* 36, 201, 1966.

67. **Van Rensburg, S., Purchase, I., Rose, E., and Roach, W.,** Structural alterations in rat esophagus after ingestion of Transkei diet, *S. Afr. Med. J.,* 48, 2361, 1974.

68. **Sandler, D., Sandler, R., and Horney, L.,** Primary liver cancer mortality in the United States, *J. Chron. Dis.,* 36, 227, 1983.

69. **Kew, M. and Geddes, E.,** Hepatocellular carcinoma in rural Southern Africa Blacks, *Medicine,* 61, 98, 1982.

70. **Lai, C., Lam, K., Wong, K., Wu, P., and Todd, D.,** Clinical features in Hong Kong, *Cancer,* 47, 2746, 1981.

71. Hong Kong Government, Hong Kong Annual Department Report, Hong Kong Government Printer, Hong Kong, 1985.

72. **Yu, C. M., Mack, T., Hanisch, R., Peters, R. L., Henderson, B. E., and Pike, M. C.,** Hepatitis, alcohol consumption, cigarette smoking, and hepatocellular carcinoma in Los Angeles, *Cancer Res.,* 43, 6077, 1983.

73. **Austin, H., Delzell, E., Grufferman, S., Levine, R., Morrison, A. S., Stolley, P. D., and Cole, P. A.,** Case-control study of hepatocellular carcinoma and the hepatitis B virus, cigarette smoking, and alcohol consumption, *Cancer Res.,* 46, 962, 1986.

74. **Oshima, A., Tsukuma, H., Hiyama, T., Fujimoto, I., Yamano, H., and Tanaka, M.,** Follow-up study of HB$_s$Ag-positive blood donors with special reference to effect of drinking and smoking on development of liver cancer, *Int. J. Cancer,* 34, 775, 1984.

75. **Inaba, Y., Maruchi, N., Matsuda, M., Yoshihara, N., and Yamamoto, S.,** A case-control study in liver cancer and liver cirrhosis in Yamanashi perfecture, *Jpn. J. Public Health,* 26, 362, 1981.

76. **Hakulinen, T., Lehtimaki, L., Lehtonen, M., and Teppo, L.,** Cancer morbidity among two male cohorts with increased alcohol consumption in Finland, *J. Natl. Cancer Inst.,* 52, 1711, 1974.

77. **Jensen, O. M.,** Cancer morbidity and causes of death among Danish brewery workers, *Int. J. Cancer,* 23, 454, 1979.

78. **Schmidt, W. and Popham, R. E.,** The role of drinking and smoking in mortality from cancer and other causes in male alcoholics, *Cancer,* 47, 1031, 1981.

79. **Hirayama, T.,** A large-scale cohort study on the relationship between diet and selected cancers of digestive organs, *Banbury Rep.,* 7, 409, 1981.

80. **Kono, S., Ikeda, M., Tokudome, S., Nishizumi, M., and Kurastune, M.,** Cigarette smoking, alcohol, and cancer mortality: a cohort study of male Japanese physicians, *Gann,* 78, 1323, 1987.

81. **Shibata, A., Hirohata, T., Toshima, H., and Tashiro, H.,** The role of drinking and cigarette smoking in the excess deaths from liver cancer, *Gann,* 77, 287, 1986.

82. **Yu, M. C. and Henderson, B. E.,** Correspondence re: Harland Austin et al. A case-control study of hepatocellular carcinoma and the hepatitis B virus, cigarette smoking, and alcohol consumption, *Cancer Res.,* 46, 962, 1986; *Cancer Res.,* 47, 654, 1987.

83. **Yu, H., Harris, R. E., Kabat, G. C., and Wynder, E. L.,** Cigarette smoking, alcohol consumption, and primary liver cancer: a case-control study in the U.S.A., *Int. J. Cancer,* 42, 325, 1988.

84. **Tanaka, K., Hirohata, T., and Takeshita, S.,** Blood transfusion, alcohol consumption, and cigarette smoking in causation of hepatocellular carcinoma: a case-control study in Fukuoka, Japan, *Gann,* 79, 1075, 1988.

85. **Ohnishi, K., Iida, S., Iwama, S., Goto, N., Nomura, F., Takashi, M., Mishima, A., Kono, K., Kimura, K., Musha, H., Kotota, K., and Okuda, K.,** The effect of habitual alcohol intake in the development of liver cirrhosis and hepatocellular carcinoma: relation to hepatitis B surface antigen carriage, *Cancer,* 49, 672, 1982.

86. **Ohnishi, K., Terabayashi, H., Unuma, T., Takahashi, A., and Okuda, K.,** Effects of habitual alcohol intake and cigarette smoking on the development of hepatocellular carcinoma, *Alcohol.: Clin. Exp. Res.,* 11, 45, 1987.

87. **Helske, T.,** Carriers of hepatitis B antigen and transfusion hepatitis in Finland, *Scand. J. Haematol. Suppl.,* 22, 1, 1974.

88. **Hardell, L., Bengtsson, N. O., Jonsson, U., Eriksson, S., and Larsson, L. G.,** Aetiological aspects of primary liver cancer with special regard to alcohol, organic solvents and acute intermittent porphyria — an epidemiologic investigation, *Br. J. Cancer,* 50, 389, 1984.

89. **Villa, E., Baldini, G. M., Pasquinelli, C., Malegari, M., Cariani, E., Chirico, G., and Manenti, F.,** Risk factors for hepatocellular carcinoma in Italy. Male sex, hepatitis B virus, nonA, nonB infection, and alcohol, *Cancer,* 62, 611, 1988.

90. **Karhunen, P. J. and Penttila, A.,** Preneoplastic lesions of human liver, *Hepato-gastroenterol.,* 34, 10, 1987.

91. **Busby, W. F. and Wogan, G. N.,** *Aflatoxins in Chemical Carcinogens,* Searle, C. E., Ed., American Chemical Society, Washington, D.C., 1984, 945.

92. **Van Rensburg, S. J., Cook-Mozaffari, P., Van Schalkwyk, D. J., Van Der Watt, J. J., Vincent, T. J., and Purchase, I. F.,** Hepatocellular carcinoma and dietary aflatoxin in Mozambique and Transkei, *Br. J. Cancer,* 51, 713, 1985.

93. **Groopman, J. D., Cain, L. G., and Kensler, T. W.,** Aflatoxin exposure in human populations: measurements and relationship to cancer, *Crit. Rev. Toxicol.,* 19, 113, 1988.
94. **Wogan, G. N.,** Dietary risk factors for primary hepatocellular carcinoma, *Cancer Detect. Prev.,* 14, 209, 1989.
95. **Walker, E. A., Castegnaro, M., Garren, L., Touissaint, G., and Gowalski, B.,** Intake of volatile nitrosamines from consumption of alcohols, *J. Natl. Cancer Inst.,* 63, 947, 1979.
96. **Masuda, Y., Mori, K., Hirshata, T., and Kuratsune, M.,** Carcinogenesis in the esophagus, III. Polycyclic hydrocarbons and phenois in whisky, *Gann,* 57, 549, 1966.
97. **Wehman, H. J., Plantholt, B. A.,** Asbestos fibrils in beverages. I, *Gin. Bull. Environ. Contam. Toxicol.,* 11, 267, 1974.
98. **Magee, P. N. and Barnes, J. M.,** Carcinogenic nitroso compounds, *Adv. Cancer Res.,* 10, 163, 1967.
99. **Druckrey, H., Preussmann, R., Ivankovic, S., and Schmahl, D.,** Organotrophe carcinogene Wirkungen bei 65 verschiedenen *N*-nitroso-verbindungen an BD-ratten, *Z. Krebsforsch.,* 69, 103, 1967.
100. **Ender, F. and Ceh, L.,** Occurrence of nitrosamines in food stuffs for human and animal consumption, *Food Cosmet. Toxicol.,* 6, 569, 1968.
101. **Fazio, T., Damico, J. N., Howard, J. W., White, R. H., and Watts, J. O.,** Gaschromatographic determination and mass spectrometric confirmation on *N*-nitrosodimethylamine in smoke-processed marine fish, *J. Agric. Food Chem.,* 19, 250, 1971.
102. **Sen, N. P.,** The evidence for the presence of dimethylnitrosamine in meat products, *Food Cosmet. Toxicol.,* 10, 219, 1972.
103. **Wasserman, A. E., Fiddler, W., Doerr, R. C., Osman, S. F., and Dooley, J. D.,** Dimethylnitrosamine in frankfurters, *Food Cosmet. Toxicol.,* 10, 681, 1972.
104. **Panalaks, T., Iyengar, J. R., and Sen, N. P.,** Nitrate, nitrite and dimethylnitrosamine in cured meat products, *J. Assoc. Off. Anal. Chem.,* 56, 621, 1973.
105. **Walker, E. A., Castegnaro, M., Garren, L., Toussaint, G., and Gowelski, B.,** Intake of volatile nitrosamines fron consumption of alcohols, *J. Natl. Cancer Inst.,* 63, 947, 1979.
106. **Cook, P.,** Cancer of the esophagus in Africa, *Br. J. Cancer,* 25, 853, 1971.
107. **Diller, R. B.,** Cancer of the esophagus and alcoholic drinks in East Africa, *Lancet,* 1, 743, 1972.
108. **Fong, Y. Y. and Walsh, E. O. F.,** Carcinogenic nitrosamines in cantonese salt-dried fish, *Lancet,* 2, 1032, 1971.
109. **Fong, Y. Y. and Chan, W. C.,** Nitrate, nitrite, dimethylnitrosamine, and *N*-Nitrosopyrrolidine in some Chinese food products, *Food Cosmet. Toxicol.,* 15, 143, 1977.
110. **Fong, L. Y. Y., Ho, J. H. C., and Huang, D. P.,** Preserved food as possible cancer hazards, W. A. Rats fed salted fish have mutagenic urine, *Int. J. Cancer,* 23, 542, 1975.
111. **Fong, L. Y. Y., Huang, D. P., Lau, S. K. D., and Ho, J. H. C.,** The salmonella/ mammalian mutagenicity test to detect chemical mutagens in Chinese preserved foods, in *Food and Nutritional Biochemistry in Asia and Oceania,* Khor, H. I., Ed., 2nd Federation of Asian and Oceanian Biochemists Symposium, Kuala Lumpur, Malaysia, 1980, 157.
112. **Kaplan, H. S. and Tsuchitani, P. J.,** *Cancer in China,* Alan R. Liss, New York, 1978.
113. International Agency for Research on Cancer, *N-Nitroso Compounds: Occurrence, Biological Effects and Relevance to Human Cancer,* IARC, Lyon, France, 1984.
114. **Sander, J., Schweinsberg, F., and Menz, H. Y.,** Untersuchungen uber die entstehung cancerogener nitrosamine in Magen, *Hoppe-Seyler's Z. Physiol. Chem.,* 349, 1691, 1968.
115. **Sen, N. P., Smith, D. C., and Schwinghamer, L.,** Formation of *N*-nitrosamines from secondary amines and nitrite in human and animal gastric juice, *Food Cosmet. Toxicol.,* 7, 301, 1969.

116. **Wang, J. L., Lu, S. H., and Li, M. M.,** Determination of nitrates and nitrites in well-water from Yaocun Commune, Linxian County, Honan Province, (transl.), *Chin. J. Oncol.,* 1, 201, 1979.

117. **Li, M., Li, P., and Li, B.,** Recent progress in research on esophageal cancer in China, *Adv. Cancer Res.,* 33, 173, 1980.

118. **Fong, L. Y. Y., Lee, J. S. S., Chan, W. C., and Newberne, P. M.,** Zinc deficiency and the induction of oesophageal tumors in rats by benzylmethylamine and sodium nitrite, in *N-Nitroso Compounds: Occurrence and Biological Effects,* Bartsch, H., Castegnaro, M., O'Neill, I. K., Okada, M., and Davis, W., Eds., IARC, Lyon, France, 1982, 679.

119. **Li, M., Lu, S., Ji, C., Wang, M., Cheng, S., and Jin, C.,** Formation of carcinogenic N-nitroso compounds in cornbread inoculated with fungi, *Sci. Sin.,* 22, 471, 1979(a).

120. **Li, M. H., Lu, S. H., Ji, C., Wang, M. Y., Cheng, S. J., and Jin, C. L.,** A new nitrosamine in moldy food: N-1-methylacetonyl-N-3-methylbutylnitrosamine, *Sci. Sin.,* 22, 401, 1979(b).

121. **Lu, S. H., Wang, Y. L., and Lu, M. H.,** Effect of fungi on formation of carcinogenic nitrosamines and their precursors in food, (transl.), *Acta Acad. Med. Sin.,* 2, 24, 1980.

122. **Magee, P. N. and Barnes, J. M.,** Carcinogenic nitroso compounds, *Adv. Cancer Res.,* 10, 163, 1967.

123. **Magee, P. N., Nicoll, J. W., Pegg, A. E., and Swann, P. F.,** Alkylation intermediates in nitrosamine metabolism, *Biochem. Soc. Trans.,* 3, 62, 1975.

124. **Goth, R. and Rajewsky, M. F.,** Persistence of O⁶-ethylguanine in rat brain DNA, *Proc. Natl. Acad. Sci. U.S.A.,* 70, 639, 1974.

125. **Nicoll, J. W., Swann, P. F., and Pegg, A. E.,** Effect of dimethylnitrosamine on persistence of methylated guanines in rat liver and kidney DNA, *Nature (London),* 254, 261, 1975.

126. **Margison, G. P. and Kleihues, P.,** Chemical carcinogenesis in the nervous system. Preferential accumulation of O⁶-methylguanine in the rat brain DNA during repetitive administration of N-methyl-N-nitrosourea, *Biochem. J.,* 148, 521, 1975.

127. **Lawley, P. D.,** Methylation of DNA by carcinogens: some applications of chemical analytical methods, in *Screening Tests in Chemical Carcinogenesis,* Montesano, R., Bartsch, H., and Tomatis, L., Eds., IARC Scientific Publication No. 12, Lyon, France, 1976, 181.

128. **Kleihues, P. and Margison, G. P.,** Exhaustion and recovery of repair excision of O⁶-methylguanine from rat liver DNA, *Nature (London),* 259, 153, 1976.

129. **Pegg, A. E. and Nicoll, J. W.,** Nitrosamine carcinogenesis: the importance of the persistence in DNA of alkylated bases in the organotropism of tumor induction, in *Screening Tests in Chemical Carcinogenesis,* Montesano, R., Bartsch, H., and Tomatis, L., Eds., IARC Scientific Publication No. 12, Lyon, France, 1976, 571.

130. **Pegg, A. E.,** Formation and metabolism of alkylated nucleosides: possible role in carcinogenesis by nitroso compounds and alkylating agents, *Adv. Cancer Res.,* 25, 195, 1977.

131. **Cox, R. and Irving, C. C.,** Selective accumulation of O⁶-methylguanine in DNA of rat bladder epithelium after intravesical administration of N-methyl-N-nitrosourea, *Cancer Lett.,* 3, 265, 1977.

132. **Pegg, A. E. and Hui, G.,** Removal of methylated purines from rat liver DNA after administration of dimethylnitrosamine, *Cancer Res.,* 38, 2011, 1978.

133. **Singer, B.,** N-nitroso alkylating agents: formation and persistence of alkyl derivatives in mammalian nucleic acids as contribution factors in carcinogenesis, *J. Natl. Cancer Inst.,* 62, 1329, 1979.

134. **Hirani-Hojatti, S., Milligan, J. R., and Archer, M. C.,** Activation of the human c-Ha-ras-1 proto-oncogene by *in vitro* reaction with N-nitroso-methyl(acetoxymethyl)amine, in *The Relevance of N-Nitroso Compounds to Human Cancer: Exposures and Mechanisms,* Bartsch, H., O'Neill, I., and Schultz-Hermann, R., Eds., IARC Scientific Publication No. 84, Lyon, France, 1987, 26.

135. **Gan, L. S., Skipper, P. L., and Peng, X.,** Serum albumin adducts in the molecular epidemiology of aflatoxin carcinogenesis: correlation with aflatoxin B, intake and urinary excretion of aflatoxin M_1, *Carcinogenesis,* 9, 1323, 1988.

136. **Gu, J. R., Hu, L. F., Cheng, Y. C., and Wan, D. F.,** Oncogenesis in primary hepatic cancer, *J. Cell Physiol.,* Suppl. 4, 13, 1986.

137. **McMohan, G., Davis, E., and Wogan, G. N.,** Characterization of c-ki-ras oncogene alleles by direct sequencing of enzymatically-amplified DNA from carcinogen-induced tumors, *Proc. Natl. Acad. Sci. U.S.A.,* 84, 4974, 1987.

138. **Liebowitz, M. J., McAllister, W. T., and Strohl, W. A.,** Advances in cancer: viruses as causes of human cancer, *N.J. Med.,* 83, 603, 1986.

139. **Wynder, E. L., Bross, I. J., and Feldman, R. M. A.,** Study of the etiological factors in cancer of the mouth, *Cancer,* 10, 1300, 1957.

140. **Fry, H. J. B.,** Syphilis and malignant disease: a serological study, *Br. J. Hyg.,* 29, 313, 1929.

141. **Levin, M. L., Kress, L. C., and Goldstein, H.,** Syphilis and cancer: reported syphilis prevalence among 7761 cancer patients, *N.Y. State J. Med.,* 42, 1737, 1942.

142. **Rapp, F.,** Transformation by herpes simplex viruses, in *Cold Spring Harbor Conference on Cell Proliferation,* Vol. 7(A), Essex, M., Todaro, G., and Hausen, H. Z., Eds., Cold Spring Harbor, N.Y., 1980, 63.

143. **Shillitoe, E. J., Greenspan, J. S., and Silverman, S.,** Neutralizing antibody to herpes simplex virus type 1 in patients with oral cancer, *Cancer,* 49, 2315, 1982.

144. **Scully, C., Prime, S., and Maitland, N.,** Papiltomaviruses: their possible role in oral disease, *Oral Surg.,* 60, 166, 1985.

145. **Lack, E., Vawter, G. F., Smith, H. G., Healy, G. B., Lancaster, W. D., and Jenson, A. B.,** Immunohistochemical localization of human papilloma virus in squamous pap-illomes of the larynx, *Lancet,* 2, 592, 1980.

146. **Syrjanen, K. J.,** Bronchial squamous cell carcinomas associated with epithelial changes identical to condylmatous lesions of the uterine cervis, *Lung,* 158, 131, 1980.

147. **Syrjanen, K. J.,** Histological changes identical to those of condylmatous lesions found in oesophageal squamous cell carcinomas, *Arch. Geschwulstforsch,* 4, 203, 1982.

148. **Syrjanen, K. J. and Syrjanen, S. M.,** Histological evidence for the presence of con-dylmatous epithelial lesions in association with laryngeal squamous cell carcinoma, *ORL,* 43, 181, 1981.

149. **Syrjanen, K. J., Pyrhonen, S., Syrjanen, S. M., and Lamberg, M. A.,** Immuno-histological demonstration of human papilloma virus (HPV) antigens in oral squamous cell lesions, *Br. J. Oral Surg.,* 21, 147, 1983.

150. **Eisenberg, E., Rosenberg, B., and Krutchkoff, D. J.,** Verrucous carcinoma: a possible viral pathogenesis, *Oral Surg.,* 59, 52, 1985.

151. **Loning, T., Reichart, P., Staquet, M. J., Becker, J., and Thivolet, J.,** Occurrence of papilloma virus structural antigens in oral papillomas and leukoplakias, *J. Oral. Pathol.,* 13, 155, 1984.

152. **Geer, D. A., Lee, Y. M., Brooks, V. P., and Berenberg, J. L.,** Primary liver cancer in a referral hospital in Hawaii, *J. Surg. Oncol.,* 35, 235, 1987.

153. **Gibson, J. P., Wu, P. C., Ho, J. C., and Lauder, I. J.,** HB_sAg, hepatocellular carcinoma and cirrhosis in Hong Kong: a necropsy study 1963–1976, *Br. J. Cancer,* 42, 370, 1980.

154. **Peters, R. L., Afroudakis, A. P., and Tatter, D.,** The changing incidence of association of hepatitis B with hepatocellular carcinoma in California, *Am. J. Clin. Pathol.,* 68, 1, 1977.

155. **Thompson, J. G.,** Primary carcinoma of the liver in the three ethnic groups in Capetown, *Acta U.I.C.C.,* 17, 632, 1961.

156. **Stuart, H. L.,** *Geographic Distribution of Hepatic Cancer in Primary Hepatoma,* Bur-dette, W. J., Ed., University of Utah Press, Salt Lake City, 1965.

157. **Lam, K. C., Yu, M. C., Leung, J. W. C., and Henderson, B. E.,** Hepatitis B virus and cigarette smoking: risk factors for hepatocellular carcinoma in Hong Kong, *Cancer Res.,* 42, 5246, 1982.

158. **Beasley, R. P., Hwang, L. Y., Lin, C. C., and Chien, C. S.,** Hepatocellular carcinoma and hepatitis B virus: a prospective study of 22,707 men in Taiwan, *Lancet,* 2, 1129, 1981.

159. **Lingao, A. L., Domingo, E. O., and Nishioka, K.,** Hepatitis B virus profile of hepatocellular carcinoma in the Phillipines, *Cancer,* 48, 1590, 1981.

160. **MacNab, G. M., Urbanowicz, J. M., Geddes, E. W., and Kew, M. C.,** Hepatitis B surface antigen and antibody in Bantu patients with primary hepatocellular cancer, *Br. J. Cancer,* 33, 544, 1976.

161. **Simons, M. J., Yap, E. H., Yu, M., and Shanmugaratnam, K.,** Australia antigen in Singapore. Chinese patients with hepatocellular carcinoma and comparison groups: influence of technique sensitivity on differential frequencies, *Int. J. Cancer,* 10, 320, 1972.

162. **Tong, M. J., Sun, S. C., Shaeffer, B. T., Chang, N. K., Lo, K. J., and Peters, R. T.,** Hepatitis-associated antigen and hepatocellular carcinoma in Taiwan, *Ann. Intern. Med.,* 75, 687, 1971.

163. **Hsu, H. C., Lin, W. S., and Tsai, M. J.,** Hepatitis B surface antigen and hepatocellular carcinoma in Taiwan: with special reference to types and localization of HB_sAg in tumor cells, *Cancer,* 52, 1825, 1983.

164. **Trichopoulos, D., Tabor, E., Gerety, R. J., Xirouchaki, E., Sparros, L., and Munoz, N.,** Hepatitis B and primary hepatocellular carcinoma in a European population, *Lancet,* 2, 1217, 1978.

165. **Nomura, A., Stemmerman, G. N., and Wasnich, R. D.,** Presence of hepatitis B surface antigen before primary hepatocellular carcinoma, *JAMA,* 247, 2247, 1982.

166. **Sandlow, L. J. and Spellberg, M. A.,** Primary hepatic carcinoma: its incidence and relationship to HB_sAg, *Am. J. Gastroenterol.,* 74, 512, 1980.

167. **Brechot, C., Hadchouel, M., and Scotto, J.,** State of hepatitis B virus DNA in hepatocytes of patients with hepatitis B surface antigen-positive and -negative liver diseases, *Proc. Natl. Acad. Sci. U.S.A.,* 78, 3906, 1981.

168. **Wu, T. C., Tong, M. J., Hwang, B., Lee, S. D., and Hu, M. M.,** Primary hepatocellular carcinoma and hepatitis B infection during childhood, *Hepatology,* 7, 46, 1987.

169. **Brechot, C., Nalpas, Courouce, A. M., Duhamel, G., Callard, P., Carnot, F., Tiollais, P., and Berthelot, P.,** Evidence that hepatitis B virus has a role in liver-cell carcinoma in alcoholic liver disease, *N. Engl. J. Med.,* 306, 1384, 1982.

170. **Trichopoulos, D., Kremastinou, J., and Tzonou, A.,** Does hepatitis B virus cause hepatocellular carcinoma?, in *Factors in Human Carcinogenesis,* Armstrong, B. and Bartsch, H., Eds., IARC Scientific Publication No. 39, International Agency for Research on Cancer, Lyon, France, 1982, 317.

171. **Prince, a. M. and Alcabes, P.,** The risk of development of hepatocellular carcinoma in hepatitis B virus carriers in New York. A preliminary estimate using death-records matching, *Hepatology,* 2, 15S, 1982.

172. **Arthur, M. J. P., Hall, A. J., and Wright, R.,** Hepatitis B, hepatocellular carcinoma, and strategies for prevention, *Lancet,* 1, 607, 1984.

173. **Iuma, T., Saitoh, N., Nobutomo, K., Nambu, M., and Sakuma, K.,** A prospective cohort study of hepatitis B surface antigen carriers in a working population, *Gann,* 75, 571, 1984.

174. **Yeh, F. S., Mo, C. C., Luo, S., Henderson, B. E., Tong, M. J., and Yu, M. C.,** A serological case-control study of primary hepatocellular carcinoma in Guangxi, China, *Cancer Res.,* 45, 872, 1985.

175. **Hall, A. J., Winter, P. O., and Wright, R.,** Mortality of hepatitis B positive blood donors in England and Wales, *Lancet,* 1, 91, 1985.

176. **Trichopoulos, D., Day, N. E., Kaklamani, E., Tzonou, A., Munoz, N., Zavitsanos, X., Koumantaki, Y., and Trichopoulou, D.,** Hepatitis B virus, tobacco smoking and ethanol consumption in the etiology of hepatocellular carcinoma, *Int. J. Cancer,* 39, 45, 1987.

177. **Cook-Mozaffari, P. and Van Rensburg, S. J.,** Cancer of the liver, *Br. Med. Bull.,* 40, 342, 1984.

178. **Resnick, R. H., Stone, K. S., and Antonioli, D.,** Primary hepatocellular carcinoma following nonA, nonB post transfusion hepatitis, *Dig. Dis. Sci.,* 28, 908, 1983.

179. **Gilliam, J. H., Geisinger, K. R., and Richter, J. E.,** Primary hepatocellular carcinoma after chronic nonA, nonB hepatics, *Ann. Intern. Med.,* 101, 794, 1984.

180. **Kiyosawa, K., Akahoma, Y., Nagata, A., and Futura, S.,** Hepatocellular carcinoma after nonA, nonB post-transfusion hepatitis, *Am. J. Gastroenterol.,* 78, 777, 1987.

181. **Kuo, G., Choo, Q. L., Alter, H. J., Gitnick, G. L., Redeker, A. G., Purcell, R. H., Miyamura, T., Dienstag, J. L., Alter, J. J., Stevens, C. E., Tegtmeier, G. E., Bonino, F., Colombo, M., Lee, W. S., Kuo, C., Berger, K., Shuster, J. R., Overby, L. R., Bradley, D. W., and Houghton, M.,** An assay for circulating antibodies to a major etiologic virus of human nonA, nonB hepatitis, *Science,* 244, 362, 1989.

182. **Choo, Q. L., Kuo, G., Weiner, A. J., Overby, L. R., Bradley, D. W., and Houghton, M.,** Isolation of a cDNA clone derived from a blood-borne nonA nonB viral hepatitis genome, *Science,* 244, 359, 1989.

183. **Esteban, J. I., Esteban, R., Viladomiu, L., Lopez-Talavera, J. C., Gonzalez, A., Hernandez, J. M., Roget, M., Vargas, V., Genesea, J., Buti, M., Guardia, J., Houghton, M., Choo, Q. L., and Kuo, G.,** Hepatitis C virus antibodies among risk groups in Spain, *Lancet,* 1, 294, 1989.

184. **Bruix, J., Barrera, J. M., Calvet, X., Ercilla, G., Costa, J., Sanchez-Tapias, J. M., Ventura, M., Vall, M., Bruguera, M., Bru, C., Castillo, R., and Rodes, J.,** Prevalence of antibodies to hepatitis C virus in Spanish patients with hepatocellular carcinoma and hepatic cirrhosis, *Lancet,* 2, 1004, 1989.

185. **Colombo, M., Kuo, G., Choo, Q. L., Donato, M. F., Del Ninno, E., Tommasini, M. A., Dioguardi, N., and Houghton, M.,** Prevalence of antibodies to hepatitis C virus in Italian patients with hepatocellular carcinoma, *Lancet,* 2, 1006, 1989.

186. **Simonetti, R. G., Cottone, M., Craxi, A., Pagliaro, L., Rapicetta, M., Chionne, P., and Costantino, A.,** Prevalence of antibodies to hepatitis C virus in hepatocellular carcinoma, *Lancet,* 2, 1338, 1989.

187. **Hasan, F., Jeffers, L., de Madina, M., Reddy, R., Parker, T., Schiff, E., Houghton, M., Choo, Q. L., and Kuo, G.,** Hepatitis C (HCV) associated hepatocellular carcinoma, *Hepatology,* 10, 608, 1989.

188. **Tremolada, F., Benvegnu, L., Casarin, C., Pontisso, P., Tagger, A., and Alberti, A.,** Antibody to hepatitis C virus in hepatocellular carcinoma, *Lancet,* 1, 300, 1990.

189. **Chiaramonte, M., Farinati, F., Fagiuoli, S., Ongaro, S., Aneloni, V., De Maria, N., and Naccarato, R.,** Antibody to hepatitis C virus in hepatocellular carcinoma, *Lancet,* 1, 301, 1990.

190. **Dazza, M. C., Meneses, L. V., Girard, P. M., Villaroel, C., Brechot, C., and Larouze, B.,** Hepatitis C virus antibody and hepatocellular carcinoma, *Lancet,* 2, 1216, 1990.

191. **Vargas, V., Castells, L., and Esteban, J. I.,** High frequency of antibodies to the hepatitis C virus among patients with hepatocellular carcinoma, *Ann. Intern. Med.,* 112, 232, 1990.

192. **Alter, M. J., Mares, A., Hadler, S. C., and Maynard, J. E.,** The effect of underreporting on the apparent incidence and epidemiology of acute viral hepatitis, *Am. J. Epidemiol.,* 125, 133, 1987.

193. **Seeff, L. B.,** *Alcohol and Viral Hepatitis (VH),* (Abstr. 586), 5th Congr. Int. Soc. Biomed. Res. Alcohol, University of Toronto, Canada, 1990.

194. **Ishii, K., Sata, M., Furudera, S., Kumashiro, R., Abe, H., Tanikawa, K., and Yokoyama, T.,** Studies on anti-HCV in alcoholic patients with chronic hepatitis and hepatocellular carcinoma, (Abstr. 383), 5th Congr. Int. Soc. Biomed. Res. Alcohol, University of Toronto, Toronto, 1990.

195. **Nalpas, B., Driss, F., Hamelin, B., Pal, S., Brechot, C., and Berthelot, P.,** Strong association between HCV and HBV infection in HCC and alcoholic liver disease, (Abstr. 387), 5th Congr. Int. Soc. Biomed. Res. Alcohol, University of Toronto, Toronto, 1990.

196. **Pares, A., Barrera, J. M., Caballeria, J., Ercilla, G., Bruguera, M., Caballeria, L., Castillo, R., and Rodes, J.,** Hepatitis C virus antibodies in chronic alcoholics: Association with the severity of liver injury, (Abstr. 392), 5th Congr. Int. Soc. Biomed. Res. Alcohol, University of Toronto, Toronto, 1990.

197. **Shafritz, D. A. and Kew, M. C.,** Identification of integrated hepatitis B virus DNA sequences in human hepatocellular carcinomas, *Hepatology,* 1, 1, 1981.

198. **Prince, A. M.,** Hepatitis B virus and hepatocellular carcinoma: molecular biology provides further evidence for an etiologic association, *Hepatology,* 1, 73, 1981.

199. **Larouze, B., London, W. T., Saimot, G., Werner, H. G., Lustbader, E. D., Payet, M., and Blumberg, B. S.,** Host responses to hepatitis B infection in patients with primary hepatic carcinoma and their families. A case-control study in Senegal, West Africa, *Lancet,* 2, 534, 1976.

200. **Wynder, E. L. and Klein, W. E.,** Possible role of riboflavin deficiency in epithelial neoplasia. I. Epithelial changes of mice in simple deficiency, *Cancer,* 18, 167, 1965.

201. **Bradshaw, E. and Schonland, M.,** Esophageal and lung cancers in Natal African males in relation to certain socio-economic factors, *Br. J. Cancer,* 23, 275, 1969.

202. **Warwick, G. P.,** Some aspects of the epidemiology and etiology of esophageal cancer with particular emphasis on the Transkei, South Africa, *Adv. Cancer Res.,* 17, 81, 1973.

203. **Mahboubi, E., Kmet, J., Cook, P. J., Day, N. E., Ghadirian, P., and Salmasizadeh, S.,** Esophageal cancer studies in the Caspian Littoral of Iran: the Caspian Cancer Registry, *Br. J. Cancer,* 28, 197, 1973.

204. Joint Iran-International Agency for Research on Cancer Study Group. Esophageal cancer studies in the Caspian Littoral of Iran: results of population studies — a Prodrome, *J. Natl. Cancer Inst.,* 59, 1127, 1977.

205. **Newberne, P. M.,** Diet and nutrition, *Bull. N.Y. Acad. Med.,* 54, 385, 1978.

206. **Cook-Mozaffari, P. J., Azordegan, F., Day, N. E., Ressicaud, A., Sabai, C., and Aramesh, B.,** Esophageal cancer studies in the Caspian Littoral of Iran: results of a case control study, *Br. J. Cancer,* 39, 293, 1979.

207. **Yang, S. C.,** Research on esophageal cancer in China, a review, *Cancer Res.,* 40, 2633, 1980.

208. **Leonard, T. K., Mohs, M. E., Ho, E. E., and Watson, R. R.,** Nutrient intakes: cancer causation and prevention, *Prog. Food Nutr. Sci.,* 10, 237, 1986.

209. **Lieber, C. S., Seitz, H. K., Garro, A. J., and Worner, T.,** Alcohol-related diseases and carcinogenesis, *Cancer Res.,* 39, 2863, 1979.

210. **Armstrong, B. K.,** The role of diet in human carcinogenesis with special reference to endometrial cancer, in *Origins of Human Cancer, Book A, Incidence of Cancer in Humans,* Hiatt, H. H., Watson, J. D., and Wristen, J. A., Eds., Cold Spring Harbor Laboratory, Cold Spring Harbor, N.Y., 1977, 557.

211. **Hayes, J. R. and Campbell, R. C.,** Nutrition as a modifier of chemical carcinogenesis, in *Carcinogenesis-A Comprehensive Survey,* Vol. 5, Slaga, T. J., Ed., Raven Press, New York, 1980, 207.

212. **Moor, T. A.,** *Vitamin A,* Elsevier, Amsterdam, 1957.

213. **Hirayama, T.,** Changing patterns of cancer in Japan with special references to the decrease in stomach cancer mortality, in *Origins of Human Cancer, Book A, Incidence of Cancer in Humans,* Hiatt, H. H., Watson, J. D., and Wristen, J. A., Eds., Cold Spring Harbor Laboratory, Cold Spring Harbor, N.Y., 1977, 55.

214. **Maugh, T. H.,** Vitamin A: potential protection from carcinogens, *Science,* 186, 1198, 1974.
215. **Sporn, M. B., Dunlop, N. M., Newton, D. L., and Smith, J. M.,** Prevention of chemical carcinogenesis by vitamin A and its synthetic analogs (retinoids), *Fed. Proc.,* 35, 1332, 1976.
216. **Colditz, G. A., Branch, L. G., Lipnick, R. J., Willett, W. C., Rosner, B., Posner, B. M., and Hennekens, D. H.,** Increased green and yellow vegetable intake and lowered cancer deaths in an elderly population, *Am. J. Clin. Nutr.,* 41, 32, 1985.
217. **Wahi, P. N., Kehar, U., and Lahiri, B.,** Factors influencing oral and oropharyngeal cancer in India, *Br. J. Cancer,* 19, 646, 1965.
218. **Ibrahim, N. A., Jafarey, N. A., and Zuberi, S. J.,** Plasma vitamin ''A'' and carotene levels in squamous cell carcinoma of oral cavity and oro-pharynx, *Clin. Oncol.,* 3, 203, 1977.
219. **Editorial,** Vitamin A and cancer, *Lancet,* 1, 575, 1980.
220. **Mellow, M. H., Layne, E. A., Lipman, T. O., Kaushik, M., Hostetler, C., and Smith, J. C.,** Plasma zinc and vitamin A in human squamous carcinoma of the esophagus, *Cancer,* 51, 1615, 1983.
221. **Lasnitzki, I.,** The effect of excess vitamin A on the embryonic rat esophagus in culture, *J. Exp. Med.,* 118, 1, 1963.
222. **Chu, E. and Malmgren, R.,** An inhibitory effect of vitamin A on the induction of tumors of forestomach and cervix in the Syrian hamster by carcinogenic polycyclic hydrocarbons, *Cancer Res.,* 25, 884, 1964.
223. **Port, C., Sporn, M., and Kaufman, D.,** Prevention of lung cancers in hamsters by 13-cis-retinoic acid, *Proc. Am. Assoc. Cancer Res.,* 16, 21, 1975.
224. **Moon, R., Grubbs, C., Sporn, M., et al.,** Retinyl acetate inhibits mammary carcinogenesis induced by N-methyl-N-nitrosourea, *Nature (London),* 267, 620, 1977.
225. **Smith, J. C., McDaniel, E. G., Fan, F. F., and Halsted, J. A.,** Zinc: a trace element essential in vitamin A metabolism, *Science,* 181, 954, 1973.
226. **Kramer, A. J. and Petering, D. H.,** Tumor-host metabolism. The central role of metallothionein, *Biol. Trace Element Res.,* 5, 303, 1983.
227. **Fong, L. Y., Sivak, A., and Newberne, P. M.,** Zinc deficiency and methylbenzylnitrosamine-induced esophageal cancer in rats, *J. Natl. Cancer Inst.,* 61, 145, 1978.
228. **Gabrial, G. N. and Newberne, P. M.,** Zinc deficiency, alcohol and esophageal cancer, in *Trace Substances in Environmental Health,* Hempill, D. D., Ed., Proc. University Missouri's 13th Ann. Conf. Trace Substances Environ. Health, Columbia, Missouri, 1979, 315.
229. **Abdulla, M., Biorklund, A., Mathur, A., et al.,** Zinc and copper levels in whole blood and plasma from patients with squamous cell carcinomas of head and neck, *J. Surg. Oncol.,* 12, 107, 1979.
230. **Atukorala, S., Basu, T. K., Dickerson, J. W. T., Donaldson, D., and Sakula, A.,** Vitamin A, zinc and lung cancer, *Br. J. Cancer,* 40, 927, 1979.
231. **Lin, J. H., Chan, W. C., Fong, Y. Y., and Newberne, P. M.,** Zinc levels in serum, hair and tumors from patients with esophageal cancer, *Nutr. Rep. Int.,* 15, 635, 1977.
232. **Newberne, P. M. and Schrager, T.,** Promotion of gastrointestinal tract tumors in animals: dietary factors, *Environ. Health Persp.,* 50, 71, 1983.
233. **Ahlbom, H. E.,** Simple achlorhydric anaemia, Plummer-Vinson syndrome and carcinoma of the mouth, pharynx and oesophagus in women, *Br. Med. J.,* 2, 331, 1936.
234. **Ahlbom, H. E.,** Predisponierende faktorenfur platten epithelkarzinom in mund hals and speiserohre, *Acta Radiol.,* 18, 163, 1937.
235. **Wynder, E. L. and Fryer, J. H.,** Etiologic considerations of Plummer-Vinson (Paterson-Kelly) syndrome, *Ann. Intern. Med.,* 49, 1106, 1950.
236. **Watts, J. M.,** The importance of the Plummer-Vinson syndrome in the actiology of carcinoma of the upper gastrointestinal tract, *Postgrad. Med. J.,* 37, 523, 1961.

237. National Research Council, Committee on Diet, Nutrition and Cancer, *Diet, Nutrition, and Cancer,* Assembly of Life Sciences, NRC, National Academy Press, Washington, D.C., 1982.

238. **Shamberger, R. J.,** Minerals and Cancer, in *Nutrition and Cancer,* Shamberger, R. J., Ed., Plenum Press, New York, 1984, 195.

239. **Siassi, F.,** Iron and esophageal cancer: Iron status of children in the patient and control households, (Abstr.) XIII Int. Congr. Nutr., Brighton, U.K., 1985, 133.

240. **Van Fleet, J. F. and Watson, R. R.,** Effect of selenium and vitamin E on resistance to infectious disease, in *Nutrition, Disease Resistance, and Immune Function,* Watson, R. R., Ed., Marcel Dekker, New York, 1984, 299.

241. **Clark, L. C.,** The epidemiology of selenium and cancer, *Fed. Proc.,* 44 (Abstr.), 2584, 1985.

242. **Schrauzer, G. N., White, D. A., and Schneider, C. J.,** Cancer mortality correlation studies. III. Statistical associates with dietary selenium intakes, *Bioinorg. Chem.,* 7, 23, 1977.

243. **Beach, R. S., Gershwin, M. E., and Hurley, L. S.,** Zinc, copper, and manganese in immune function and experimental oncogenesis, *Nutr. Cancer,* 3, 172, 1982.

244. **Helzlsouer, K. J.,** Selenium and cancer prevention, *Sem. Oncol.,* 10, 305, 1983.

245. **Mettlin, C., Miller, A. B., Wynder, E. L., and Willett, W. C.,** Diet and cancer: what can be reasonably recommend?, *Data Centrum,* 1, 45, 1984.

246. **Jacobs, A. and Cavill, I.,** The oral lesions of iron deficiency anaemia: pyridoxine and riboflavin status, *Br. J. Haematol.,* 14, 291, 1968.

247. **Toskes, P. P., Smith, G. W., Bensinger, T. A., Gianella, R. A., and Conrad, M. E.,** Folic acid abnormalities in iron-deficiency: the mechanism of decreased serum folate levels in rats, *Am. J. Clin. Nutr.,* 27, 355, 1974.

248. **Vitale, J. J., Briotman, S. A., Varrousek-Jakuba, F., Rodday, P. W., and Gottlieb, L. S.,** The effects of iron deficiency and the quality and quantity of fat on chemically-induced cancer, *Adv. Exp. Med. Biol.,* 91, 229, 1978.

249. **Harrison, R. J.,** Vitamin B_{12} levels in erythrocytes in hypochromic anaemia, *J. Clin. Pathol.,* 24, 698, 1971.

250. **Editorial,** Vitamin A and teratogenesis, *Lancet,* 1, 319, 1985.

251. **Mirvish, S. S., Wallcave, L., Eagen, M., and Shubik, P.,** Ascorbate-nitrite reaction: possible means of blocking the formation of carcinogenic *N*-nitroso compounds, *Science,* 177, 65, 1972.

252. Coordinating Group for Research on the Etiology of Esophageal Cancer of North China, *The epidemiology of esophageal cancer in North China and preliminary results in the investigation of its etiological factors,* paper presented at the 11th Int. Cancer Congr., Bucalossi, P., Veronesi, U., and Cascinelli, Eds., Excerpta Medica, Amsterdam, 1975.

253. **Wynder, E. L. and Chan, P. C.,** Possible role of riboflavin deficiency in epithelial neoplasia. II. Effect of skin tumor development, *Cancer,* 26, 1221, 1970.

254. **Thurnham, D. I., Munoz, N., Lu, J., Crespi, M., and Wahrendorf, J.,** Nutritional intervention studies in a high-risk area for oesophageal cancer in China, paper presented at XIII Int. Congr. Nutr., (Abstr.), Brighton, U.K., 1985, 211.

255. **Diaz Gomez, M. I., Swann, P. F., and Magee, P. N.,** The absorption and metabolism in rats of small oral doses of dimethylnitrosamine, *Biochem. J.,* 164, 497, 1977.

256. **Swann, P. F.,** Metabolism of nitrosamines: observations on the effect of alcohol on nitrosamine metabolism and on human cancer, *Banbury Report,* Vol. 12, Cold Spring Harbor Press, Cold Spring, NY, 1982, 53.

257. **Swann, P. F., Coe, A. M., and Mace, R.,** Ethanol and dimethylnitrosamine and dimethylnitrosamine metabolism in the rat. Possible relevance to the influence of ethanol on human cancer incidence, *Carcinogenesis,* 5, 1337, 1984.

258. **Schmahl, D., Thomas, C., Sattler, W., and Scheld, G. F.,** Experimental studies of syncarcinogenesis. III. Attempts to induce cancer in rats by administering dimethylnitrosamine and CCl₄ (or ethyl alcohol) simultaneously. In addition, an experimental contribution regarding "alcoholic cirrhosis," *Z. Krebsforsch.,* 66, 526, 1965.

259. **Schmahl, D.,** Investigations on esophageal carcinogenicity by methyl-phenyl-nitrosamine and ethyl alcohol in rats, *Cancer Lett.,* 1, 215, 1976.

260. **Habs, M. and Schmahl, D.,** Inhibition of the hepatocarcinogenic activity of dimethylnitrosamine (DENA) by ethanol inrats, *Hepato-Gastroenterol.,* 28, 242, 1981.

261. **Teschke, R., Minzlaff, M., Oldiges, H., and Frenzel, H.,** Effect of chronic alcohol consumption on human incidence due to dimethylnitrosamine administration, *J. Cancer Res. Clin. Oncol.,* 106, 58, 1983.

262. **Schwarz, M., Buchmann, A., Wiesbeck, G., and Kinz, W.,** Effect of ethanol on early nitrosamine carcinogenesis in rat liver, *Cancer Lett.,* 20, 305, 1983.

263. **Radlike, M. J., Stemmen, K. L., Brown, P. G., Larson, E., and Bingham, E.,** Effect of ethanol and vinyl chloride on the induction of liver tumours: preliminary report, *Environ. Health Perspect.,* 21, 153, 1977.

264. **Yamamoto, R. S., Korzis, J., and Weisburger, J. H.,** Chronic ethanol ingestion and the hepatocarcinogenicity of *N*-hydroxy-*N*-2-fluorenylacetamide, *Int. J. Cancer,* 2, 337, 1967.

265. **Yanagi, S., Yamashita, M., Hiasa, Y., and Kamiya, T.,** Effect of ethanol on hepatocarcinogenesis initiated in rats with 3′-methyl-4-dimethylaminoazobenzene in the absence of liver injuries, *Int. J. Cancer,* 44, 681, 1989.

266. **Mufti, S. I., Becker, G., and Sipes, I. G.,** Effect of chronic dietary ethanol consumption on the initiation and promotion of chemically-induced esophageal carcinogenesis in experimental rats, *Carcinogenesis,* 10, 313, 1989.

267. **Phillips, J. C., Lake, B. G., Gangolli, S. D., Grasso, P., and Lloyd, A. G.,** Effects of pyrazole and 3-amino-1,2,4-triagote on the metabolism and toxicity of dimethylnitrosamine in the rat, *J. Health Cancer Inst.,* 58, 629, 1977.

268. **Schwarz, M., Appel, K. E., Schrenk, D., and Kunz, W.,** Effect of ethanol on microsomal metabolism of dimethylnitrosamine, *J. Cancer Res. Clin. Oncol.,* 97, 233, 1980.

269. **Takada, A., Nei, J., Takase, S., and Matsuda, Y.,** Effects of ethanol on experimental hepatocarcinogenesis, *Hepatology,* 6, 65, 1986.

270. **Driver, H. E. and McLean, A. E. M.,** Dose-response relationships for initiation of rat liver tumours by dimethylnitrosamine and promotion by phenobarbitone or alcohol, *Fd. Chem. Toxic.,* 24, 242, 1986.

271. **Mufti, S. I. and Sipes, I. G.,** A reduction in mixed function oxidases and in tumor promoting effects of ethanol in a NDEA-initiated hepatocarcinogenesis model, *Adv. Exp. Med. Biol.,* 283, 347, 1991.

272. **Szebeni, J., Eskelson, C. D., Mufti, S., Watson, R. R., and Sipes, I. G.,** Inhibition of ethanol induced ethane exhalation by carcinogenic pretreatment of rats 12 months earlier, *Life Sci.,* 39, 2589, 1986.

273. **Mufti, S. I.,** Free radicals generated in ethanol metabolism may be responsible for tumor promoting effects of ethanol, *Adv. Exp. Med. Biol.,* 283, 777, 1991.

274. **Mufti, S. I. and Eskelson, C. D.,** Lack of tumor-promoting effects of ethanol in a hepatocarcinogenesis model and association of free radicals generation by ethanol with its tumor promoting effects, submitted.

275. **Mufti, S. I. and Eskelson, C. D.,** Alcohol related cancers may be inhibited by dietary vitamin E, *Ann. N.Y. Acad. Sci.,* 625, 824, 1991.

276. **Odeleye, O., Eskelson, C. D., Mufti, S. I., and Watson, R. R.,** Vitamin E reduction of lipid peroxidation products in rats fed cod liver oil and ethanol, *Alcohol,* 8, 273, 1991.

277. **Copeland, E. S.,** A National Institutes of Health Workshops report, free radicals in promotion — a chemical pathology study section workshop, *Cancer Res.,* 43, 5631, 1983.
278. **Weinstein, I. B.,** Synergistic interactions between chemical carcinogens, tumor promoters, and viruses and their relevance to human liver cancer, *Cancer Detect. Prev.,* 14, 253, 1989.

Chapter 11

ALCOHOL AND HEPATIC CARCINOGENESIS

Akira Takada, Shujiro Takase, and Mikihiro Tsutsumi

TABLE OF CONTENTS

5761-6/93/$0.00 + $.50
187

I. INTRODUCTION

The epidemiological link between cancer and alcoholism indicated that excessive alcohol intake increases the risk of cancer of the liver, upper alimentary tract, colon, and lung.[1-3] However, in the case of liver cancer this has usually been attributed not to ethanol per se, but rather to the ensuing cirrhosis.[4-6] Several recent reports[2,7,8] have emphasized the specific role of ethanol in the development of hepatocellular carcinoma (HCC). The possible mechanisms whereby alcohol abuse may promote the development of hepatic cancer are

1.   Hepatocellular injury by ethanol
2.   An increase in the conversion of carcinogen by induction of microsomal enzymes due to chronic ethanol consumption
3.   The "preneoplasia" hypothesis for Mallory body pathogenesis which may relate to a genetically controlled neoplastic characteristic of the cells
4.   Promoter action of ethanol itself, or the release from inhibitory stimulus for hepatocytic regeneration by ethanol which may act as a promoter for the development of hepatic cancer
5.   Deficiency of nutrients such as vitamin A and methyl radical, which may relate to the control mechanism of cell growth or carcinogenesis

However, there is little experimental evidence to support a direct pathogenic role of alcohol abuse in the development of HCC

The oncogenic role of hepatitis B virus (HBV) infection in the development of HCC has been widely accepted. In our own experience,[10] the incidence of HCC was higher among HBV carriers who were heavy drinkers than in nondrinkers. Among heavy drinkers, HCC developed at a younger age. Ohnishi et al.[11] also reported similar observations. These results suggest that alcohol may promote the development of cancer induced by HBV. Recently, detection techniques for hepatitis C virus (HCV) have been developed,[12-16] and a high prevalence of HCV markers in alcoholic patients with HCC has been reported.[17-19] These results also suggest that alcohol may promote the development of cancer induced by HCV. However, a pathogenetic correlation between HCC induced by viruses and alcohol abuse has not yet been demonstrated. A national survey in Japan[20] revealed that the number of alcoholic cirrhotic patients with hepatic cancer increased very quickly in recent years. However, the reason for this increase is also obscure.

In this chapter, the etiopathogenic relationships between alcohol abuse and HCC will be briefly reviewed, and our own results concerning these problems will be discussed.

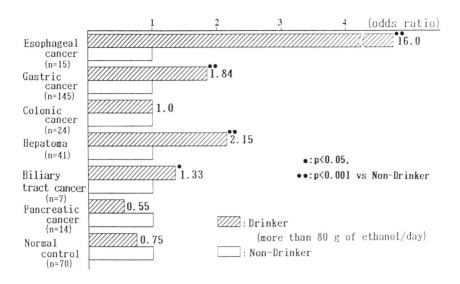

FIGURE 1. Relative risk factor of drinking for development of alimentary tract cancer. A case-control study. The odds ratios for esophageal, gastric, biliary tract, and hepatic cancer were significantly higher in drinkers.

II. EPIDEMIOLOGIC STUDIES

All prospective and retrospective case-control studies in Western countries indicate that the incidence of HCC among alcoholics is above expected normal levels.[1,3,7,21] In our own analysis, the relative risk factor of HCC, as well as esophageal cancer and gastric cancer, was significantly higher in drinkers (Figure 1), indicating the same situation for the risk of alcohol abuse on the development of HCC in Japan. Recent epidemiologic studies emphasize the high-risk scores of HBV infection and history of blood transfusion, or nonA, nonB hepatitis, in addition to alcohol consumption and cigarette smoking, for the development of HCC.[22-25] Although a proportion of alcohol drinkers with HCC may also have HBs antigen or history of blood transfusion, pathogenetic correlations between these risk factors are not well known.

III. PREVALENCE OF HCC IN ALCOHOLIC CIRRHOSIS

Variable prevalence of HCC in alcoholic cirrhosis has been reported. Generally, low incidences (2 to 7%) have been reported in Western countries. However, Parker[26] and Lee[5] reported relatively high incidences (33 and 30%). In Japan, the number of alcohol drinkers with HCC has recently increased. A national survey by Takeuchi et al.[20] revealed that prevalence of HCC in alcoholic cirrhosis increased at the rate of 1.27% per year during ten years

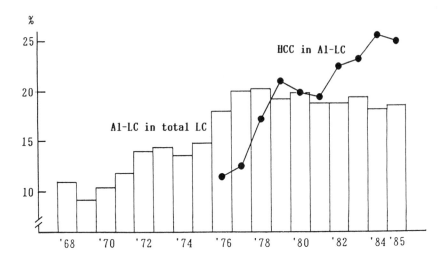

FIGURE 2.   Serial changes in the annual incidence of alcoholic cirrhosis in total cirrhosis and of hepatocellular carcinoma in alcoholic cirrhosis in Japan. A national survey. Incidence of hepatocellular carcinoma in alcoholic cirrhosis increased sharply during the last 10 years.

from 1976 to 1985 (Figure 2). In 1985, the incidence reached 25%. This value is close to the incidence of HCC in type B or C viral cirrhosis (about 30 to 50%), and higher than those from Western countries. However, Gerber et al.[27] reported that the incidence in North America has recently reached 15%. These results suggested that the incidence of HCC in alcoholic cirrhosis tended to increase throughout the world. This tendency may be partially related to the prolongation of the survival time of patients by the improvement of therapy for alcoholic cirrhosis. It is well-known that HCC of alcoholics is usually found in macronodular cirrhosis. This also indicates the importance of longer survival time of cirrhotic patients in the development of HCC.

After the report of Lee,[5] some studies emphasized the pathogenetic relationship between development of HCC and abstinence from alcohol. However, the effects of abstinence on the development of HCC were variable.[4,5] Stimulation of hepatocyte regeneration, as in partial hepatectomy, acts as a promoter of chemically induced hepatic cancer. It was shown that ethanol, either administered acutely or chronically, clearly inhibits hepatocyte regeneration.[28,29] Therefore, release from the inhibitory effect of ethanol on hepatocyte regeneration by abstinence may have the same effect as the stimulation of hepatocyte regeneration. From these observations, the possibility exists that the release from the inhibitory effect of alcohol on hepatocyte regeneration may promote the development of hepatic cancer. The elevation of alpha-fetoprotein after abstinence was considered as evidence of the increase in the stimulus on hepatocyte regeneration.[30] However, contrary results have been also reported.[31] In our own experience,[32] elevation of alpha-feto-protein after abstinence was not evident, and abstinence from alcohol was not related to the development of HCC.[10] In Japan, a large number of conflicting results concerning the relationships between abstinence and development of HCC have been reported. Recently, Ohta et al.[33] carefully analyzed the relationships between HCC and abstinence, and they pointed out that all parameters, such as incidence of HCC, duration of drinking, duration for development of HCC from cirrhosis, and ages of HCC, were not different between patients who abstained and those who continued drinking. From these results, it seemed unlikely that abstinence may be directly related to the development of HCC, and other factors appear more important. Unuma et al.[34] followed-up patients with alcoholic cirrhosis who stopped drinking completely for a long time, and found that over 80% of the patients eventually died of HCC. These results indicated that the most important determining factor for prognosis of cirrhosis in abstinents is the development of HCC, at least in Japan. In patients who abstained completely, hepatocellular damage by alcohol can be excluded, and therefore, the possibility that cirrhosis itself is the cause of death may decrease. Consequently, incidence of HCC may increase.

IV. MECHANISM OF THE DEVELOPMENT OF HCC IN ALCOHOLICS

It has been considered that development of HCC may be attributed merely to ensuing cirrhosis. Recently, attention has been focused on the specific role of ethanol itself in the development of HCC. It has been reported that some cases of HCC developed at the stage of alcoholic fibrosis without cirrhosis.[35] This fact suggests that ethanol itself may play some pathogenetic role in the development of HCC. However, evidence to confirm the etiopathogenesis of alcohol in the development of HCC is still lacking, although many attractive theories have been proposed.

A. HEPATOCYTE INJURY BY ETHANOL

The concept that HCC may be attributed to ensuing cirrhosis has been widely accepted. However, for the acceptance of this theory, the mechanism whereby HCC develops in cirrhosis should be made clear. Recently, pathogenetic relationships between HBV infection and the development of HCC have been emphasized. However, development of HCC is not only specific to type B cirrhosis, but HCC developed equally in nonA, nonB cirrhosis.[10] HCC also frequently developed in other types of cirrhosis, such as Budd-Chiari syndrome and hemochromatosis. Cirrhosis should be considered as a kind of precancer state, even without relation to viral infection. Therefore, alcoholic cirrhosis is one of the risk factors for the development of HCC, even if a specific role of ethanol for the development of HCC is absent. It is true that alcoholic fibrosis patients without detectable virus markers can develop cirrhosis, and finally, HCC. These facts indicate that HCC in some patients may be attributed to ensuing cirrhosis without any other specific pathogenesis.

B. INCREASE IN CONVERSION OF PROCARCINOGEN TO CARCINOGEN

Many chemical agents usually reveal cancer-producing action after metabolism to more active forms *in vivo*. Conversion of procarcinogen to carcinogen occurs by the action of a drug metabolizing enzyme (cytochrome P-450) in the liver microsome. It is well known that cytochrome P-450 is induced by chronic alcohol consumption. Therefore, the possibility exists that induction of cytochrome P-450 by chronic alcohol consumption may increase the conversion of procarcinogen to carcinogen, and may favor the development of liver cancer. However, experimental evidence to confirm the pathogenetic correlation between alcohol abuse and HCC is almost lacking, although many experimental studies were based on the assumption of an increased conversion of procarcinogen to carcinogen.[36] This lack of experimental evidence may be attributed mainly to the competitive inhibition of microsomal procarcinogen activation by ethanol. Similar results have been reported,[37] showing that the simultaneous feeding of a chemical carcinogen and phenobarbital, a potent inducer of cytochrome P-450, reduced the hepato-carcinogenetic effect of the carcinogen.

Recently, it became clear that P-450 II E1 is a specific isoenzyme of cytochrome P-450 induced by ethanol.[38,39] P-450 II E1 may be also the only enzyme which metabolizes nitrosodimethylamine (NDMA) at a very low concentration.[40] NDMA is a procarcinogen, and human beings are exposed to a very low dose of environmental NDMA during their lifetimes. Therefore, the possibility that induction of P-450 II E1 by alcohol abuse may accelerate the carcinogenic action of a very small dose of NDMA, can be considered. However, there is no experimental evidence to confirm this possibility at the present time.

C. PROMOTER ACTION OF ETHANOL

It seems improbable that ethanol or its metabolites may act on the liver as direct carcinogens or procarcinogens. Chemically, ethanol does not fit the profile of tumor initiators or procarcinogens, and is negative in both the Ames mutagenicity test[41] and the sister chromatid exchange test.[42] Phenobarbital, a potent inducer of drug-metabolizing enzymes, shows a clear promoter action on experimental carcinogenesis.[37,43,44] Alcohol is also one of the inducers of drug-metabolizing enzymes. Therefore, we tried to explore the possibility that alcohol may promote the development of experimental carcinogenesis in the same manner as phenobarbital.[45] Several studies[46,47] indicated no promoting action of ethanol in chemical hepato-carcinogenesis. However, the conditions for ethanol-feeding were not so strict in previous experiments. We used the Porta model[48] modifying the concentration of ethanol-sucrose mixture to 20% ethanol and 10% sucrose solution for ethanol-feeding in which rats consumed 35% of total calories as ethanol.[49] In conjunction with the Pitot model of multistage hepato-carcinogenesis,[43] it was found that numbers and areas of enzyme-altered focus (EAF) were significantly increased in chronically alcohol-treated rats. These changes were similar to those in the phenobarbital-treated rats. In the alcohol- and phenobarbital-treated groups, the numbers of visible nodules were also significantly increased. The visible nodules showed preneoplastic histologic changes. These results indicate that ethanol in alcoholic beverages may act as a promoting agent for induction of HCC.

D. MALLORY BODY AND HCC

Mallory body is one of the hallmarks of alcoholic liver injury, and the bodies are also found in the liver with HCC. Experimentally, Mallory bodies developed in chronically griseofulvin-treated mice and HCC is also found in these animals.[50] In the hepatocytes developing Mallory bodies, histologically detectable gamma-glutamyl transpeptidase (GGT) activity was observed from the early stage of development.[51] GGT is one of the markers of enzyme-altered focus during the development of experimental hepatic carcinogenesis. From these results, French et al.[52] theorized that the Mallory body may be a phenotypical expression of carcinogenesis of hepatocytes. Nakanuma et al.[53] reported that incidence of Mallory bodies was high in the hepatocytes of the liver with HCC, and that incidence of HCC was significantly higher in cirrhosis with Mallory bodies than in those without Mallory bodies. Although these results may lend some support to the French's[52] theory, our own analysis did not support this pathogenetic theory.

E. NUTRITIONAL FACTORS

Various nutritional deficiencies are known to be encountered in patients with alcoholic liver disease. It is also well known that chronic alcoholism in rats increased the dietary requirement for methyl, and that choline deficiency enhances the action of several hepato-carcinogens.[54] Recently, Porta et al.[55] found that chronic alcohol consumption did enhance the hepato-carcinogenicity of diethylnitrosamine (DEN) in rats fed a marginally methyl-deficient diet, and strongly suggested, therefore, that the action of ethanol on hepato-carcinogenicity was mediated through the exacerbation of methyl deficiency. Vitamin A plays an important role for cell growth and differentiation, and has inhibitory effects on carcinogenesis.[36] Vitamin A content in the liver decreases in alcoholic liver disease.[56] Recently, Leo et al.[57] reported that the metabolism of vitamin A is modified by ethanol. These results suggest the possibility that hepato-carcinogenesis may be enhanced by vitamin A deficiency due to alcohol abuse, although there is no experimental evidence on this point.

As mentioned above, many studies on experimental hepato-carcinogenesis have been reported. However, the applicability of the experimental results to human HCC remains to be determined.

V. HCC AND HBV INFECTION IN ALCOHOLICS

It has been recently considered that the HBV infection is the most important etiopathogenic factor of HCC. Molecular hybridization analysis identified HBV-DNA integrated into the cellular genome of HCC tissue from HBV carriers, and gave strong evidence of the hepato-carcinogenicity of HBV.[58-60] Furthermore, there is even an animal model of HCC caused by another hepadna virus.[61,62] The excitement created by the association of HBV infection with HCC around the world, and detection of HBV-DNA in HCC of some human alcoholics have created a great deal of confusion, and have overshadowed the etiopathogenic role of chronic alcoholism in HCC.[63,64] For example, Brechot et al.[64] have reported integrated HBV-DNA sequences in HCC in six of eight (75%) patients negative for all HBV markers, as well as twenty of twenty (100%) HBs Ag-negative patients with alcoholic cirrhosis. Although these results suggested that the real pathogenic factor of cirrhosis and HCC in chronic alcoholics could be the HBV infection rather than alcoholism per se, their data were quite surprising because they studied alcoholic patients in France where HBV infection is not endemic. Conversely, recent studies in HCC in Japan, where HBV infection is high, showed HBV-DNA integration in only a minority of HCC from HBs Ag-negative patients.[65,66] The high frequency of HBV-DNA integration noted by Brechot et al.[63,64] into the liver of patients seronegative for markers of HBV with or without alcohol liver disease, and its role in the pathogenesis of cirrhosis and HCC, has been questioned by other investigators.[67-69] In a more recent study[70] of HCC and cirrhotic tissue from HBs Ag-negative chronic alcoholic patients in Western countries, no HBV-DNA integration could be detected in any of the patients, Horiike et al.[71] also reported that HBV integration was found frequently in HBs Ag-positive HCC patients, but the integration could not be detected in HCC of HBs Ag-negative alcoholic patients in Japan.

Some alcoholic patients with HCC have also HBV infection, and these two risk factors may be found independently. However, how independent chronic alcoholism is from the development of HCC is still an unresolved problem. The prevalence of HBV markers in Japanese alcoholics was not different from that in nonalcoholics, indicating that HBV infection and alcoholism are independent, at least in Japan.[72] On the other hand, it seems likely that there may be some pathogenic relationships between the two risk factors for the development of HCC. Ohnishi et al.[11] reported that incidence of HCC was significantly higher among chronic HBV carriers who were drinkers than among HBV carriers who were nondrinkers. Among drinkers, HCC developed at younger ages. From these results, they assumed that hepatic cell injury caused by alcohol may enhance the development of HCC caused by HBV. We[9,10] have also reported similar results. However, these results could also be explained by the promoter action of ethanol itself. Numerous studies concerning the relationship between alcoholism and HBV infection in the development of HCC have been reported in Japan. In most of these studies, the tendency that HBV-related HCC was found more frequently at younger ages in drinkers than in nondrinkers was recognized. However, statistically significant evidence was documented in very few, suggesting that further detail in studies with large numbers of patients will be needed to confirm the etiopathogenic relation between these two risk factors for the development of HCC.

VI. HCC AND HCV INFECTION IN ALCOHOLICS

The role of HBV infection in the development of HCC has been emphasized. However, we have pointed out that the incidence of HCC in nonA, nonB cirrhosis was nearly similar to that in HBV-related cirrhosis.[10] These results indicate that viral infection other than HBV is also important for the development of HCC. Recently, detection methods were developed for HCV markers.[12-16] From the results on anti-100-3 protein antibodies (HCV-Ab), Nishioka et al.[73] pointed out that in Japan, HCV infection is more important for etiopathogenesis of HCC than HBV infection, and emphasized that a recent large increase of HCC in Japan was caused by increase in HCV-related HCC, but not in HBV-related HCC. Reports which document high prevalence of HCV-Ab in alcoholic liver disease, especially in cirrhosis and HCC, are rapidly increasing throughout the world.[17-19,74-76] As in the case of HBV infection, confusion has been created on the etiopathogenic relationships between chronic alcoholism and HCV infection in the development of HCC.

We have recently developed a method to detect the HCV-ribonucleic acid (RNA) genome (NS-5 domain) itself from the patient's plasma.[15,16] Detection rates of HCV markers (HCV-Ab and HCV-RNA) in alcoholic patients are shown in Figure 3. HCV markers were seldom found in alcoholic fibrosis and alcoholic hepatitis, indicating that these types of alcoholic liver disease were caused purely by alcohol. On the other hand, HCV markers were found in many cases of chronic hepatitis HCC in heavy drinkers. In alcoholic cirrhosis, the incidence of HCV markers was about 30%. These incidences were compared with those in nonA-, nonB-related liver disease of nondrinkers. In HCC, the incidence of HCV markers was not different between alcoholics and nonalcoholics. However, the detection rate of HCV-RNA in alcoholic HCC patients was higher than that of nonalcoholics. The detection rates of HCV-RNA decreased in parallel with the progression of liver disease in nonalcoholics. On the other hand, the rates tended to increase in alcoholics with the progression of liver disease. These differences in the pattern of prevalence of HCV markers suggest that chronic alcohol consumption may

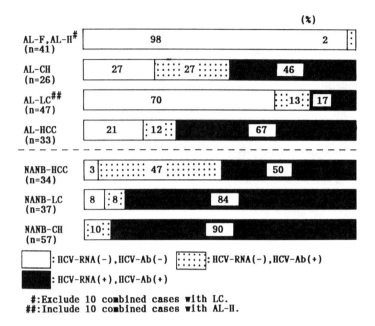

FIGURE 3.   Prevalence of HCV markers by the stage of liver disease: comparison between alcoholic and nonA- nonB-related liver disease. Patterns of the prevalence of HCV markers in each type of alcoholic liver disease were somewhat different from those in nonA- nonB-related liver disease. Prevalence of HCV-RNA in HCC of alcoholics was higher than in that of nonalcoholics.

modify the HCV replication and the development of HCC induced by HCV. In two patients with chronic hepatitis of heavy drinker, HCV-RNA became nondetectable in their plasma after abstinence with clear improvement of clinical symptoms. In one patient, HCV-Ab also disappeared after abstinence (Figure 4). Disappearance of HCV-RNA from plasma of patients with chronic liver disease was observed only by the treatment with interferon, but never observed naturally, except for these two patients. These results indicate that alcohol abuse may enhance the replication of HCV. HCV-RNA genome can be divided into two types, namely, K1-PT and K2.[77] The ratios of K1-PT type to K2 type were about 8:2 in all types of HCV-related liver disease in nonalcoholics. On the other hand, only K1-PT type can be detected in HCC of drinkers, except for one patient (Figure 5). This difference in the pattern of the type of HCV-RNA also suggests that alcohol abuse may modify the development of HCC related to HCV.

Serial changes of liver histology in patients with different types of alcoholic liver disease were analyzed in relation to the results of HCV markers, retrospectively. In 24 patients with alcoholic fibrosis and 2 patients with minimal change of liver histology, about one third (7 patients) progressed to

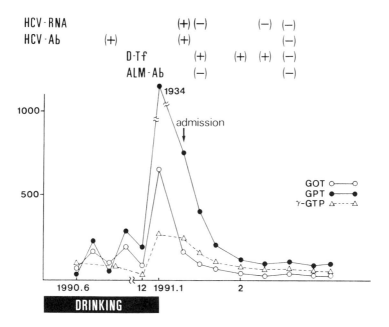

FIGURE 4. Clinical course of a patient with chronic hepatitis of heavy drinker following abstinence. Both HCV-RNA and HCV-Ab disappeared after abstinence from alcohol, with marked improvement of clinical symptoms. D-Tf: desialo-transferrin, ALM-Ab: alcohol-altered liver membrane antibody.

cirrhosis during 2- to 7-year periods. In these patients, HCV markers and HBs Ag were all negative, HCC was found in one case (Figure 6). In this case, alcohol may play the main etiopathogenic role in the development of HCC. All of the 3 patients with alcoholic hepatitis and about two-thirds of patients (8 out of 14 cases) with chronic hepatitis of heavy drinkers developed cirrhosis during relatively short periods (1- to 6-year periods). Development of cirrhosis was not related to the presence or absence of HCV markers. HCC developed in 4 patients with chronic hepatitis, although the presence of cirrhosis was not confirmed in 2 cases. These 4 patients were positive for HCV markers (Figures 7 and 8). These results indicate that alcoholics with alcoholic hepatitis and chronic hepatitis are the high-risk groups for the development of cirrhosis, and that chronic hepatitis patients are a high-risk group for the development of HCC. Although the risks are low in alcoholic fibrosis, some patients may develop cirrhosis, and few of them may develop HCC. From these results and the incidence of HCV markers in each type of alcoholic liver disease, it is possible to infer the progression to cirrhosis and HCC in alcoholics as shown in Figure 9. About half of the cases of cirrhosis may develop from alcoholic hepatitis and alcoholic fibrosis, and the remaining half may develop from chronic hepatitis. Over 80% of HCC patients may develop from chronic hepatitis. These presumptions strongly suggest that

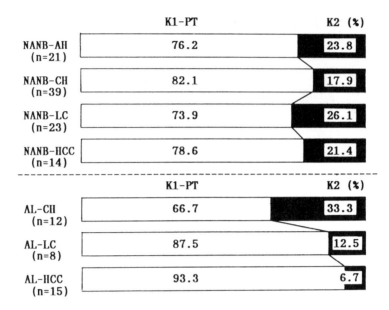

FIGURE 5.   Distribution of the different types of HCV-RNA by the stage of liver disease: comparison between alcoholic and nonA- nonB-related liver disease. The patterns were somewhat different between both diseases. In alcoholic HCC, K1 type was detected in only one patient. The other patients were K1-PT type.

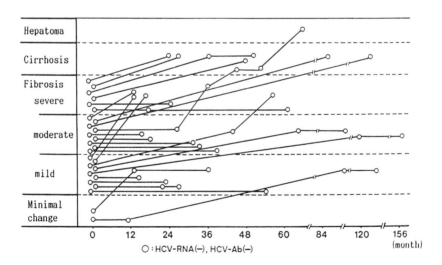

FIGURE 6.   Serial changes in liver histology in patients with alcoholic fibrosis or minimal change of liver histology. Progression to cirrhosis was observed in about one third of patients during 2- to 7-year periods. In one case, HCC developed. Virus markers were all negative in these patients.

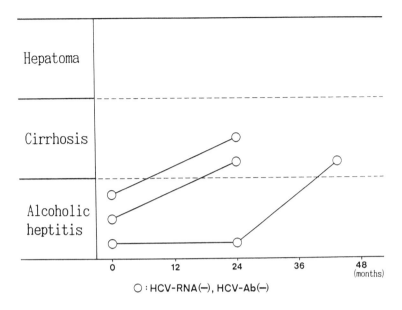

FIGURE 7. Serial changes in liver histology in patients with alcoholic hepatitis. All patients developed cirrhosis during 1- to 6-year periods. However, HCC was not found.

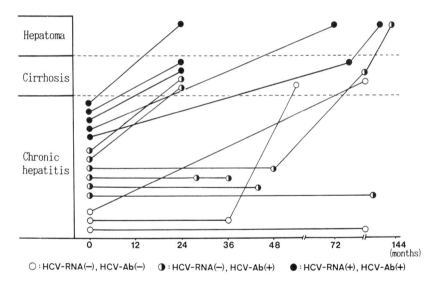

FIGURE 8. Serial changes in liver histology in patients with chronic hepatitis of heavy drinker. About half of the patients developed cirrhosis during 1- to 6-year periods. HCC was found in 4 cases. In these 4 cases, HCV markers were positive.

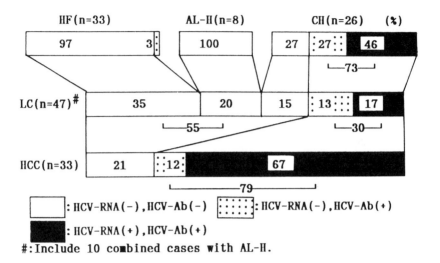

FIGURE 9. A schematic illustration of the progression of alcoholic liver disease, assumed mainly from prevalence of HCV markers. About half of cirrhosis patients and most of HCC patients may have originated from chronic hepatitis of heavy drinker.

heavy drinkers with chronic hepatitis and patients with HCV-related alcoholic cirrhosis are very high-risk groups for the development of HCC, and that alcohol abuse plays an etiopathogenic role in the development of HCC related to HCV infection.

VII. EFFECTS OF ALCOHOL ON HCC INDUCED BY VIRUSES

From our recent clinical studies, it became clear that most of the alcoholic patients with HCC are infected with hepatitis viruses. It seems quite possible, therefore, that alcohol abuse may enhance the development of HCC induced by viruses. In order to clarify the role of alcohol in the development of HCC induced by virus, we have reexamined the course and HCV markers in cirrhotic patients admitted to our department in the last 20 years. Among 369 cirrhotic patients, 126 had HCC (34.1%). Among these 126 HCC patients, both HBs Ag, and HCV markers were negative in only 9 patients (7.1%). In the remaining 117 cases, either HBs Ag or HCV markers were positive (Table 1). In alcoholic cirrhotic patients who were negative for all viral markers, the incidence of HCC was only 9.6%. On the other hand, in the virus markers-positive cirrhotic patients, the incidence of HCC was between 36 and 50%. In 48 male alcoholic patients with HCC, virus markers were positive in 43 patients (89.6%), a negative in only 5 patients (10.4%). These results suggest a minimal etiopathogenic role of alcohol per se in the development of HCC. Incidence of HCC among alcoholic cirrhotic patients who are positive for virus markers tended to be higher than in nonalcoholic cirrhotic patients who

TABLE 1
Incidence of Hepatocellular Carcinoma in Cirrhotic Patients with Different Etiologies

Etiology of cirrhosis	Number of patients with HCC in cirrhosis	%
Alcohol	5/52 (5/52)[a]	9.6 (9.6)[a]
HBV-related		
Drinker	16/33 (16/33)[a]	48.5[b] (48.5)[a]
Nondrinker	28/73 (21/50)[a]	38.4[b] (42.0)[a]
HCV-related		
Drinker	27/54 (27/52)[a]	50.0[b] (51.9)[a]
Nondrinker	46/128 (33/76)[a]	35.9[b] (43.4)[a]
Others	4/29 (0/0)[a]	13.8 (0)[a]
Total	126/369 (102/262)	34.1 (38.9)[a]

[a]   ( ), Male patients only.
[b] $p < 0.01$ vs. alcohol group.

are also positive for HBV and HCV markers. However, the difference was not statistically significant. The number of HCC patients positive for HCV markers was larger than that of HBV carriers (73 vs. 44), suggesting that HCV infection is more etiologically important than HBV for HCC in Japan.

The ages of HCC patients tended to be younger in HBV carriers than in other types of HCC patients. The ages of HCC alcoholics also tended to be younger than those in nonalcoholics in HCV carriers. However, the ages in HBV carriers were not different between drinkers and nondrinkers in this analysis (Table 2). Ages of HCC patients of HCV carriers may be related to the ages at HCV infection. Duration from the time of blood transfusion to the time of HCC diagnosis was compared between heavy drinkers and nondrinkers. The average duration was about 20 years, and there was no difference in the duration between heavy drinkers and nondrinkers (Table 3).

From these analyses, the enhancing effects of alcohol on the development of HCC induced by viruses are not clearly evident. Therefore, prevalence of HCC in patients with cirrhosis was analyzed by the multiple logistic-regression analysis.[78] The estimated relative risk for HCC development in cirrhotic patients was 8.2 and 8.3 times higher in HBV and HCV carriers, respectively, than in virus markers-negative alcoholics (Table 4). The odds ratios were 5.2 times in HBV carriers and 3.8 times in nonalcoholic HCV carriers, compared to those in the noncarrier alcoholics. These differences were statistically significant. The interactions between the variables (HBV and alcohol or HCV and alcohol) were also calculated. The calculated interactions between HCV and alcohol for the development of HCC were clearly recognizable ($p < 0.03$) as shown in Table 4. However, the interactions between HBV and alcohol were not clearly evident ($p < 0.29$). The logistic curves are shown in

TABLE 2
Ages of Patients with Hepatocellular Carcinoma Developed in Cirrhosis with Different Etiologies

Etiology of cirrhosis	Number of patients	Ages (average ± SD[c])	
Alcohol	5 (5)[a]	62.0 ± 9.9	(62.0 ± 9.9)[a]
HBV-related			
Drinker	16 (16)[a]	55.6 ± 9.0	(55.6 ± 9.0)[a]
Nondrinker	28 (21)[a]	55.7 ± 11.4[b]	(53.9 ± 14.7)[a]
HCV-related			
Drinker	27 (27)[a]	60.3 ± 7.4	(60.3 ± 7.4)[a]
Nondrinker	46 (33)[a]	62.5 ± 8.7	(61.1 ± 13.6)[a]
Others	4 (0)[a]	65.7 ± 9.1	
Total	126 (102)	58.6 ± 11.8	(59.7 ± 9.3)[a]

[a] ( ), Male patients only.
[b] $p < 0.05$ vs. alcohol group.
[c] SD, Standard deviation.

TABLE 3
Duration from the Time of Blood Transfusion to the Time of Diagnosis of Hepatocellular Carcinoma in HCV Carriers

Alcohol intake	Number of patients	Duration (Average years ± SD[a])
Drinkers	4	21.8 ± 5.4
Nondrinkers	14	20.4 ± 7.6
Male patients	8	21.8 ± 8.0

[a] SD, Standard deviation.

Figure 10. The curves showed that the probabilities of HCC in cirrhosis of virus carriers are higher in alcoholics than in the corresponding nonalcoholics between the ages of 20 to 80. Odds ratios for development of HCC in virus-carrier alcoholics were compared to those in nonalcoholic virus carriers. The calculated odds ratio for HCC development in alcoholics with HCV-related cirrhosis was significantly higher than that of the corresponding nonalcoholics (2.9 times, $p < 0.05$). The odds ratio for HCC development in alcoholics with HBV-related cirrhosis was 1.6 times higher than that of the corresponding nonalcoholics. However, this difference was not statistically significant ($p > 0.05$). These results indicate that chronic alcoholism enhances the development of HCC caused by both HBV and HCV, especially by HCV. The multiple logistic-regression analysis clearly showed that both risk factors of alcohol and HCV infection are etiopathogenically dependent, and alcohol

TABLE 4
Logistic Regression Coefficients of Prevalence of Hepatocellular Carcinoma in 369 Cirrhotic Patients with Different Etiologies

Variables	Beta	Standard error	p values
Intercept	− 4.8066	0.8316	0.0001
Age	0.0485	0.0126	0.0001
HBV nondrinker	1.6442	0.5357	0.0021
HCV nondrinker	1.3438	0.5176	0.0094
HBV drinker	2.1064	0.5952	0.0004
HCV drinker	2.1276	0.5505	0.0001
HBV × alcohol[a]	0.4622	0.4372	0.2905
HCV × alcohol[a]	0.7838	0.3451	0.0231

Note: Beta is the coefficient of the following formula:

$$\frac{1-p}{p} \ (Odds) = {}_c\beta_o + \beta_{Age} + \beta_{HBV} + \beta_{HCV} + \beta_{HBV+Al} + \beta_{HCV+Al}$$

[a] Interaction of both variables.

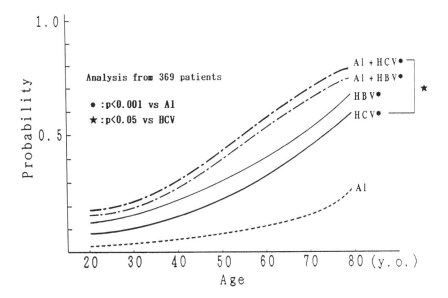

FIGURE 10. Logistic curves illustrating the probabilities of HCC in liver cirrhosis with different etiologies, calculated from the logistic model during the ages of 20 to 80. The probabilities of HCC in cirrhosis of virus carriers were higher in drinkers than in the corresponding nondrinkers. Statistical significance was evaluated from the odds ratios for HCC development in each group. The ratio in drinkers was significantly higher than in that of the corresponding nondrinkers.

abuse enhances the development of HCC related to HCV infection. On the other hand, etiopathogenic dependence of alcohol to HBV-induced HCC was not supported statistically by the present analysis, suggesting that alcohol may act only as a promoter for the development of HCC-induced HBV. Although the precise mechanism of the interactions between alcohol abuse and HCV infection on the development of HCV-related HCC is not known at the present time, the enhancing effects of alcohol on the HCV replication or the modifying effects of alcohol on the oncogenicity of HCV may be important in this matter.

VIII. SUMMARY

Although many attractive theories and experimental data concerning the hepato-carcinogenicity of alcohol have been present, recent clinical data, including HCV analysis, clearly showed that the etiopathogenic role of alcohol per se in the development of HCC is minimal. In most patients, HCC was related to hepatitis viral (HBV or HCV) infection. Our results suggested that, etiopathogenically, HCV infection is more closely related to HCC in heavy drinkers than is HBV infection. Alcoholic patients with HCV markers, especially HCV-RNA, should stop drinking or start interferon treatment to prevent HCC development. The results of our study strongly suggested that alcohol abuse enhances the development of HCC related to hepatitis virus infection, through the interactions with the replication and oncogenicity of HCV, and through the promoter action superimposed on HBV oncogenicity. The recent rapid increase of HCC in alcoholic cirrhotic patients in Japan may be related to the increase in alcohol consumption, to the increase of blood transfusion which increases the chances for HCV infection, and to the improvement of therapy for alcoholic cirrhosis. In the increase of HCC in heavy drinkers, the enhancing effects of alcohol may be very important.

ACKNOWLEDGMENTS

We are grateful to Dr. Masao Ishizaki, Department of Hygiene, for his help in the multiple logistic-regression analysis. We are also grateful to Dr. Eduardo A. Porta (Hawaii University) for his English edition of this manuscript. This work was supported in part by a Grant-in-Aid for Cooperative Research A02304040 from the Ministry of Education, Science, and Culture of Japan.

REFERENCES

1. **Tuyns, A. J.,** Epidemiology of alcohol and cancer, *Cancer Res.,* 39, 2840, 1979.
2. **Lieber, C. S., Seitz, H. K., Garro, A. J., and Worner, T. M.,** Alcohol-related diseases and carcinogenesis, *Cancer Res.,* 39, 2863, 1979.
3. **Potter, J. D., McMichael, A. J., and Hartshorne, J. M.,** Alcohol and beer consumption in relation to cancers of bowel and lung: an extended correlation analysis, *J. Chron. Dis.,* 35, 833, 1982.
4. **Leevy, C. M., Gellene, R., and Ning, M.,** Primary liver cancer in cirrhosis of the alcoholic, *Ann. N.Y. Acad. Sci.,* 114, 1026, 1964.
5. **Lee, F. I.,** Cirrhosis and hepatoma in alcoholics, *Gut,* 7, 77, 1966.
6. **Omata, M., Ashcavai, M., Liew, C. T., and Peters, R. L.,** Hepatocellular carcinoma in the U.S.A., etiologic considerations. Localization of hepatitis B antigens, *Gastroenterology,* 76, 279, 1979.
7. **Lehmann, F. G. and Wegener, T. R.,** Etiology of liver cancer: controlled prospective study in liver cirrhosis, *J. Toxicol. Environ. Health,* 5, 281, 1979.
8. **Dourdourekas, D., Villa, F., Szanto, P. B., and Steigmann, F.,** Hepatocellular carcinoma: relation to alcohol, HB-antigen and alpha-fetoprotein, *Am. J. Gastroenterol.,* 63, 307, 1975.
9. **Takada, A., Takase, S., Takeuchi, J., Ohta, Y., Tsujii, T., Ikegamin, F.,** Pathophysiology of liver cirrhosis with different etiologies, in *Etiology and Prognosis of Liver Cirrhosis,* Ohta, Y. and Harada, T., Eds, Nankodo, Tokyo, 1984, 173 (in Japanese).
10. **Nei, J., Takase, S., Matsuda, Y., and Takada, A.,** Alcohol and hepatocellular carcinoma, *Alcohol Metabolism and the Liver,* 6, 134, 1987 (in Japanese).
11. **Ohnishi, K., Iida, S., Iwama, S., Goto, N., Nomura, F., Takashi, M., Mishima, A., Kono, K., Kimura, K., Musha, H., Kolota, K., and Okuda, K.,** The effect of chronic habitual alcohol intake on the development of liver cirrhosis and hepatocellular carcinoma: relation to hepatitis B surface antigen carriage, *Cancer,* 49, 672, 1982.
12. **Choo, Q. L., Kuo, G., Weiner, A. J., Overby, L. R., Bradley, D. W., and Houghton, M.,** Isolation of a cDNA clone derived from a blood-borne nonA, nonB viral hepatitis genome, *Science,* 244, 359, 1989.
13. **Kuo, G., Choo, Q. L., Alter, H. J., Gitnick, G. L., Redeker, A. G., Purcell, R. H., Miyamura, T., Dienstag, J. L., Alter, M. J., Stevens, C. E., Tegtmeier, G. E., Bonino, F., Colombo, M., Lee, W.-S., Kuo, C., Berger, K., Shuster, J. R., Overby, L. R., Bradley, D. M., and Houghton, M.,** An assay for circulating antibodies to a major etiologic virus of human nonA, nonB hepatitis, *Science,* 244, 362, 1989.
14. **Arima, T., Mori, C., Takamizawa, A., Shimomura, H., and Tsuji, T.,** A cDNA clone encoding a peptide highly specific for hepatitis C infection, *Gastroenterol. Jpn.,* 25, 218, 1990.
15. **Enomoto, N., Takase, S., Takada, A., and Date, T.,** Detection of hepatitis C virus genomes from patient's plasma using PCR method, *Gastroenterol. Jpn.,* 25, 404, 1990.
16. **Enomoto, N., Takada, N., Takase, S., Takada, A., and Date, T.,** Hepatitis C virus RNA genome in plasma of patients with nonA, nonB hepatitis, *Gastroenterol. Jpn.,* 26, 42, 1991.
17. **Bruix, J., Barrera, J. M., Calvet, X., Ercilla, G., Costa, J., Sanchez-Tapias, J. M., Ventura, M., Vall, M., Bruguera, M., Bru, C., Castillo, R., and Rodes, J.,** Prevalence of antibodies to hepatitis C virus in Spanish patients with hepatocellular carcinoma and hepatic cirrhosis, *Lancet,* 2, 1004, 1989.
18. **Nalpas, B., Driss, F., Pol, S., Hamelin, B., Housset, C., Brechot, C., and Berthelot, P.,** Association between HCV and HBV infection in hepatocellular carcinoma and alcoholic liver disease, *J. Hepatol.,* 12, 70, 1991.
19. **Takada, N., Enomoto, N., Takase, S., Takada, A.,** Alcoholic liver disease and hepatitis C virus infection, *Alcohol Metabolism and the Liver,* 10, 200, 1991 (in Japanese).

20. **Takeuchi, J., Okudaira, M., Takada, A., Ohta, Y., Tsujii, T., Itoh, S., Fujisawa,. K., Tanikawa, K., and Hasumura, Y.,** The incidence of alcoholic liver disease in Japan (1976–1985), *Jpn. J. Gastroenterol.,* 84, 1623, 1987 (in Japanese).

21. **MacDonald, R. A.,** Primary carcinoma of the liver. A clinicopathologic study of 108 cases, *Arch. Inter. Med.,* 99, 266, 1957.

22. **Austin, H., Delzell, E., Grufferman, S., Levin, R., Morrison, A. S., Stolley, P. D., and Cole, P.,** A case-control study of hepatocellular carcinoma and the hepatitis B virus, cigarette smoking, and alcohol consumption, *Cancer Res.,* 46, 962, 1986.

23. **Mayans, M. V., Calvet, X., Bruix, J., Bruguera, M., Costa, J., Esteve, J., Bosch, E. X., and Rodes, J.,** Risk factors for hepatocellular carcinoma in Catalonia, Spain, *Int. J. Cancer,* 46, 378, 1990.

24. **Villa, E., Baldini, G. M., Pasquinelli, G., Melegari, M., Cariani, E., DiChirico, E., and Manenti, F.,** Risk factors for hepatocellular carcinoma in Italy. Male sex, hepatitis B virus, nonA nonB infection, and alcohol, *Cancer,* 62, 611, 1988.

25. **Tsukuma, H., Hiyama, T., Oshima, A., Sobue, T., Fujimoto, I., Kasugai, H., Kojima, J., Sasaki, Y., Imaoka, S., Horuchi, N., and Okuda, S.,** A case-control study of hepatocellular carcinoma in Osaka, Japan, *Int. J. Cancer,* 45, 231, 1990.

26. **Parker, R. G. F.,** The incidence of primary hepatic carcinoma in cirrhosis, *Proc. Roy. Soc. Med.,* 50, 145, 1957.

27. **Gerber, M. A., Thung, S., and Popper, H.,** Pathology of alcoholic liver injury. Update 1981 and problems, in *New Trends in Hepatology,* Oda, T. and Okuda, K., Eds., Medical Tosho, Tokyo, 1986, 8.

28. **Takada, A., Nei, J., Tamino, H., and Takase, S.,** Effects of malotilate on ethanol-inhibited hepatocyte regeneration in rats, *J. Hepatol.,* 5, 336, 1987.

29. **Diehl, A. M., Thorgeirsson, S. S., and Steer, C. J.,** Ethanol inhibits liver regeneration in rats without reducing transcripts of key protooncogenes, *Gastroenterology,* 99, 1105, 1990.

30. **Bloomer, J. R., Waldmann, T. A., McIntire, K. R., and Klatskin, G.,** Alpha-fetoprotein in nonneoplastic hepatic disorders, *JAMA,* 233, 38, 1975.

31. **Noble, T. E., Galdabini, J., Resnick, R. M., and Alpert, E.,** Alcoholic liver disease. Absence of alpha-fetoprotein elevations in the recovery phase, *Dig. Dis. Sci.,* 25, 248, 1980.

32. **Enyama, K., Takada, A.,** Metabolic changes of proteins in alcoholic liver injury. in *Alcoholic Liver Disease: Clinical Characteristics in Japan,* Takeuchi, J., Ed., Asakurashoten, Tokyo, 1988, 252 (in Japanese).

33. **Ohta, Y. and Michitaka, K.,** Hepatocellular carcinoma and drinking, in *Feature, Course and Prognosis of Alcoholic Liver Injury,* Okumura, M., Takada, A., and Tanikawa, K., Eds., Kokusai Ishoshuppan, Tokyo, 1990, 233 (in Japanese).

34. **Unuma, N., Muto, H., Shiina, H., Itoh, Y., Tagawa, K., and Takanashi, R.,** Analysis of 129 heavy drinkers who developed hepatocellular carcinoma. Especially to the relation to abstinence and histology of the non-cancer tissues, *Alcohol Metabolism and the Liver,* 6, 164, 1987 (in Japanese).

35. **Nishimura, M., Tazawa, J., Sakai, H., Uchihara, M., Hasumura, Y., Takeuchi, J., Maeda, M., Koyama, H., and Kanayama, M.,** Clinicopathological study on hepatocellular carcinoma in heavy drinkers, *Alcohol Metabolism and the Liver,* 6, 155, 1987 (in Japanese).

36. **Lieber, C. S., Garro, A., Leo, M. A., Mak, K. M., and Worner, T.,** Alcohol and cancer, *Hepatology,* 5, 1005, 1986.

37. **Peraino, C., Fry, R. J., and Staffeldt, E.,** Reduction and enhancement by phenobarbital of hepatocarcinogenesis induced in the rat by 2-acetylaminofluorene, *Cancer Res.,* 31, 1506, 1971.

38. **Johansson, I., Ekstrom, G., Scholte, B., Puzycki, D., Jornvall, H., and Ingelman-Sundberg, M.,** Ethanol-, fasting- and aceton-inducible cytochromes P-450 in rat liver: regulation and characteristics of enzymes belonging to the IIB and IIE gene subfamilies, *Biochemistry,* 27, 1925, 1988.

39. **Koop, D. R. and Coon, M. J.,** Ethanol oxidation and toxicity: role of alcohol P-450 oxygenase, *Alcohol.: Clin. Exp. Res.,* 10, 44, 1986.

40. **Thomas, P. E., Bandiera, S., Maines, S. L., Ryan, D. E., and Levin, W.,** Regulation of cytochrome P-450j, a high-affinity N-nitrosodimethylamine demethylase, in rat hepatic microsomes, *Biochemistry,* 26, 2280, 1987.

41. **McCann, J., Choi, E., Yamasaki, E., and Ames, B. N.,** Detection of carcinogens as mutagens in the Salmonella/microsome test: assay of 300 chemicals, *Proc. Natl. Acad. Sci. U.S.A.,* 72, 5135, 1975.

42. **Obe, G. and Ristow, H.,** Mutagenic, cancerogenic and teratogenic effects of alcohol, *Mutat. Res.,* 65, 229, 1979.

43. **Pitot, H., Barsness, L., Goldsworthy, T., and Kitagawa, T.,** Biochemical characterization of stages of hepatocarcinogenesis after a single dose of diethylnitrosamine, *Nature (London),* 271, 456, 1978.

44. **Kitagawa, T. and Sugano, H.,** Enhancing effect of phenobarbital on the development of enzyme-altered islands and hepatocellular carcinomas initiated by 3'-methyl-4-(dimethylamino) azobenzene or diethylnitrosamine, *Gann,* 69, 679, 1978.

45. **Takada, A., Nei, J., Takase, S., and Matsuda, Y.,** Effects of ethanol on experimental hepatocarcinogenesis, *Hepatology,* 6, 65, 1986.

46. **Schwarz, M., Buchmann, A., Wiesbeck, G., and Kunz, W.,** Effect of ethanol on early stages in nitrosamine carcinogenesis in rat liver, *Cancer Lett.,* 20, 305, 1983.

47. **Ikawa, E., Tsuda, H., Sakata, T., Masui, T., Satoh, K., Sato, K., and Ito, N.,** Modification potentials of ethyl alcohol and acetaldehyde on development of preneoplastic glutathione S-transferase P-form-positive liver cell foci initiated by diethylnitrosamine in the rat, *Cancer Lett.,* 31, 53, 1986.

48. **Porta, E. A. and Gomez-Dumm, C. L.,** A new experimental approach in the study of chronic alcoholism. I. Effects of high alcohol intake in rats fed a commercial laboratory diet, *Lab. Invest.,* 18, 352, 1968.

49. **Takeuchi, J., Takada, A., Kato, Y., Hasumura, Y., Ikegami, F., and Matsuda, Y.,** Hepatic changes in chronic alcoholic rats following periodic acute alcoholic intoxications, *Am. J. Clin. Nutr.,* 24, 628, 1971.

50. **Denk, H., Gschnait, F., and Wolff, K.,** Hepatocellular hyalin (Mallory bodies) in long-term griseofulvin-treated mice: a new experimental model for the study of hyalin formation, *Lab. Invest.,* 32, 773, 1975.

51. **Tazawa, J., Irie, T., and French, S. W.,** Mallory body formation runs parallel to gamma-glutamyl transferase induction in hepatocytes of griseofulvin-fed mice, *Hepatology,* 3, 989, 1983.

52. **French, S. W.,** The Mallory body: structure, composition, and pathogenesis, *Hepatology,* 1, 76, 1981.

53. **Nakanuma, Y. and Ohta, G.,** Is Mallory body formation a preneoplastic change? A study of 181 cases of liver bearing hepatocellular carcinoma and 82 cases of cirrhosis, *Cancer,* 55, 2400, 1985.

54. **Rogers, A. E. and Newberne, P. M.,** Lipotrope deficiency in experimental carcinogenesis, *Nutr. Cancer,* 2, 104, 1980.

55. **Porta, E. A., Markell, N., and Dorado, R. D.,** Chronic alcoholism enhances hepatocarcinogenicity of diethylnitrosamine in rats fed a marginally methyl-deficient diet, *Hepatology,* 5, 1120, 1985.

56. **Leo, M. A. and Lieber, C. S.,** Hepatic vitamin A depletion in alcoholic liver injury, *N. Engl. J. Med.,* 307, 597, 1982.

57. **Leo, M. A. and Lieber, C. S.,** New pathways of vitamin A metabolism and their interaction with ethanol and carcinogens, in *Biomedical and Social Aspects of Alcohol and Alcoholism,* Kuriyama, K., Takada, A., and Ishii, H., Eds., Excerpta Medica, Amsterdam, 1988, 809.

58. **Shafritz, D. A. and Lieberman, H. M.,** The molecular biology of hepatitis B virus, *Annu. Rev. Med.,* 35, 219, 1984.

59. **Tiollais, P., Purcel, C., and Dejean, A.,** The hepatitis B virus, *Nature (London),* 317, 489, 1985.

60. **Ganem, D. and Varmus, H. E.,** The molecular biology of the hepatitis B viruses, *Annu. Rev. Biochem.,* 56, 651, 1987.

61. **Summers, J., Smolec, J. M., and Snyder, R.,** A virus similar to human hepatitis B virus associated with hepatitis and hepatoma in woodchucks, *Proc. Natl. Acad. Sci. U.S.A.,* 75, 4533, 1978.

62. **Popper, H., Roth, L., Purcell, R. H., Tennant, B. C., and Gerin, J. L.,** Hepato-carcinogenicity of the woodchuck hepatitis virus, *Proc. Natl. Acad. Sci. U.S.A.,* 84, 866, 1987.

63. **Brechot, C., Degos, F., Lugassy, C., Thiers, V., Zafrani, S., Franco, D., Bismuth, H., Trepo, C., Benhamou, J.-P., Wands, J., Isselbacher, K., Tiollais, P., and Berthelot, P.,** Hepatitis B virus DNA in patients with chronic liver disease and negative tests for hepatitis B surface antigen, *N. Engl. J. Med.,* 312, 270, 1985.

64. **Brechot, C., Nalpas, B., Courouce, A. M., Duhamel, G., Callard, P., Carnot, F., Tiollais, P., and Berthelot, P.,** Evidence that hepatitis B virus has a role in liver-cell carcinoma in alcoholic liver disease, *N. Engl. J. Med.,* 306, 1384, 1982.

65. **Hino, O., Kitagawa, T., and Sugano, H.,** Relationship between serum and histochemical markers for hepatitis B virus and rate of viral integration in hepatocellular carcinomas in Japan, *Int. J. Cancer,* 35, 5, 1985.

66. **Imazeki, F., Omata, M., Yokosuka, O., and Okuda, K.,** Integration of hepatitis B virus DNA in hepatocellular carcinoma, *Cancer,* 58, 1055, 1986.

67. **Harrison, T. J., Anderson, M. G., Murray-Lyon, I. M., and Zuckerman, A. J.,** Hepatitis B virus DNA in the hepatocyte. A series of 160 biopsies, *J. Hepatol.,* 2, 1, 1986.

68. **Fowler, M. J., Greenfield, C., Chu, C.-M., Karayiannis, P., Dunk, A., Lok, A. S., Lai, C. L., Yeoh, E. K., Monjardino, J. P., Wankyd, B. M., and Thomas, H. C.,** Integration of HBV DNA may not be a prerequisite for the maintenance of the state of malignant transformation. An analysis of 110 liver biopsies, *J. Hepatol.,* 2, 218, 1986.

69. **Pontisso, P., Stenico, D., Diodati, G., Marin, G., Caldironi, M. V., Giacchino, R., Realdi, G., and Alberti, A.,** HBV-DNA sequences are rarely detected in the liver of patients with HBsAg-negative chronic active liver disease and with hepatocellular carcinoma in Italy, *Liver,* 7, 211, 1987.

70. **Walter, E., Blum, H. E., Meier, P., Huonker, M., Schmid, M., Maier, K. P., Offensperger, W. B., Offensperger, S., and Gerok, W.,** Hepatocellular carcinoma in alcoholic liver disease: no evidence for a pathogenetic role of hepatitis B virus infection, *Hepatology,* 8, 745, 1988.

71. **Horiike, N., Michitaka, K., Onji, M., Murota, T., and Ohta, Y.,** HBV-DNA hybridization in hepatocellular carcinoma associated with alcohol in Japan, *J. Med. Virol.,* 28, 189, 1989.

72. **Takino, T., Sakanaka, T., Yuki, T., Ogawa, D., Toyoda, E., Takamori, S., Takahashi, T., and Masuda, M.,** The clinical study on liver diseases in alcoholics, *Acta, Hepatol. Jpn.,* 15, 18, 1974 (in Japanese).

73. **Nishioka, K., Watanabe, J., Furuta, S., Tanaka, E., Iino, S., Suzuki, H., Tsuji, T., Yano, M., Kuo, G., Choo, Q. L., Houghton, M., and Oda, T.,** A high prevalence of antibody to the hepatitis C virus in patients with hepatocellular carcinoma in Japan, *Cancer,* 67, 429, 1991.

74. **Brillanti, S., Barbara, L., Miglioli, M., and Bonino, F.,** Hepatitis C virus: a possible cause of chronic hepatitis in alcoholics, *Lancet,* 2, 1390, 1989.

75. **Colombo, M., Kuo, G., Choo, Q. L., Donato, M. F., DelNinno, E., Tommasini, M. A., Dioguardi, N., and Houghton, M.,** Prevalence of antibodies to hepatitis C virus in Italian patients with hepatocellular carcinoma, *Lancet,* 2, 1006, 1989.

76. **Pares, A., Barrera, J. M., Caballeria, J., Ercilla, G., Bruguera, M., Caballeria, L., Castillo, R., and Rodes, J.,** Hepatitis C virus antibodies in chronic alcoholic patients: association with severity of liver injury, *Hepatology,* 12, 1295, 1990.

77. **Enomoto, N., Takada, A., Nakao, T., and Date, T.,** There are two major types of hepatitis C virus in Japan, *Biochem. Biophys. Res. Commun.,* 170, 1021, 1990.

78. **Truett, J., Cornfield, J., and Kannel, W.,** A multivariate analysis of the risk of coronary heart disease in Framingham, *J. Chron. Dis.,* 20, 511, 1967.

Chapter 12

ETHANOL AND COLORECTAL CANCER

Helmut K. Seitz and Ulrich A. Simanowski

TABLE OF CONTENTS

5761-6/93/$0.00 + $.50

I. EPIDEMIOLOGY

In 1974 Breslow and Enstrom[1] were the first to raise the possibility of an association between beer consumption and the occurrence of rectal cancer. In a retrospective study, average annual age-adjusted cancer mortality rates from 1950 to 1967 were correlated with per capita consumption of spirits, wine, and beer, estimated from tax receipts in 41 states of the United States and in 24 other countries. The strongest single association found was between rectal, but not colon, cancer and beer consumption.[2] Other retrospective cohort studies followed, confirming these data. McMichael et al.[3] analyzed time trends in cancer mortality from 1921 in the United States, England and Wales, Australia, and New Zealand, in relation to changes in per capita consumption of alcohol. For rectal cancer, and to a lesser extent for colon cancer, the most consistent correlate in comparison across time, and between place, sex, and age-group, was again beer intake. Similar observations have been made by Knox[4] who analyzed alcohol intake and chief causes of mortality in 20 different countries, including European countries, the U.S., Canada, and Japan; by Kono and Ikeda,[5] who found, in a retrospective study based on geographic correlations between standardized mortality ratios and alcohol consumption, over time, correlated with subsequent changes in rectal cancer, particularly among younger age groups. Finally, in a more recent study, a high-lifetime intake of beer and total alcohol was associated with an increased risk of rectal cancer, and this was independent of either socioeconomic status or diet.[6] At an individual level, various case-control studies have collected data on alcohol consumption and large bowel cancer. From 1979 to 1981, 419 patients with colon and rectal cancer and 732 controls were questioned regarding diet and alcohol.[7] Cancer cases were a population-based series reported in the South Australian Central Cancer Registry, were 30 to 74 years of age, and were residents in metropolitan Adelaide. Total alcohol intake (but not specifically beer) was associated with increased risk of both colon and rectal cancer in women. In addition, in both sexes, there was an increased risk of large intestinal cancer associated with spirit consumption. Three further case-control studies also reported an increased risk for cancer of both colon and rectum in relation to beer intake,[8-10] and two other studies failed to show an association at all,[11,12] whereas one study showed an increased risk for rectal cancer only.[13] A Japanese study also failed to detect a relationship between beer consumption and rectal cancer.[14] However, in Japan, beer consumption is low,[15] and rectal cancer might, therefore, be more related to exposure variables of greater interindividual heterogeneity. Unfortunately, some case-control studies have treated large bowel cancer as a single entity without differentiation between colon and rectum.[16-18] In these studies, only Higginson[16] observed a higher risk of rectal cancer for beer drinkers. Furthermore, two follow-up studies in Norway, one of the over 12,000 middle-aged men, the other of approximately 1700 male alcoholics, have also observed such an increased risk for beer consumers.[8,19]

In two recent studies of brewery workers, no excess risk of bowel cancer was inferred in the Copenhagen study,[20] whereas in Dublin, a twofold excess of rectal cancer was observed with beer consumption.[21] However, reexamination of the Danish data suggests that there may have been some increased risk for this group of brewery workers relative to that of social class peers.[18] Another possible explanation for the controversial results between the Copenhagen and Dublin studies was the fact that Danish beers have a significantly lower dimethylnitrosamine content than Irish beers.[22] In addition, more recently, an eighteen-year follow-up of 6230 Swedish brewery workers showed a significant increased risk of rectal cancer, while colonic carcinogenesis was not affected.[23]

Subsequently, two prospective studies have been performed in the United States with respect to alcohol consumption and large bowel cancer. In Hawaii, 8006 subjects were followed for an average of approximately 14 years. The study showed an approximate threefold risk of developing rectal, but not colon cancer, when 1 l or more of beer was ingested regularly every day.[24] Similar results were published from Southern California, where 11,888 residents of a retirement community were followed up for $4^1/_2$ years. Here daily alcohol drinkers experienced a nearly twofold increase in risk for rectal cancer.[25] Furthermore Klatsky et al.[26] studied the incidence of cancers of the colorectum in 106,203 men and women who supplied data at Northern California Kaiser Permanente Facilities, about use of alcoholic beverages from 1978 to 1984. The data suggest that total alcohol use, but no one specific beverage type, is associated with increased risk of rectal cancer. It seems highly interesting that chronic beer consumption also is a risk factor for precancerous lesions, such as colonic adenomas, especially in older subjects.[27]

Taking all these data from retrospective, prospective, and case-control studies together, chronic alcohol consumption seems to be associated with a small but significant increase of cancer risk for the rectum, but far less for the colon. This increased risk seems mainly due to beer consumption, although alcohol itself may also affect rectal carcinogenesis. In this context it should be noted that small amounts of nitrosamines have been found in beers.[28]

II. ANIMAL EXPERIMENTS

Ethanol per se is not a carcinogen.[29] However, when administered to animals in combination with a chemical carcinogen, ethanol may be cocarcinogenic for some organs under certain experimental conditions, especially when given before or together with the carcinogen, or it may act as a tumor promoter when administered after tumor initiation.[30] Factors which influence the effect of ethanol on carcinogenesis in animals include the type of carcinogen used, as well as the dose, duration, and means of carcinogen and ethanol administration.[31]

Table 1 summarizes the results of chronic ethanol ingestion on chemically induced colorectal carcinogenesis in rats. In two of the nine studies, ethanol

TABLE 1
Effect of Ethanol on Chemically Induced Colorectal Carcinogenesis in Rats

Carcinogen	Ethanol administration	Ethanol effect	Ref.
DMH, s.c.	6% l.d. (36% total calories), preinduction	Increased rectal but not colonic tumors	37
DMH, s.c.	5% d.w., induction	No effect	32
DMH, s.c.	5% d.w., preinduction/induction	No effect	33
DMH, s.c.	6% l.d. (36% total calories), preinduction	No effect	38
AMMN, i.r.	6% l.d. (36% total calories), preinduction/induction	Increased rectal tumors	42
AM, s.c.	l.d. (9%, 18% total calories ethanol) (12%, 23% total calories beer), preinduction/ induction	High ethanol inhibits tumors in the right but not in the left colon, while low ethanol enhances tumors in the left colon but not in the right colon. No effect of beer.	34
AM, s.c.	l.d. (11%, 22%, 33% total calories), preinduction/induction/postinduction	Inhibition of tumor development in the left but less in the right colon. Higher ethanol intake has a stronger inhibitory effect. No effect when ethanol is given in the postinduction phase.	35
AM, s.c. (high dose)	l.d. (33% total calories), preinduction/induction	Inhibition	36
AMMN, i.r.	i.g. (4.8 g/kg b.wt./day), preinduction/induction	Increased rectal tumors. Carcinogenesis was further stimulated when cyanamide, an acetaldehyde dehydrogenase inhibitor was additionally administered.	43

Note: DMH, 1,2-dimethylhydrazine; AMMN, azetoxymethyl-methylnitrosamine; AM, azoxymethane; s.c., subcutaneously; i.r., intrarectally; l.d., liquid diets; d.w., drinking water; i.g., intragastrically.

was given in the drinking water, and the results of these experiments have, therefore, to be questioned.[32,33] When the two procarcinogens, dimethylhydrazine (DMH) and azoxymethane (AOM), have been used to induce colorectal tumors, different results have been reported, mainly depending on the experimental conditions. In these studies it is important to note that both compounds need metabolic activation by cytochrome P-450-dependent microsomal enzymes to become carcinogenic. The results of these studies depend on the ethanol dose used, and on the timing of ethanol administration.[34-37] It must be emphasized that in one experiment with DMH, ethanol ingestion only enhanced tumor development in the rectum (last 5 cm), but not in the remaining large intestine.[37] In this study, ethanol was given during acclimatization and initiation, but at the time of procarcinogen application, ethanol was not present in the body. In a similar study by McGarrity et al.,[38] these results could not be confirmed.

The conclusions derived from those experiments with DMH and AOM are

1. The modulation of experimental colonic tumorigenesis by chronic dietary beer and ethanol consumption is due to alcohol rather than to other beverage constituents.
2. The tumorigenesis in the right and left colorectum is affected differently by alcohol, and may depend on the levels of alcohol consumption. Thus, high alcohol intake (18 to 33% of total calories) inhibits carcinogenesis in the right colon and has little or no effect on the left colon, while lower ethanol consumption (9 to 12% of total calories) enhances tumor development in the left colon without effect on the right colon.
3. Ethanol affects carcinogenesis during the preinduction and/or induction phase, including carcinogen metabolism, but not during the postinduction phase (promotion).
4. An interaction between ethanol and procarcinogen metabolism does occur, and this may influence tumor incidences.

In addition, in two more recent animal experiments, the primary carcinogen acetoxymethyl-methylnitrosamine (AMMN) was used to induce rectal tumors. This carcinogen does not need metabolic activation to exert its carcinogenic power, and is applied locally to the rectal mucosa of rats.[39] The animals were endoscopied regularly,[40,41] and tumor occurrence was registered. Alcohol was given continuously before (preinduction) and during tumor initiation, and during tumor promotion. Since chronic ethanol administration, given either as a liquid diet or intragastrically, accelerates the appearance of rectal tumors induced by AMMN,[42,43] it seems most likely that alcohol enhances carcinogenesis, at least in part, by local mechanisms in the rectal mucosa and not only by increasing the activation of procarcinogens.

III. POSSIBLE MECHANISMS BY WHICH ETHANOL MAY AFFECT COLORECTAL CARCINOGENESIS

Ethanol may increase the susceptibility of various tissues to chemical carcinogenesis by a variety of mechanisms, such as activation of chemical procarcinogens, altering the metabolism and/or distribution of carcinogens, interference with the repair of carcinogen-mediated DNA alkylation and the immune response, stimulating cellular regeneration, and exacerbation of dietary deficiencies (Figure 1).[22,30,44] With respect to the effect of ethanol on colorectal carcinogenesis, two factors may be of particular interest, namely increased activation of procarcinogens and local ethanol-mediated effects in

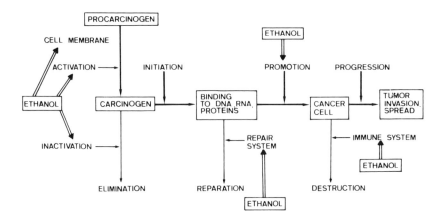

FIGURE 1. Simplified scheme of two step carcinogenesis and possible effects of ethanol. (From Seitz, H. K. and Simanowski, U. A., in *Colorectal Cancer. From Pathogenesis to Prevention,* Seitz, H. K., Simanowski, U. A., and Wright, N. A., Eds., Springer-Verlag, Berlin, 1989, 181. With permission.)

the rectal mucosa, leading to tissue injury and hyperregeneration which favor carcinogenesis.

A. EFFECT OF ETHANOL ON THE ACTIVATION OF PROCARCINOGENS

Many environmental carcinogens exist in their procarcinogenic form and require metabolic activation by microsomal cytochrome P-450-dependent enzymes.[45] The activated procarcinogens exhibit a high capacity to bind to macromolecules such as DNA, ribonucleic acid (RNA), or proteins, and thus lead to initiation of the carcinogenic process. Induction of microsomal enzyme activities increases the mutagenic effect of many compounds in the Ames salmonella mutagenesis assay.[46] Since the extent of metabolic activation of various secondary carcinogens can be correlated with microsomal enzyme activities,[47,48] factors such as environmental pollutants, drugs, and diet, which can influence the activity of this enzyme system, are also expected to affect tumor formation in animals exposed to carcinogens. In the light of this fact, it seems important that ethanol is a well-known microsomal enzyme "inducer" leading to enhanced procarcinogen activation in the liver and in other tissues,[49-53] but probably not in the colon.[54] Both ethanol and procarcinogens are metabolized via cytochrome P-450-dependent microsomal pathways, and therefore interactions between the two compounds occur (Figure 2).

If ethanol and a procarcinogen are present at the same time, ethanol inhibits the activation of the procarcinogen (Figure 2B), and carcinogenesis may also be inhibited. During chronic ethanol consumption, microsomal enzyme activity increases, and microsomal ethanol oxidation is enhanced. Under these conditions, the activation of the procarcinogen is still inhibited (Figure

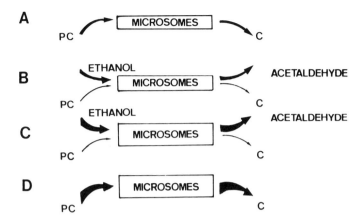

FIGURE 2. Interaction between microsomal metabolism of ethanol and procarcinogens: (A) In the normal situation, a procarcinogen [PC] is activated by microsomes to its active metabolite. In the presence of ethanol, the microsomal activation of PC to ultimative carcinogens [C] is inhibited (B), while ethanol is metabolized to acetaldehyde. Chronic ethanol ingestion increases microsomal cytochrome P-450 and microsomal enzyme activity. Thus, in the presence of ethanol, microsomal ethanol oxidation is enhanced, and procarcinogen activation is still inhibited (C). Following withdrawal of ethanol, procarcinogen activation is enhanced (depending on the time interval between the last drink and procarcinogen exposure), due to microsomal enzyme induction (D). (From Seitz, H. K. and Simanowski, U. A., in *Colorectal Cancer. From Pathogenesis to Prevention,* Seitz, H. K., Simanowski, U. A., and Wright, N. A., Eds., Springer-Verlag, Berlin, 1989, 181. With permission.)

2C). However, when ethanol is withdrawn from the organism at this stage of microsomal enzyme induction, an increased activation of the procarcinogen occurs (Figure 2D), possibly resulting in an enhancement of carcinogenesis. Thus, it has been shown that ethanol inhibits the hepatic microsomal activation of AOM[55] and of dimethylnitrosamine (DMN),[55,56] while activation of these two procarcinogens is strikingly enhanced following chronic ethanol consumption when ethanol is withdrawn.[55,57]

The conversion of AOM to methylazoxymethanol (MAM) is catalyzed by a microsomal cytochrome P-450-dependent *N*-hydroxylase in the liver[58] and in the colon.[59-61] Pretreatment of animals with microsomal enzyme inducers such as phenobarbital, chrysene,[58] or ethanol[55] leads to an increased metabolism of AOM to carbon monoxide, probably through an induction of the microsomal enzyme. On the other hand, agents which inhibit DMH metabolism[62] also inhibit DMH-induced colorectal carcinogenesis *in vivo.*[63] It therefore seems possible that the effect of ethanol observed in the animal experiment with DMH and AOM can be attributed, at least in part, to the alcohol-related changes in the metabolism of the procarcinogen. In the light of these facts, it is understandable that high-ethanol intake leading to high-ethanol blood concentrations results in an inhibition of colorectal carcinogenesis, and low-alcohol intake does not. The presence of ethanol during tumor initiation also inhibits tumor development,[35] while its absence at a stage of enzyme induction enhances the carcinogenic process.[37] However, it is not clear why ethanol, under certain experimental conditions, stimulates tumor occurrence in the left colon and rectum, but not in the right colon.[34,37] An excellent summary on the activation of colonic procarcinogens by colonic microsomal enzymes has been recently prescribed by Strobel et al.[64]

Another enzyme possibly involved in DMH metabolism is alcohol dehydrogenase (ADH). It has been suggested by Schoenthal[65] that the conversion of MAM to the diazonium ion is enzymatically catalyzed by ADH. This concept is supported by the observation that the incidence of DMH- or MAM-induced intestinal tumors is paralleled by the activity of intestinal mucosal ADH.[66] Both tumor yield and ADH activity are highest in the large intestine and in the duodenum, but low in the jejunum or ileum.[66,67] Furthermore, ADH inhibitors, such as pyrazole[68,69] or butylated hydroxyanisole (BHA), inhibit both colonic carcinogenesis and colonic ADH activity.[70] However, it was shown recently by Fiala et al.,[71] in the ADH-lacking deer mouse, that MAM can also be metabolized by a nonADH pathway. Thus, the inhibitory effect of BHA and pyrazole on chemically induced colonic carcinogenesis was possibly due to an inhibition of microsomal cytochrome P-450-dependent enzyme activities,[72,73] and not to their effect on ADH.

B. LOCAL MECHANISMS

The fact that chronic ethanol ingestion enhances rectal carcinogenesis induced by the local application of the primary carcinogen, AMMN, which does not require metabolic activation, suggests that alcohol also acts by local mechanisms in the rectal mucosa, and not by enhancing the activation of procarcinogens alone.[42,43]

Bile acids, which may be involved as tumor promoters in colorectal carcinogenesis,[74] do not play an important role in ethanol-associated colorectal cancer, since chronic ethanol consumption, although increasing biliary bile acid output,[75] does not change fecal bile-acid excretion and pattern.[37,76]

However, one important feature in intestinal carcinogenesis is the change in mucosal cell-renewal modulating response to chemical carcinogens.[77] Utilizing the metaphase arrest technique with vincristine, cell proliferation was selectively increased in the rectal mucosa of chronically ethanol-fed rats when compared to controls.[78] A similar stimulatory effect of alcohol on cell regeneration has already been reported for the esophagus, where ethanol also acts as a cocarcinogen.[79] A concomitant increase in the proliferative compartment of the crypt toward the intestinal lumen appears to be predictive of increased susceptibility to chemical carcinogens.[80] Cell regeneration is triggered by polyamines, and their synthesis is regulated by the activity of ornithine decarboxylase (ODC). ODC activity was found to be significantly enhanced after chronic ethanol consumption, but falls rapidly in the colonic mucosa after cessation of the ethanol intake.[43,81] Most recent studies from our laboratory show an additional age-dependent effect of ethanol on rectal cell regeneration. The ethanol-stimulating effect on crypt cell production rate increases strikingly with age.[82]

The rectal hyperproliferation observed after alcohol ingestion may be of secondary compensatory nature, since light microscopy of rectal mucosa from alcoholics reveals superficial cell damage, which returns to normal following alcohol abstinence for two weeks,[83] and also since the life span of functional epithelial cells in the rectal crypt is reduced.[78]

Some gastrointestinal hormones such as gastrin, enteroglucagon (EG), and peptide YY may cause hyperregeneration in the intestinal mucosa. Acute and chronic ethanol consumption increases serum concentrations of EG,[84] which could lead to an additional stimulation of cell regeneration in the colon without explaining the difference in cell turnover between the right and the left colon following ethanol ingestion.

It has been suspected that acetaldehyde (AA), a rather toxic metabolite of ethanol, may cause the rectal tissue injury observed in the alcoholic. Significantly high concentrations of AA have been found in the distal colon after alcohol application.[85] These AA concentrations were significantly elevated compared to the proximal colon and to the liver when calculated per gram of tissue. In addition, increased ADH activity has been found in the mucosa derived from the distal colon when compared to the proximal large intestine,[37] which may favor AA accumulation through ethanol oxidation. However, it seems impossible that the colonic ADH with its low activity is capable of producing the striking accumulation of AA in the rectum. It is therefore hypothesized that bacterial production of AA, especially in the distal colon (where the highest bacteria counts occur), may be responsible for the AA formation, and that the observed ADH activity in the mucosal cytoplasm may be due, at least in part, to a contamination by bacterial ADH. This theory is supported by the fact that various aldehydes, including AA, can be detected *in vitro* following incubation of feces with ethanol.[86]

Most recent data on the effect of ethanol on AMMN-induced rectal cancer further support the concept that AA is involved in ethanol-associated rectal carcinogenesis. Furthermore, mucosal AA concentration in the rectum and in the colon was paralleled by fecal bacterial counts, which suggests the concept that bacteria produce AA.

Animals that received ethanol and cyanamide, a potent AA-dehydrogenase inhibitor, exhibited an earlier occurrence of rectal tumors compared to animals that received ethanol alone.[53] In these experiments, AA concentrations were significantly elevated in the serum and in the colonic mucosa following the application of cyanamide. A possible pathogenesis sequence of ethanol-associated rectal carcinogenesis is illustrated in Figure 3.

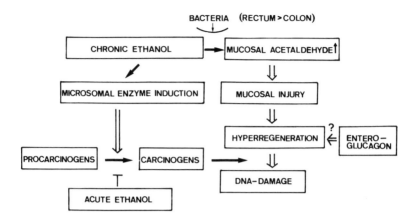

FIGURE 3.   Hypothesis of ethanol-associated rectal cocarcinogenesis.

IV. CONCLUSION

The effect of chronic ethanol consumption on chemically induced colo-rectal carcinogenesis is complex, and varies with the experimental conditions. Although conflicting results have been reported, ethanol may have a cocar-cinogenic effect on the distal colon or rectum in animal experiments. Ethanol may both enhance and inhibit colorectal carcinogenesis by:

1.   Interfering with the activation of procarcinogens
2.   Stimulating carcinogenesis by local mechanisms possibly mediated by AA

ACKNOWLEDGMENTS

Original studies have been supported by the Deutsche Forschungsge-meinschaft (Se 333 /1, 2, 4-1, 6-1, 2), and by the Gerhardt Katsch Studienfond der Deutschen Gesellschaft für Verdauungs- und Stoffwechselerkrankungen.

REFERENCES

1.   **Breslow, N. E. and Enstrom, J. E.,** Geographic correlations between mortality rates and alcohol, tobacco consumption in the United States, *J. Natl. Cancer Inst.,* 53, 631, 1974.
2.   **Enstrom, J. E.,** Colorectal cancer and beer drinking, *Br. J. Cancer,* 35, 674, 1977.
3.   **McMichael, A. J., Potter, J. D., and Hetzel, B. S.,** Time trends in colorectal cancer mortality in relation to food and alcohol consumption: USA, UK, Australia, and New Zealand, *Int. J. Epidemiol.,* 8, 295, 1979.

4. **Knox, E. G.,** Foods and diseases, *Br. J. Prevent. Soc. Med.,* 31, 71, 1977.

5. **Kono, S. and Ikeda, M.,** Correlation between cancer mortality and alcoholic beverages in Japan, *Br. J. Cancer,* 40, 449, 1979.

6. **Freudenheim, J. L., Graham, S., Marshall, J. R., Haughes, B. P., and Wilkinson, G.,** Life time alcohol intake and risk of rectal cancer in Western New York, *Nutr. Cancer,* 13, 101, 1990.

7. **Potter, J. D. and McMichael, A. J.,** Diet and cancer of the colon and rectum: a case control study, *J. Natl. Cancer Inst.,* 76, 557, 1986.

8. **Bjelke, E.,** Epidemiological Studies of Cancer of the Stomach, Colon and Rectum, Thesis, University of Michigan, Ann Arbor, 1973.

9. **Kato, I., Tominaga, S., and Ikari, A.,** A case control study of male colorectal cancer in Aichi Prefecture, Japan: with special reference to occupational activity lecel, drinking habits and family history, *Jpn. J. Cancer Res.,* 81, 115, 1990.

10. **Wynder, E. L. and Shigematsu, T.,** Environmental factors of cancer of the colon and rectum, *Cancer,* 20, 1520, 1967.

11. **Graham, S., Dayal, H., Swanson, M., Mittelman, A., and Wilkinson, G.,** Diet in the epidemiology of cancer of the colon and rectum, *J. Natl. Cancer Inst.,* 61, 709, 1978.

12. **Kabat, G. C., Howson, C. P., and Wynder, E. L.,** Beer consumption and rectal cancer, *Int. J. Epidemiol.,* 15, 494, 1986.

13. **Kune, S., Kune, G. A., and Watson, L. F.,** Case-control study of alcoholic beverages as etiological factors: the Melbourne colorectal cancer study, *Nutr. Cancer,* 9, 43, 1987.

14. **Wynder, E. L., Kajitani, T., Ishakawa, S., Dodo, H., and Takano, A.,** Environmental factors of the cancer of the colon and rectum. II. Japanese epidemiological data, *Cancer,* 23, 1210, 1969.

15. International Statistics on Alcoholic Beverages, Vol. 27, Finnish Foundation for Alcohol Studies, Helsinki, 1977.

16. **Higginson, J.,** Etiological factors in gastrointestinal cancer in man, *J. Natl. Cancer Inst.,* 37, 527, 1966.

17. **Pernu, J.,** An epidemiological study on cancer of the digestive organs and respiratory system, *Ann. Med. Int. Fenn.,* Suppl. 49, 33, 1, 1960.

18. **Potter, J. D., McMichael, A. J., and Hartshorne, J. M.,** Alcohol and beer consumption in relation to cancers of bowel and lung: an extended correlation analysis, *J. Chronic Dis.,* 35, 833, 1982.

19. **Sundby, P.,** *Alcoholism and mortality,* Rutgers Center on Alcohol Studies, New Brunswick, 1967, p. 107.

20. **Jensen, O. M.,** Cancer morbidity and cause of death among Danish brewery workers, *Int. J. Cancer,* 23, 454, 1979.

21. **Dean, G., MacLennan, R., McLoughlin, H., and Shelley, E.,** The cause of death of blue collar workers at a Dublin brewery 1954–1973, *Br. J. Cancer,* 40, 581, 1979.

22. **Lieber, C. S., Garro, A. J., Leo, M. A., Mak, K. M., and Worner, T. M.,** Alcohol and cancer, *Hepatology,* 6, 1005, 1986.

23. **Carstensen, J. M., Bygren, L. O., and Hatschek, T.,** Cancer incidence among Swedish brewery workers, *Int. J. Cancer,* 45, 393, 1990.

24. **Pollack, E. S., Nomura, A. M. Y., Heilbrun, L. K., Stemmermann, G. N., and Green, S. B.,** Prospective study of alcohol consumption and cancer, *N. Engl. J. Med.,* 310, 617, 1984.

25. **Wu, A. H., Paganini-Hill, A., Ross, R. K., and Henderson, B. E.,** Alcohol, physical activity and other risk factors for colorectal cancer: a prospective study, *Br. J. Cancer,* 55, 687, 1987.

26. **Klatsky, A. L., Armstrong, M. A., Friedman, G. D., and Hiatt, R. A.,** The relations of alcoholic beverage use to colon and rectal cancer, *Am. J. Epidemiol.,* 128, 1007, 1988.

27. **Kikendall, J. W., Bowen, P. E., Burgess, M. B., Magnetti, C., Woodward, J., and Langenberg, P.,** Cigarettes and alcohol as independent risk factors for colonic adenomas, *Gastroenterology,* 97, 660, 1989.

28. **Spiegelhalder, B., Eisenbrand, G., and Preussmann, R.,** Contamination of beer with trace quantities of N-nitrosodimethylamine, *Food Cosmet. Toxicol.,* 17, 29, 1979.

29. **Ketcham, A. S., Wexler, H., and Mantel, N.,** Affects of alcohol in mouse neoplasia, *Cancer Res.,* 23, 667, 1963.

30. **Seitz, H. K. and Simanowski, U. A.,** Alcohol and carcinogenesis, *Annu. Rev. Nutr.,* 8, 99, 1988.

31. **Seitz, H. K.,** Ethanol and carcinogenesis, *Alcohol Related Diseases in Gastroenterology,* Seitz, H. K. and Kommerell, B., Eds., Springer-Verlag, 1985, 192.

32. **Howarth, A. E. and Pihl, E.,** High fat diet promotes and causes distal shift of experimental rat colonic cancer — beer and alcohol do not, *Nutr. Cancer,* 6, 229, 1985.

33. **Nelson, R. L. and Samelson, S. L.,** Neither dietary ethanol nor beer augments experimental colon tumors in rats, *Dis. Colon Rectum,* 28, 460, 1985.

34. **Hamilton, S. R., Hyland, J., McAvinchey, D., Chaudhry, Y., Hartka, L., Kim, H. T., Cichon, P., Floyd, J., Turjman, N., Kessie, G., Nair, P. P., and Dick, J.,** Effects of chronic dietary beer and ethanol consumption on experimental colonic carcinogenesis by azoxymethane in rats, *Cancer Res.,* 47, 1551, 1987.

35. **Hamilton, S. R., Sohn, O. S., and Fiala, E. S.,** Effects of timing and quantity of chronic dietary ethanol consumption on azoxymethane-induced colonic carcinogenesis and azoxymethane metabolism in Fischer 344 rats, *Cancer Res.,* 47, 4305, 1987.

36. **Hamilton, S. R., Sohns, O. S., and Fiala, E. S.,** Inhibition by dietary ethanol of experimental colonic carcinogenesis induced by high-dose azoxymethane in F344 rats, *Cancer Res.,* 48, 3313, 1988.

37. **Seitz, H. K., Czygan, P., Waldherr, R., Veith, S., Raedsch, R., Kässmodel, H., and Kommerell, B.,** Enhancement of 1,2-dimethylhydrazine induced rectal carcinogenesis following chronic ethanol consumption in the rat, *Gastroenterology,* 86, 886, 1984.

38. **McGarrity, T. J., Pfeiffer, L. P., Colony, P. C., and Pegg, A. E.,** The effects of chronic ethanol administration on polyamine content during DMH-induced colorectal carcinogenesis in the rat, *Carcinogenesis,* 9, 2093, 1988.

39. **Wiessler, M.,** Chemie der nitrosamine. II. Synthese a-funktioneller dimethylnitrosamine, *Tetrahedron Lett.,* 30, 2575, 1975.

40. **Merz, R., Wagner, I., Habs, M., and Schmähl, D.,** Endoscopic diagnosis of chemically induced autochthonous colonic tumors in rats, *Hepatogastroenterology,* 28, 53, 1981.

41. **Narisawa, T., Wong, C. Q., and Weisburger, J. H.,** Evaluation of endoscopic examination of colon tumors in rats, *Dig. Dis.,* 20, 928, 1975.

42. **Garzon, F. T., Simanowski, U. A., Berger, M. R., Schmähl, D., Kommerell, B., and Seitz, H. K.,** Acetoxymethyl-methylnitrosamine (AMMN) induced colorectal carcinogenesis is stimulated by chronic alcohol consumption, *Alcohol Alcohol,* Suppl. 1, 501, 1987.

43. **Seitz, H. K., Simanowski, U. A., Garzon, F. T., Rideout, J. M., Peters, T. J., Koch, A., Berger, M. R., Einecke, H., and Maiwald, M.,** Possible role of acetaldehyde in ethanol-related rectal cocarcinogenesis in the rat, *Gastroenterology,* 98, 406, 1990.

44. **Seitz, H. K. and Simanowski, U. A.,** Ethanol and gastrointestinal carcinogenesis, *Alcohol.: Clin. Exp. Res.,* 10, 33, 1986.

45. **Guengerich, F. P.,** Polymorphism of cytochrome P-450 in humans, *Trends Pharmacol. Sciences,* 10, 107, 1989.

46. **Ames, B. N., McCann, J., and Yamasaki, E.,** Methods for detecting carcinogens and mutagens with the salmonella/mammalian-microsomes mutagenicity test, *Mutat. Res.,* 31, 347, 1975.

47. **Conney, A. G.,** Induction of microsomal enzymes by foreign chemicals and carcinogenesis by polycyclic hydrocarbons, *Cancer Res.,* 42, 4875, 1982.

48. **Felton, J. S. and Nebert, D. W.**, Mutagenesis of certain activated carcinogens *in vitro* associated with genetically mediated increases in monooxygenase activity and cytochrome P-450, *J. Biol. Chem.*, 250, 6769, 1975.

49. **Lieber, C. S.**, Ethanol metabolism and pathophysiology of alcoholic liver disease, in *Alcohol Related Diseases in Gastroenterology*, Seitz, H. K. and Kommerell, B., Eds., Springer-Verlag, Berlin, 1985, 19.

50. **Seitz, H. K. and Simanowski, U. A.**, Metabolic and nutritional effects of alcohol, in *Nutritional Toxicology*, Vol. II, Hathcock, J. N., Ed., Academic Press, New York, 1987, 63.

51. **Seitz, H. K., Garro, A. J., and Lieber, C. S.**, Effect of chronic ethanol ingestion on intestinal metabolism and mutagenicity of benzo[α]pyrene, *Biochem. Biophys. Res. Commun.*, 85, 1061, 1978.

52. **Seitz, H. K., Garro, A. J., and Lieber, C. S.**, Sex-dependent effect of chronic ethanol consumption in rats on hepatic microsome mediated mutagenicity of Benzo[α]pyrene, *Cancer Lett.*, 13, 97, 1981.

53. **Seitz, H. K., Garro, A. J., and Lieber, C. S.**, Enhanced pulmonary and intestinal activation of procarcinogens and mutagens after chronic ethanol consumption in the rat, *Eur. J. Clin. Invest.*, 11, 33, 1981.

54. **Seitz, H. K., Bösche, J., Czygan, P., Veith, S., and Kommerell, B.**, Microsomal ethanol oxidation in the colonic mucosa of the rat: effect of chronic ethanol ingestion, *Arch. Pharmacol.*, 310, 81, 1982.

55. **Sohn, O. A., Fiala, E. S., Puz, C., Hamilton, S. R., and Williams, G. M.**, Enhancement of rat liver microsomal metabolism of azoxymethane to methylazoxymethanol by chronic ethanol administration: similarity to the microsomal metabolism of *N*-nitrosomethylamine, *Cancer Res.*, 47, 3123, 1987.

56. **Peng, R., Yong-Tu, Y., and Yang, C. S.**, The induction and competitive inhibition of a high affinity microsomal nitrosodimethylamine demethylase by ethanol, *Carcinogenesis*, 3, 1457, 1982.

57. **Garro, A. J., Seitz, H. K., and Lieber, C. S.**, Enhancement of dimethylnitrosamine metabolism and activation to a mutagen following chronic ethanol consumption in the rat, *Cancer Res.*, 41, 120, 1981.

58. **Fiala, E. S.**, Investigations into the metabolism and mode of action of the colon carcinogen 1,2 DMH and azoxymethane, *Cancer*, 40, 4236, 1977.

59. **Glauert, H. P. and Bennink, M. R.**, Metabolism of 1,2-dimethylhydrazine by cultured rat colon epithelial cells, *Nutr. Cancer*, 5, 78, 1983.

60. **Oravec, C. T., Jones, C. A., and Huberman, E.**, Activation of the colon carcinogen DMH in a rat colon cell-mediated mutagenesis assay, *Cancer Res.*, 46, 5068, 1986.

61. **Wargovich, M. J. and Felkner, I. C.**, Metabolic activation of DMH by colonic microsomes: a process influenced by dietary fat, *Nutr. Cancer*, 4, 146, 1982.

62. **Fiala, E. S., Bobota, G., Kulakis, C., Wattenberg, W., and Weisburger, J. H.**, Effects of disulfiram and related compounds on the metabolism *in vivo* of the colon carcinogen 1,2-dimethylhydrazine, *Biochem. Pharmacol.*, 26, 1763, 1977.

63. **Wattenberg, L. W.**, Inhibition of dimethylhydrazine-induced neoplasia of the large intestine by disulfiram, *J. Natl. Cancer Inst.*, 54, 1005, 1975.

64. **Strobel, H. W., Hammard, D. K., and White, T. B.**, Colonic microsomal enzymes and their role in colorectal cocarcinogenesis, in *Colorectal Cancer*, Seitz, H. K., Simanowski, U. A., and Wright, N. A., Eds., Springer-Verlag, Berlin, 1989, 217.

65. **Schoenthal, R.**, The mechanism of cocarcinogenic nitro- and related compounds, *Br. J. Cancer*, 28, 436, 1973.

66. **Grab, D. J. and Zedeck, M. S.**, Organ specific effects of the carcinogen methylazoxymethanol related to the metabolism by nicotinamide adenosine dinucleotide dependent dehydrogenases, *Cancer Res.*, 37, 4182, 1977.

67. **Mezey, E.**, Intestinal function in chronic alcoholism, *Ann. N.Y. Acad. Sci.*, 252, 215, 1975.

68. **Zedeck, M. S.**, Colon carcinogenesis and the role of dehydrogenase activity: inhibition of tumorigenesis by pyrazole, *Prev. Med.*, 9, 346, 1980.

69. **Zedeck, M. S. and Tan, Q. H.**, Effect of pyrazole on tumor induction by methylazoxymethanol (MAM) acetate: relationship to metabolism of MAM, *Pharmacologist*, 20, 174, 1978.

70. **Wattenberg, L. W. and Sparnens, V. L.**, Inhibitory effects of butylated hydroxyanisole on methylazoxymethanol acetate-induced neoplasia of the large intestine and on nicotinamide adenine dinucleotide dependent alcohol dehydrogenase activity in mice, *J. Natl. Cancer Inst.*, 63, 219, 1979.

71. **Fiala, E. S., Caswell, N., Sohn, O. S., Felder, M. R., McCoy, G. D., and Weisburger, J. H.**, Non-alcohol dehydrogenase-mediated metabolism of methylazoxymethanol in the deer mouse. Peromyscus maniculatus, *Cancer Res.*, 44, 2885, 1984.

72. **Fiala, E. S., Kulakis, C., Christiansen, G., and Weisburger, J. H.**, Inhibition of the metabolism of the colon carcinogen azomethane by pyrazole, *Cancer Res.*, 38, 4515, 1978.

73. **Stohs, S. J. and Wu, C. L. J.**, Effect of various xenobiotics and steroids on aryl hydrocarbon hydroxylase of intestinal and hepatic microsomes from male rats, *Pharmacology*, 25, 237, 1982.

74. **Cohen, B. I. and Deschner, E. E.**, The role of bile acid in colorectal carcinogenesis, in *Colorectal Cancer*, Seitz, H. K., Simanowski, U. A., Wright, N. A., Eds., Springer-Verlag, Berlin, 1989, 125.

75. **Sieg, A. and Seitz, H. K.**, Increased production, hepatic conjugation, and biliary secretion of bilirubin in the rat following chronic ethanol consumption, *Gastroenterology*, 93, 261, 1987.

76. **Cohen, B. I. and Raicht, R. F.**, Sterol metabolism in the rat: effect of alcohol on sterol metabolism in two strains of rats, *Alcoholism*, 5, 225, 1981.

77. **Simanowski, U. A., Wright, N. A., and Seitz, H. K.**, Increased cellular regeneration in colorectal carcinogenesis, in *Colorectal Cancer*, Seitz, H. K., Simanowski, U. A., and Wright, N. A., Eds., Springer-Verlag, Berlin, 1989, 225.

78. **Simanowski, U. A., Seitz, H. K., Baier, B., Kommerell, B., Schmidt-Gayk, H., and Wright, N. A.**, Chronic ethanol consumption selectively stimulates rectal cell proliferation in the rat, *Gut*, 27, 278, 1986.

79. **Mak, K. M., Leo, M. A., and Lieber, C. S.**, Effect of ethanol and vitamin A deficiency on epithelial cell proliferation and structure in the rat esophagus, *Gastroenterology*, 93, 362, 1987.

80. **Lipkin, M.**, Biomarkers in the identification of high risk groups, in *Colorectal Cancer*, Seitz, H. K., Simanowski, U. A., and Wright, N. A., Eds., Springer-Verlag, Berlin, 1989, 73.

81. **Hamilton, S. R. and Luk, G. D.**, Induction of colonic mucosal ornithine decarboxylase activity by chronic dietary ethanol consumption in the rat, *Gastroenterology*, (Abstr.), 92, 1423, 1987.

82. **Simanowski, U. A., Suter, P., Russell, R. M., and Seitz, H. K.**, Cell regeneration in the rat rectum is strikingly enhanced with age, *Alcohol.: Clin. Exp. Res.*, 14, 444, 1990.

83. **Brozinski, S., Fami, K., Grosberg, J. J.**, Alcohol ingestion-induced changes in the human rectal mucosa: light and electron microscopic studies, *Dis. Colon Rectum*, 21, 329, 1979.

84. **Simanowski, U. A., Hubalek, K., Ghatei, M. A., Bloom, S. R., Polak, J. M., and Seitz, H. K.**, Effects of acute and chronic ethanol administration on the gastrointestinal hormones gastrin, enteroglucagon, pancreatic glucagon and PYY in the rat, *Digestion*, 42, 167, 1989.

85. **Seitz, H. K., Simanowski, U. A., Garzon, F. T., and Peters, T. J.,** Alcohol and cancer, *Hepatology,* 7, 616, 1987.
86. **Levitt, M. D., Doizaki, W., and Levine, A. S.,** Hypothesis: metabolic activity of the colonic bacteria influences organ injury from ethanol, *Hepatology,* 2, 598, 1982.

Chapter 13

ALCOHOL AND CANCER OF THE PANCREAS

Ruud A. Woutersen and Corjan J. T. Visser

TABLE OF CONTENTS

I. INTRODUCTION

In most Western countries, pancreatic cancer is relatively frequent.[1-3] In the United States, pancreatic cancer is the second most common gastrointestinal malignancy, and the fourth common cause of cancer death.[1,2,4] In the Netherlands, pancreatic cancer in males ranks third among gastrointestinal and fifth among all cancer deaths, while in females it ranks third and sixth, respectively.[3] The mortality rate for pancreatic cancer is similar to its incidence because of its extremely bad prognosis.[2,5,6] The bad prognosis is mainly due to the lack of early symptoms. The prognosis of pancreatic cancer may be improved by a better understanding of its etiology and pathogenesis. Up to now, however, epidemiological and toxicological studies have not identified a specific factor responsible for the development of pancreatic cancer.[2,5,7] Therefore, it is believed that dietary and lifestyle factors such as fat, protein, and alcohol, which are thought to promote the effects of environmental carcinogens, play an important role in the etiology of this highly fatal form of cancer.[1,2,7-14] In this chapter, a review will be presented of the data available to date about the role of alcohol in the development of pancreatic cancer.

II. EPIDEMIOLOGY

In a series of 280 cases of pancreatic cancer, Dörken[15] observed that 30 (11%) had a history of regular to heavy alcohol consumption. This finding was confirmed by Burch and Ansari,[16] who reported that 54 (65%) of 83 patients with pancreatic cancer diagnosed in the New Orleans Veterans Hospital between 1960 and 1966 had an average daily consumption of 57 to 85 g of alcohol.

These findings have stimulated epidemiologists to investigate the possible relationship between alcohol consumption and pancreatic cancer. In the present chapter these studies will be reviewed.

A. CORRELATION STUDIES

In a state-by-state comparison of cancer mortality and alcohol consumption in the United States, Breslow and Enstrom[17] reported significant correlations (males 0.42; females 0.61) between per capita consumption of alcohol and pancreas cancer mortality.

Kondo and Ikeda[18] reported a positive correlation between consumption of saki or whiskey with pancreatic cancer mortality, but they found no association between alcohol consumption and esophageal cancer, where the risk has been demonstrated to be strong.

Hinds and co-workers[19] studied the incidence rate of pancreatic cancer from the Hawaii Tumor Registry for five ethnic groups in Hawaii in relation to alcohol and tobacco consumption. A marginally significant association was observed with beer consumption, which disappeared after adjustment for sex.

Other correlation studies revealed no or inconsistent correlations between alcohol and pancreatic cancer mortality rates.[18-21]

B. COHORT STUDIES (TABLE 1)

The relationship between alcohol intake and cancer at a variety of sites has been assessed in several large cohort studies. In most studies, detailed information on type of beverage, amount drunk, and smoking was not available. Tobacco smoke is a cause of cancer at sites such as the pancreas, that may also be related to alcohol consumption.[22] Most of the cohort studies have been of the retrospective (historical) type, comparing cancer incidence in groups with high-alcohol intake with that of the general population.

Nine prospective cohort studies have been reported in which the risk at many different sites was examined in persons with high-alcohol intake.[23-32] None reported a significant number of pancreas cancer cases over that expected.

Klatsky et al.[33] found a significantly elevated risk in a cohort study of members of a health plan. They found six pancreatic cancer deaths in "heavy" drinkers (six or more drinks daily) compared to two cases in nondrinkers (relative risk, 3.0).

Adelstein et al.[28] observed only 15 cancers of the entire digestive tract among 1211 alcoholics; 11 were expected. Of 4370 Finnish alcoholics, four cases of pancreatic cancer were observed compared with two expected.[26] An analysis of proportional mortality in the 909 deaths identified among 1382 known alcoholics resulted in the observation of three deaths compared with 5.2 expected.[27] In Japan, a large population sample was surveyed and followed over time to observe more than 200 cases. While no overall effect of alcohol consumption was found, a very strong effect (relative risk, 7.2) was found among the small group of Japanese whiskey drinkers.[34-36]

Heuch et al.[37] reported a cohort of 16,713 Norwegians. Among frequent alcohol users, five pancreatic cancer cases were observed, whereas the tobacco-adjusted expected number was 1.7. Based on these findings the authors concluded that there exists a strong causal relationship between alcohol consumption and pancreatic cancer. In 1987 an IARC-working group evaluated these findings, and was unable to verify the findings of the authors. The working group noted that this fact, together with the apparent high nonparticipation rate of heavy drinkers during the formative phase of the cohort, and the conflicting evidence derived from histologically confirmed and nonconfirmed pancreatic cancer cases (among the latter, the association with alcohol intake appears to be negative), makes a causal interpretation of the findings difficult.[38] In a study among Japanese doctors, Kono et al.[39,40] concluded that alcohol drinking does not increase the risk for pancreatic cancer.

The other cohort studies summarized in Table 1 also did not demonstrate a significant association between consumption of alcoholic beverages and pancreatic cancer risk.[41-44]

TABLE 1

Summary of Results of Cohort Studies on Pancreatic Cancer and Alcohol Intake

Cohort	Definition of exposure	Results		Compared with population of	Ref.
1722 males discharged from the psychiatric department of Ulleval Hospital in Oslo with a diagnosis of alcoholism, 1925–1939	Serious and long-lasting types of chronic alcoholism	(a) O = 5, E = 3.1 (b) O = 5, E = 5.7	RR = 1.6 RR = 0.9	Norway Oslo	23
5359 males and 1119 females admitted to the Toronto Clinic of the Addiction Research Foundation, 1951–1963	History of frequent regular consumption of large amounts of alcohol	O = 1			24
922 alcoholics and 922 nonalcoholics, matched by age, sex, payroll, class, and geographical location in a U.S. company	(a) Nonalcoholics (b) Alcoholics	(a) O = 2 (b) O = 0			25
678 male and 257 female patients discharged from 4 mental hospitals with a primary or secondary diagnosis implicating abnormal drinking, London, 1953–1957	Alcoholics	O = 1			41
Males >30 years who had been listed in the registry of chronic misusers of alcohol, 1967–1970	Heavy alcohol consumers: "skid-row" alcoholics who drank mostly strong beverages, wines, and denatured alcohols	O = 4, E = 2.2	RR = 1.8		26

Description	Intake	O/E	RR	Notes	Ref
1139 males and 143 females admitted to any mental hospital in Massachusetts with a diagnosis of chronic alcoholism, 1930, 1935, and 1940	Not stated	O = 3, E = 5.1	RR = 0.6		27
1595 males and 475 females in a cohort, like Nicholls et al.,[41] but extended to all of England and Wales, 1953–1964	High alcohol intake		RR = 1.5		28
About 3600 male blue-collar workers and pensioners from a large Dublin brewery	Average of 58 g of alcohol per day	(a) O = 17, E = 14 (b) O = 17, E = 11.1	RR = 1.2 RR = 1.5	Dublin, Ireland	29
14,313 male members of the Danish Brewery Workers Union employed for at least six months in brewery, 1937–1963	Brewery workers are entitled to 2100 ml of free beer/day, i.e., 77.7 g of ethanol	O = 44, E = 40.9	RR = 1.1		30, 31
4401 males admitted to U.S. Army hospitals for alcoholism; officers were excluded, 1944–1946	65% of cohort was separated from service after hospitalization because alcohol interfered with performance of duties	O = 4, E = 5	RR = 0.9		32
Study of Hawaiian Japanese: (a) 13 cases, (b) other part of cohort	(a) Mean consumption 13.7 ml/day (b) Mean consumption 13.6 ml/day				42
9889 males admitted to the main clinical services of the Addiction Research Foundation, 1951–1970	Average daily intake of 254 ml of absolute alcohol	(a) O = 11, E = 9.2 (b) O = 11, E = 10 (c) O = 11, E = 13.3	RR = 1.2 RR = 1.1 RR = 0.8	Ontario U.S. veterans U.S. veterans with similar smoking habits	43
Kaiser-Permanente study among 1000 persons	Two or fewer drinks/day Three to five drinks/day Six or more drinks/day	(a) (b) (c)	RR = 2.5 RR = 1.5 RR = 3.0	Nondrinkers	33

TABLE 1 (continued)
Summary of Results of Cohort Studies on Pancreatic Cancer and Alcohol Intake

Cohort	Definition of exposure	Results		Compared with population of	Ref.
16,713 persons, comprising a random sample of Norwegian males (48%), emigrated Norwegian brothers (20%), and individuals with gastrointestinal (g.i.) cancer	(a) Frequent current users: at least 14 times a month	(a) O = 5, E = 1.7			37
	(b) Intermediate drinkers	(b) O = 10, E = 8.7			
	(c) Nondrinkers	(c) O = 3, E = 7.6			
Japanese prospective study, after (a) 8, (b) 9, and (c) 16 years	Men who consumed alcoholic beverages daily	(a)	RR = 1.1	Not daily drinkers	34–36
		(b)	RR = 0.9		
		(c)	RR = 0.8		
Study of Japanese doctors	(a) Nondrinkers	(a)	RR = 1.7		39, 40
	(b) Ex-drinkers	(b)	RR = 2.4		
	(c) Occasional drinkers	(c)	RR = 2.1		
	(d) Daily drinkers <27 ml	(d)	RR = 0.5		
	(e) Daily drinkers >27 ml	(e)	RR = 2.4		
	(f) Excluding daily drinkers and with correction for age and smoking	(f)	RR = 1.0		
122,894 members from North Carolina who had a multi-phasic health check-up, 1978–1984	(a) Past drinkers	(a)	RR = 2.6	Nondrinkers	44
	(b) <1 drink a day	(b)	RR = 1.3		
	(c) >1 drink a day	(c)	RR = 0.9		

Note: O, observed; E, expected; RR, relative risk; 95% confidence intervals.

C. CASE-CONTROL STUDIES (TABLE 2)

Twenty case-control studies have been reported up to now in which patients with pancreatic cancer were queried as to their lifestyle, and their responses were compared with those of people without the disease. Table 2 shows that the number of cases ranged from 18 to 901. Controls were usually hospitalized patients, and only occasionally were controls drawn from the general population. Subjects were usually classified into several categories according to alcohol intake, but the definition of these categories was not always explicitly stated. A significant positive association of alcohol consumption and pancreatic cancer was observed in four studies. Using as background data the results from a large population survey of 122,261 adults in 29 health districts in Japan, Ishii et al.[45,46] analyzed information gathered by questionnaire from 475 patients with pancreatic cancer. They reported an elevated risk in the order of 1.0 to 1.5 for those drinking alcohol, compared to nondrinkers. Their data were not adjusted for cigarette smoking.

Raymond et al.[47] reported a significant increased pancreatic cancer risk among beer drinkers. Furthermore, Durbec et al.[48] found a positive association between total alcohol intake (especially in case of wine with a high alcohol content) and pancreatic cancer risk (relative risk for drinkers vs. nondrinkers, 2.4). The risk was reduced after controlling for fat and carbohydrate intake; there was no increased risk with regular drinking of aperitives or spirits. Recently, Olson et al.[49] conducted a case-control study in the Minneapolis-St. Paul area, and observed that heavy alcohol consumption (four or more drinks per day), adjusted for several potential confounding variables, was positively associated with pancreatic cancer. Cuzick and Babiker[50] also reported evidence of a positive trend in risk of pancreatic cancer and total alcohol consumption. Moreover, they found a threefold risk of pancreatic cancer among heavy beer drinkers, and were able to demonstrate a dose-response relationship. Interestingly, they concluded that the effect of alcohol appeared to be largely confined to smokers. No significant trend with amount of alcohol was observed in nonsmokers. Wynder et al.[51,52] found a slight, dose-unrelated, nonsignificant association between alcohol intake and pancreatic cancer. Heavy drinkers (120 g ethanol/day) had tobacco-adjusted relative risks of 1.6 among men and 0.9 among women, when compared to nondrinkers. Other investigators did not observe a consistent association between alcohol intake and cancer of the pancreas.[53-63]

Interestingly, some investigators reported an inverse association between alcohol intake and the relative risk for pancreatic cancer. In a population-based case-control study in Los Angeles, Mack et al.[64] found a nonsignificant inverse association between cancer of the pancreas and alcohol intake from any source; the inverse relationship was more pronounced for table wine consumption. The data were not controlled for cigarette smoke. Norell et al.[65] performed a population-based case-control study in Sweden, and found an

Alcohol, Immunity, and Cancer

TABLE 2
Summary of Results of Case-Control Studies on Pancreatic Cancer and Alcohol Intake

Cases; controls	Definition of exposure	Results	Comparison	Ref.
Men, women (475, 122; 261)	Categories of alcohol intake	RR = 1.5	Drinkers vs. nondrinkers	45, 46
Men (100; 200) Women (42; 107)	Categorization into nondrinkers, occasional drinkers, and regular drinkers	RR = 1.3 (0.8–2.0)	Drinkers vs. nondrinkers	51
Men (901; 1770) Women (85; 3178)	Categories of wine, beer, spirits, and total alcohol	RR = 1.3 (men) RR = 0.6 (women)	Heavy drinkers vs. non-drinkers	53
Men, women (88; 336)	Mean weekly consumption (a) red wine <1270 ml/week ≥1270 ml/week (b) beer <900 ml/week ≥900 ml/week	90% CI (a) RR = 1.0 RR = 0.9 (b) RR = 0.7 RR = 2.9		47
Men (57; 57) Women (37; 37)	No clear definition	Patients drank more wine than controls, $p < 0.05$ for ≥ glasses/day		10
Men (218; 307) Women (149; 337)	(a) occasional drinkers (b) regular drinkers	(a) 1.3 (men); 0.8 (women) (b) 1.3 (men); 0.5 (women)	Drinkers vs. nondrinkers	54
Men (32; 172) Women (18; 34)	Regular drinkers: >10 g ethanol daily	RR = 0.7	Regular drinkers vs. others	55
Men (56; 112) Women (60; 120)	Categorization into alcohol intake once a day regular daily and alcohol-related problems	No association		56
Men (153; 5469) Women (122; 2525)	Daily alcohol intake >5 oz daily	RR = 1.6 (men) RR = 0.9 (women)	Drinkers vs. nondrinkers	52

Subjects	Measure	Result	Comparison	Ref.
Men (37; 100) Women (32; 99)	Daily ethanol intake in grams	RR = 2.4	Median drinkers vs. nondrinkers	48
Men (59; 72) Women (25; 29)	Habitual daily consumption	RR = 0.6	Habitual drinkers vs. others	57, 58
Men (94; 188) Women (103; 206)	Categorization into nondrinkers, drinkers (any amount of frequency)	No or inverse association		59
Men (282; 282) Women (208; 208)	Daily ethanol intake in grams; total and from various sources	<40 g/day; RR = 0.7 40–79 g/day; RR = 0.8 >79 g/day; RR = 1.2		64
Men (55; 110) Women (44; 88)	Daily ethanol consumption; (a) 0–1 g/day (b) 2–9 g/day (c) ≥10 g/day	90% CI (a) RR = 1.0 90% CI (a) RR = 1.0 (b) RR = 0.5 (c) RR = 0.5 (a) RR = 1.0 (b) RR = 0.7 (c) RR = 0.6	Drinkers vs. hospital controls Drinkers vs. population controls	65
Men (203; 890) Women (160; 344)	Weekly ethanol intake, categorization based on equivalents of numbers of beers	Male higher risk than female, but no consistent association	Drinkers vs. nondrinkers	60
Men (98; 161) Women (63; 107)	Categorization based on number of drinks/day ≥4 drinks a day	No or inverse association	Drinkers vs. nondrinkers	61
Men (212; 220)	(a) beer (b) hard-liquor (c) wine	(a) RR = 8.25 (b) RR = 3.49 (c) RR = 2.72	Drinkers vs. nondrinkers	49
Men (123; 150) Women (93; 129)	I. Beer drinkers (a) <7 pints/week (b) >7 pints/week II. Wine/spirits	I. (a) RR = 1.19 (b) RR = 3.17 II. No clear association	Drinkers vs. nondrinkers (especially smokers)	50

TABLE 2 (continued)
Summary of Results of Case-Control Studies on Pancreatic Cancer and Alcohol Intake

Cases; controls	Definition of exposure	Results	Comparison	Ref.
Men (296; 1125) Women (198; 579)	Categorization in amount and type of alcoholic beverage	No association		62
Men (148; 188)	Categorization in number of drinks/week, different types of alcoholic beverage	No or inverse association		63

Note: RR, relative risk, 95% confidence intervals (CI), except where noted.

inverse association with relative risks for frequent vs. infrequent alcohol use of 0.5 (hospital controls) and 0.7 (population controls).

D. SUMMARY OF THE EPIDEMIOLOGY

The results from correlation studies provide no consistent support for an association between alcohol consumption and risk of pancreatic cancer. Cohort studies of people with high-alcohol intake provide no significant evidence for such an association. Population-based cohort studies as well as case-control studies demonstrate inconsistent results.

The amount of alcohol intake observed in the various studies does not provide an explanation for these inconsistent results. The average alcohol intake in the studies that claimed a positive association was lower than other investigators reported in studies where no association between alcohol consumption and pancreatic cancer risk was reported. The average duration of alcohol consumption or the drinking pattern may be an important factor in this respect. The French or Italians, for example, tend to consume alcoholic beverages daily with their meals, whereas the pattern of alcohol consumption in Northern Europe or North America tends to be different.

Based on the data available at present, it can be concluded that epidemiology has failed to find a definite, consistent correlation between alcohol consumption and pancreatic cancer.

III. EXPERIMENTAL STUDIES

A. ANIMAL MODELS FOR PANCREATIC CANCER

Carcinoma of the pancreas usually refers to neoplasms arising in the exocrine pancreas, whereas neoplasms of the endocrine pancreas are collectively named islet cell tumors or apudomas.

Cubilla and Fitzgerald[66] and Morohoshi et al.[67] have classified the various types of human pancreatic exocrine tumors according to their presumed cell of origin, and concluded that 89 to 95% were of ductal or ductular origin, while only 1 to 4% were of acinar origin. The remaining 1 to 10% were classified as being of uncertain histogenesis. The great majority of human pancreatic adenocarcinomas shows the presence of tubular structures, which is interpreted as evidence that pancreatic cancer arises from ducts or ductules (Figure 1). However, no conclusive evidence is yet available for this suggestion.

It is known that spontaneous pancreatic neoplasms apparently originating from ductal or ductular epithelium are extremely rare in mammals, except in man and in hamster.[68] In contrast, tumors apparently arising from acinar cells occur in several species.[69-71] The spontaneous incidence of neoplasms of the exocrine pancreas in rats, hamsters, and most other rodents used experimentally, is generally quite low.

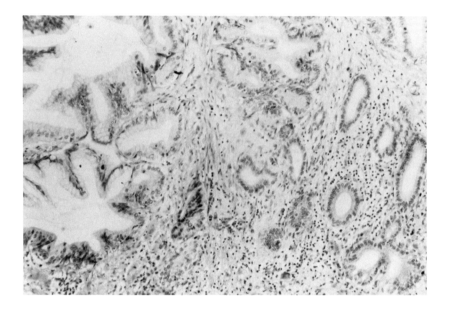

FIGURE 1.   Human pancreatic ductal cell adenocarcinoma resembling experimental ductular adenocarcinoma (compare with Figure 9). (H&E, Original magnification × 40.)

Since the early 1970s, much emphasis has been placed on the development of animal models for the study of pancreatic carcinogenesis. As a result, more than a dozen chemicals, including several oxidized derivatives of dipropyl-nitrosamine, have been identified, which induce pancreatic tumors in several rodent species.[72] Two models have been characterized in more detail than others, i.e., the azaserine-rat model,[73-76] resulting in predominantly acinar cell tumors, and the N-nitrosobis(2-oxopropyl)amine (BOP)-hamster model,[68,77-84] leading to mainly ductal type adenocarcinomas.

1. The Azaserine-Rat Model (Figures 2 through 6)

Induction of pancreatic hyperplastic nodules, adenomas, and carcinomas in rats by intraperitoneal injection of azaserine was first reported by Long-necker et al.[73,74] Adenocarcinomas or poorly differentiated carcinomas developed in the pancreas of rats repeatedly treated with azaserine as early as eleven months following initial azaserine treatment. Two months after treatment with azaserine, the earliest lesions can be found. These focal lesions have been described as atypical acinar cell foci (AACF) or nodules (AACN). The number and size of these foci/nodules increases with time following azaserine treatment. Atypical acinar cell foci are recognized in sections of pancreas by phenotypic changes comprising an increased rate of cell division, altered enzyme content of the cells, changes in nuclear size, and loss of differentiation (see Figures 2 and 3). Two different populations of atypical

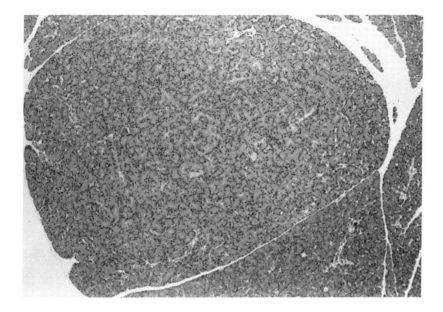

FIGURE 2. Acidophilic atypical acinar cell nodule induced in rat pancreas by azaserine. (H&E, Original magnification × 58.)

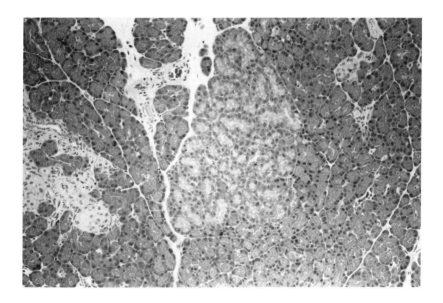

FIGURE 3. Basophilic atypical acinar cell focus induced in rat pancreas by azaserine. (H&E, Original magnification × 168.)

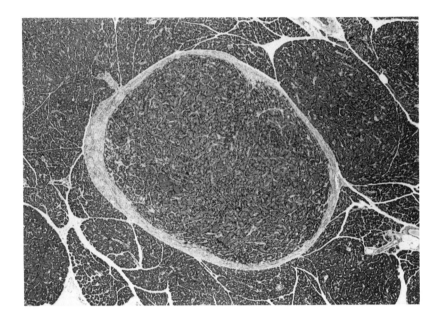

FIGURE 4.   Carcinoma *in situ* induced in rat pancreas by azaserine. Note fibrous capsule around anaplastic glandular epithelium. (H&E, Original magnification × 42.)

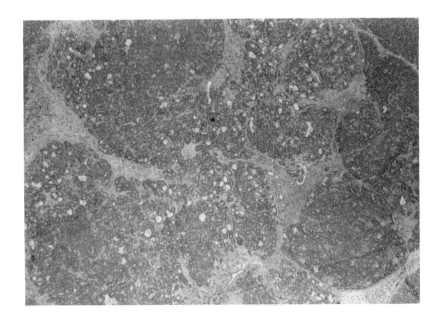

FIGURE 5.   Pancreatic acinar adenocarcinoma induced in the rat by azaserine. (H&E, Original magnification × 36.)

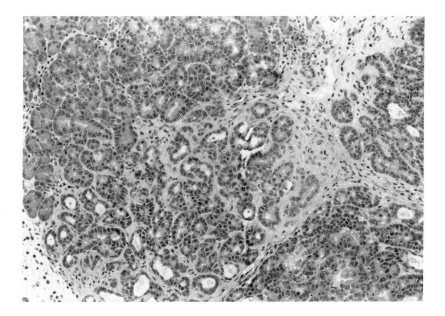

FIGURE 6. Pancreatic acinar adenocarcinoma induced in the rat by azaserine (detail from Figure 5). (H&E, Original magnification × 144.)

acinar cell foci have been characterized in hematoxylin and eosin (H&E)-stained tissue sections by their markedly basophilic or intense eosinophilic cytoplasm. The acidophilic, but not the basophilic, foci frequently show detectable secondary phenotypic changes, and are generally considered to have a high probability of progression, and hence to be related to the ultimate formation of carcinomas.[76]

2. The BOP-Hamster Model (Figures 7 through 9)

Pancreatic ductal (ductular) tumors can be induced in Syrian golden hamsters by several specific propylnitroso compounds, of which BOP has been found to have a specific pancreatropic effect with a narrow tumor spectrum in other organs (lungs, liver, gall bladder, kidneys). Pancreatic neoplasms can be induced upon repeated subcutaneous injection of BOP in doses of 10 mg/kg body weight, as early as eight weeks after the first BOP injection. After a single dose of BOP (20 mg/kg body weight) multifocal hyperplastic changes (cystic and tubular ductal complexes) are found within two months, and adenocarcinomas can be found within six months.

3. Relevance of the Animal Models to Humans

Because of the similarity of the induced tumors to those occurring in man, the BOP-hamster model has been considered to be more relevant to the

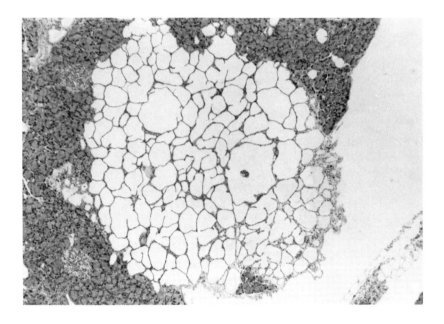

FIGURE 7. Cystic ductal complex induced in hamster pancreas by BOP. (H&E, Original magnification × 58.)

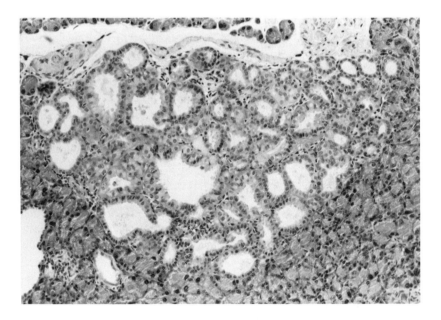

FIGURE 8. Tubular ductal complex induced in hamster pancreas by BOP. (H&E, Original magnification × 144.)

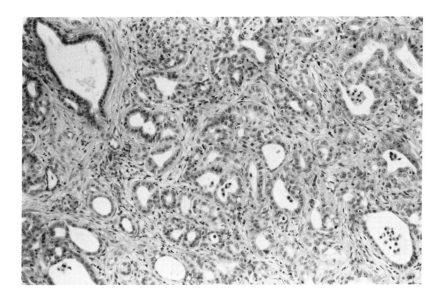

FIGURE 9. Pancreatic ductular adenocarcinoma induced in the hamster by BOP, (H&E, Original magnification × 168.)

human situation than the rat model. The histogenesis of the ductal/ductular adenocarcinomas induced in hamsters, however, is still a matter of debate in literature. In BOP-treated hamsters, many tumors are found to develop within, or in the vicinity of, islets of Langerhans in the form of intrainsular ductules. Therefore, Pour et al.[68,82] postulated that ductular and islet precursor cells are the origin of the pseudoductular lesions and, hence, of the ductular adenocarcinomas. Recently, the centroacinar cell has been suggested as the cell of origin.[85-87] Electron microscopical investigations have led to the conclusion that the ductular tumors induced in hamster pancreas by BOP, arise from existing ducts without involvement of acinar cells.[86,88,89] Other workers, however, claim that pancreatic adenocarcinomas in hamsters develop from dedifferentiated acinar cells.[90-94]

In man, only a very small percentage of tumors, namely those that have clearly recognizable acinar cell differentiation, is classified as being of acinar origin. Most other tumors contain ductlike structures and have been classified as from ductal origin. There is ultrastructural evidence, however, of acinar cell characteristics in all human pancreatic tumors.[95,96] Furthermore, acinar dysplasia appears to be common in patients with pancreatic cancer.[97]

It seems likely that factors that modulate progression of early stages of carcinogenesis may be different in lesions originating from the two different cell types. Moreover, no conclusive data are available on the role of precursor lesions in pancreatic carcinogenesis. The aforementioned observations and considerations indicate that not only the BOP-hamster, but also the azaserine-

TABLE 3
Effects of Dietary Fat and Ethanol on Putative Preneoplastic Pancreatic Foci in Rats Induced by Azaserine

		Calculated volumetric data of foci					
		Acidophilic foci			Basophilic foci		
Diet	No.	Total no. per cm³	Mean diameter (μm)	Area as % pancreas	Total no. per cm³	Mean diameter (μm)	Area as % pancreas
LF	26	588 ± 41	265 ± 8	1.07 ± 0.12	499 ± 47	113 ± 4	0.06 ± 0.01
HF	20	673 ± 60	296 ± 10	1.77 ± 0.24	786 ± 56	112 ± 3	0.09 ± 0.01
LF-E	20	777 ± 67	269 ± 8	1.64 ± 0.30	877 ± 107	97 ± 4	0.06 ± 0.01
HF-E	20	769 ± 60[c]	304 ± 15[a]	3.15 ± 0.62[b,d]	1436 ± 160[a,e]	115 ± 4[f]	0.20 ± 0.03[g]

Note: Values are means ± SEM. Data are based on H & E-stained paraffin sections. Statistics: two-way analysis of variance (two-tailed).

HF vs. LF: [a] $p < 0.01$; [b] $p < 0.001$.
E vs. tapwater: [c] $p < 0.05$; [d] $p < 0.01$; [e] $p < 0.001$.
Positive interaction between fat and ethanol: [f] $p < 0.05$; [g] $p < 0.001$.
LF, 5% corn oil; HF, 25% corn oil; E, ethanol (15% w/v).

treated rat, provide a relevant animal model to pancreatic cancer in man, and that it is worthwhile to study the modulating effects of lifestyle factors, such as alcohol, on pancreatic carcinogenesis in both hamster and rat.[98]

B. EFFECT OF ALCOHOL ON PANCREATIC CARCINOGENESIS IN ANIMALS

To our knowledge, ethanol or alcoholic beverages have not been tested for their carcinogenic potential in adequate long-term studies in mice or rats. Most of the studies that have been described in the literature cannot be used for evaluation of the carcinogenicity of alcohol, due to severe limitations in experimental design.[38] In one study, a group of 108 male and 42 female CF1 mice was given 43% ethanol in water for up to 1020 days.[99] Another group of mice was given 14% ethanol, similarly, for up to 735 days, and a further group of 100 male mice was given 19.5% as the drinking fluid for a maximum of 664 days. No difference in the incidence of tumors was found.

The results of a four-month study with azaserine-treated rats indicated that ethanol enhanced the dietary fat-promoted growth of acidophilic and basophilic atypical acinar cell foci (Table 3), pointing to a possible interaction between these two lifestyle factors.[98] In a long-term study with azaserine-treated rats, a larger, though not statistically significant, number of carcinomas was found in the high-fat (25% corn oil) + ethanol (10% in drinking water) group than in the high-fat + tap water group.[100] The larger number of carcinomas was accompanied by a lower number of adenomas (Table 4), suggesting that ethanol has the potency to enhance the development of premalignant pancreatic lesions into carcinomas. This suggestion is supported by the observation in the four-month study that 6 out of 20 rats in the high-fat + ethanol group developed a carcinoma *in situ* (see Figure 4), whereas in the high-fat-alone and the ethanol-alone group, such advanced lesions were found in one animal only.

Furthermore, it appeared that ethanol caused an increase in multiplicity, but not in incidence, of malignant tumors, pointing to an enhancing effect on the development of carcinomas in carcinoma-bearing animals.

The results obtained with BOP-treated hamsters, in a four-month study[98] as well as in a twelve-month study,[100] demonstrated that ethanol did not modulate pancreatic carcinogenesis (Tables 5 and 6). These findings are in agreement with those of Pour et al.,[101] who found that ethanol given to outbred Syrian golden hamsters in drinking water at a 5% w/v concentration, for life, beginning either before or after a single dose of BOP, had no effect on tumor induction. This observation was in contrast with the results of a previous study of this group, in which a higher concentration of ethanol (25% w/v) inhibited the development of BOP-induced pancreatic lesions.[102] The observation of Pour et al.[101] that hamsters treated with BOP and maintained on ethanol for life, exhibited a few atypical acinar cell foci, might point to the pancreatic acinar cell as the main target cell for ethanol, and not the centroacinar or ductular cell. The results in the chronic studies performed in our

TABLE 4

Number of Pancreatic Lesions in Rats Maintained on LF, HF, or HF + Ethanol Diets for 15 Months after a Single Injection with Azaserine

(Pre)neoplastic lesions observed	Number of lesions		
	LF	HF[a]	HF + E[b]
Effective number of animals	(39)	(37)	(38)
AACN (>1 mm)	175	963*	1016
Adenoma (AACN >3 mm)	33	176***	156
Total adenocarcinoma	29	57*	71
Carcinoma *in-situ*	25	35	41
Acinar cell carcinoma	4	22**	30

Note: LF, 5% corn oil; HF, 25% corn oil; E, ethanol (10% w/v). AACN, atypical acinar cell nodule. Statistics: generalized linear model (two-tailed); error is Poisson; link function is log.

[a] *p <0.05; **p <0.01; ***p <0.001 as compared to LF.
[b] HF + E has been compared with HF.

TABLE 5

Effects of Dietary Fat and Ethanol on Putative Preneoplastic Pancreatic Foci Induced in Hamsters by BOP

Post-initiation diet group	No.	Total no. per cm²	Transection area (mm² × 100)	Area as % of pancreas
Cystic foci				
LF	26	8.49 ± 0.95	3.03 ± 0.17	0.26 ± 0.03
HF	19	13.98 ± 1.89	2.90 ± 0.12	0.42 ± 0.06
LF-E	17	8.57 ± 0.98	2.55 ± 0.16	0.22 ± 0.03
HF-E	19	12.45 ± 1.46	3.32 ± 0.14	0.44 ± 0.07[a]
Ductular foci				
LF	26	7.68 ± 1.01	3.08 ± 0.18	0.24 ± 0.04
HF	19	17.78 ± 2.24	2.91 ± 0.10	0.50 ± 0.06
LF-E	17	7.68 ± 1.06	2.81 ± 0.22	0.22 ± 0.03
HF-E	19	12.70 ± 1.92	3.26 ± 0.10	0.42 ± 0.07[a]

Note: Values are means ± SEM. LF, 5% corn oil; HF, 25% corn oil; E, ethanol (15% w/v). Statistics: two-way analysis of variance (two-tailed).

HF vs. LF: [a] p <0.001; no effect of ethanol, no interaction between fat and ethanol.

institute support this hypothesis, since ethanol influenced pancreatic carcinogenesis in azaserine-treated rats but not in BOP-treated hamsters.

As has been pointed out already in Section III.A.3, it is generally accepted that the pancreatic tumors induced in hamster pancreas by BOP have a close morphological similarity with pancreatic cancer occurring in man. Therefore, the absence of an enhancing effect of ethanol on pancreatic carcinogenesis

TABLE 6
Number of Pancreatic Tumors in Hamsters Maintained on LF, HF, or HF + Ethanol Diets for 12 Months after Two Weekly Injections with BOP

	Number of lesions		
Neoplastic lesions observed	LF	HF[a]	HF + E[b]
Effective number of animals	36	38	38
Number of tumor-bearing animals	17	29	25
Total adenocarcinoma	23	37	35
carcinoma *in-situ*	17	19	22
ductal/ductular adenocarcinogenic	6	18*	13

Note: LF, 5% corn oil; HF, 25% corn oil; E, ethanol (10% w/v); AACN, atypical acinar cell nodule. Statistics: generalized linear model (two-tailed); error is Poisson; link function is log.

[a] *p* <0.05 as compared to LF.
[b] HF + E has been compared with HF.

in hamsters might be more relevant for the human situation than the enhancing effects found in the rat studies. However, an effect on pancreatic carcinogenesis via interference with the acinar cell development cannot be completely excluded.

IV. ROLE OF (CALCIFYING) PANCREATITIS

It is generally accepted that chronic alcohol abuse, whether or not in combination with a high-fat diet, is the most common cause of chronic (calcifying) pancreatitis.[46,103-108]

Several mechanisms have been proposed for the pathogenesis of alcoholic pancreatitis. There is mounting evidence from studies in both experimental animals and in humans that alcohol has a direct effect on the cells of the exocrine pancreas. Light and electron microscopy of pancreatic tissue from alcoholic patients with chronic pancreatitis, revealed dedifferentiation of acinar cells to tubular complexes.[106] In addition to the loss of acinar cells, there is loss of ductal cells. Long-term ethanol ingestion in rats (14 to 53 weeks) produced changes in acinar, centroacinar, and ductular cells. Microscopical changes comprised degeneration and atrophic changes of acinar cells, fibrosis, and intraductal protein precipitates.[109] The pseudoductular cysts are lined by cuboidal epithelium of ductal type, which may represent dedifferentiation of acinar structures or hyperplasia of centroacinar cells accompanied by atrophy of surrounding acini. A similar phenomenon has been observed in BOP-treated hamsters.[87-91]

Pour and co-workers[101] found that recurrent pancreatitis promotes tumor development in BOP-treated hamsters when it occurs after initiation, whereas

BOP given during pancreatitis had no such effect. The role of diet as a factor predisposing to alcoholic pancreatitis remains unsettled. In dogs, it has been found that a high-fat diet facilitates the development of experimental pancreatitis. This finding suggests that in alcoholics, a high fat and protein intake predispose to pancreatitis.

Jalovaara et al.[110] and Rämö et al.[111] investigated the effects of a fat-rich diet on rat pancreas, and found that both pancreatitis and ductal cell dysplasia were enhanced by long-term ethanol consumption.

The association between chronic pancreatitis and pancreatic cancer has been described by Mikal and Campbell[112] in autopsies, and by Paulino-Netto et al.[113] and Becker[114] in surgical patients. The data are, however, inadequate to draw conclusions, especially since pancreatitis may be the consequence, but not the cause, of pancreatic cancer, and moreover, both pancreatitis and pancreatic cancer could be caused by the same agent, i.e., alcohol. Rocca et al.[115] compared the cancer incidence in 172 patients affected by chronic pancreatitis in the gastroenterology unit of a hospital in Torino with data from the general population. They found an increased risk of pancreatic, as well as extrapancreatic cancer, in patients with chronic pancreatitis, compared to the general population. Although chronic pancreatitis surrounding pancreatic carcinoma is common, cancer developing in chronic pancreatitis has rarely been shown. Recently, Haas et al.[116] presented four male patients with pancreatic cancer, all of whom had previous surgery for complications of chronic pancreatitis. Chronic pancreatitis, including calcifications, was caused by alcohol in three cases. The delay between chronic pancreatitis and pancreatic carcinoma was 2 to 10 years. It has been proposed that the association of chronic pancreatitis with pancreatic cancer passes through an intermediate stage of hyperplasia, followed by metaplasia, dysplasia, carcinoma *in situ*, and, finally, adenocarcinoma.

V. CONCLUDING REMARKS

From the results presented in this chapter, it may be concluded that the epidemiological data demonstrate insufficient evidence for a causal relationship between the risk of pancreatic cancer and a high consumption of alcohol. It is, however, premature to conclude that alcohol does not play any role in the development of pancreatic cancer, although the hamster data support such reasoning. It is generally accepted that chronic alcohol abuse may be associated with chronic (calcifying) pancreatitis. Recurrent tissue damage and repair is an important phenomenon in this disease.

There is now substantial evidence that cancer might be associated to chronically injured tissue.[117] Colon cancer is frequently seen in patients with chronic colitis;[118] skin cancer may occur in burn scars,[119] and many lung tumors grow in areas of scarring.[120] A large body of animal data suggest that chronic tissue injury induced by chemical or physical agents could be a major factor in tumor development in connective tissue and epithelial tissues.[121] Malignant tumors induced in the nasal epithelium by irritating substances such as acetaldehyde and formaldehyde have been found to arise only from epithelium which is severely damaged.[122,123] Based on the data summarized in this chapter, it seems justifiable to conclude that alcohol as such is not directly, but rather indirectly, (via the induction of [calcifying] pancreatitis) responsible for the development of pancreatic cancer. This hypothesis is supported by epidemiological data suggesting a significant association between heavy beer drinking and pancreatic cancer. The stronger relationship of pancreas cancer with beer consumption than with the consumption of other alcoholic beverages raises the question as to whether the presence of a carcinogen, such as dimethylnitrosamine in beer, is important. Beer is known to be, or at least to have been, a major source of nitrosamines,[124] and beer was reported to contain more nitrosamines than other alcoholic beverages.[125] Furthermore, nitrosamines are potent pancreatic carcinogens. Moreover, some investigators claimed that the influence of alcohol on development of pancreatic cancer is much more clear in smokers than in nonsmokers. Therefore, it is possible that the nitrosamine content of cigarette smoke is also relevant to pancreatic cancer.

The present data indicate that more research is needed to elucidate the role of alcohol-induced pancreatitis, alone and in combination with a high-fat diet or cigarette smoking, in the induction of pancreatic cancer in man. Dose of exposure and response patterns have to be studied much more in detail to appreciate the real risks of drinking for the pancreas.

ACKNOWLEDGMENTS

The authors are grateful to Professor Dr. V. J. Feron and Professor Dr. R. J. J. Hermus for critical evaluation of the manuscript. Original studies have been supported by Grant CIVO 84-1 from the Dutch Cancer Society.

REFERENCES

1. **Fraumeni, J. F.,** Cancers of the pancreas and biliary tract: epidemiological considerations, *Cancer Res.,* 35, 3437, 1975.
2. **Levison, D. A.,** Carcinoma of the pancreas, *J. Pathol.,* 129, 203, 1979.
3. **Hoogendoorn, D.,** Trends in kankersterfte., *Ned. T. Geneesk.,* 127, 1661, 1983.
4. **Stephenson, H. E.,** Cancer of the pancreas and stomach: a study in contrasts, *Surgery,* 71, 307, 1972.
5. **Morgan, G. G. H. and Wormsley, K. G.,** Cancer of the pancreas, *Gut,* 18, 580, 1977.
6. **Fitzgerald, P. J.,** Pancreatic cancer, *Arch. Pathol.,* 100, 513, 1976.
7. **Wynder, E. L.,** An epidemiologic evaluation of the causes of cancer of the pancreas, *Cancer Res.,* 35, 2228, 1975.
8. **Mainz, D. and Webster, P. D.,** Pancreatic carcinoma. A review of etiologic considerations, *Dig. Dis.,* 19, 459, 1974.

9. **Gordis, L.**, Epidemiology of pancreatic cancer, in *Reviews in Cancer Epidemiology.* Vol. 1, Lilienfeld, A. M., Ed., Elsevier, Amsterdam, 1980, 84.
10. **Lin, R. S. and Kessler, I. I.**, A multifactorial model for pancreatic cancer in man. Epidemiologic evidence, *JAMA*, 245, 147, 1981.
11. **Okuda, K. and Ohnishi, K.**, Pancreatic cancer and alcohol, *Clin. Gastroenterol.*, 10, 479, 1981.
12. **MacMahon, B.**, Risk factors for cancer of the pancreas, *Cancer*, 50, 2676, 1982.
13. **Waard, F. de**, Epidemiologie en pathogenese van pancreascarcinoom., *Ned. T. Geneesk.*, 128, 245, 1984.
14. **Higginson, J. and Muir, C. S.**, Environmental carcinogenesis: misconceptions and limitations to cancer control, *J. Natl. Cancer Inst.*, 63, 1291, 1979.
15. **Dörken, H.**, Einige daten bei 280 patienten mit pancreaskrebs, *Gastroenterologia*, 102, 47, 1964.
16. **Burch, G. E. and Ansari, A.**, Chronic alcoholism and carcinoma of the pancreas: a correlative hypothesis, *Arch. Intern. Med.*, 122, 273, 1968.
17. **Breslow, N. E. and Enstrom, J. E.**, Geographic correlates between cancer mortality rates and alcohol-tobacco consumption in the United States, *J. Natl. Cancer Inst.*, 53, 631, 1974.
18. **Kono, S. and Ikeda, M.**, Correlation between cancer mortality and alcoholic beverage in Japan, *Br. J. Cancer*, 40, 449, 1979.
19. **Hinds, M. W., Kolonel, L. N., Lee, J., and Hirohata, T.**, Associations between cancer incidence and alcohol and cigarette consumption among five ethnic groups in Hawaii, *Br. J. Cancer*, 41, 929, 1980.
20. **Blot, W. J., Fraumeni, Jr., J. F., and Stone, B. J.**, Geographic correlates of pancreas cancer in the United States, *Cancer*, 42, 373, 1978.
21. **Yanai, H., Inaba, Y., Takagi, H., et al.**, Multivariate analysis of cancer mortalities for selected sites in 24 countries, *Environ. Health Perspect.*, 32, 83, 1979.
22. **IARC**, IARC Monographs on the Evaluation of the Carcinogenic Risk of Chemicals to Humans, Vol. 38, *Tobacco Smoking*, Lyon, 1986.
23. **Sundby, P.**, *Alcoholism and Mortality*, Oslo, Universitetsforlaget, 1967.
24. **Schmidt, W. and Lint, J. de**, Causes of death of alcoholics, *Q. J. Stud. Alcohol*, 33, 171, 1972.
25. **Pell, S. and D'Alonzo, C. A.**, A five-year mortality study of alcoholics, *J. Occup. Med.*, 15, 120, 1973.
26. **Hakulinen, T., Lehtimäki, L., Lehtonen, M., and Teppo, L.**, Cancer morbidity among two male cohorts with increased alcohol consumption in Finland, *J. Natl. Cancer Inst.*, 52, 1711, 1974.
27. **Monson, R. R. and Lyon, J. L.**, Proportional mortality among alcoholics, *Cancer*, 36, 1077, 1975.
28. **Adelstein, A. and White, G.**, Alcoholism and mortality, *Popul. Trends*, 6, 7, 1976.
29. **Dean, G., MacLennan, R., McLoughlin, H., and Shelley, E.**, Causes of death of blue-collar workers at a Dublin brewery, *Br. J. Cancer*, 40, 581, 1979.
30. **Jensen, O. M.**, Cancer morbidity and causes of death among Danish brewery workers, *Int. J. Cancer*, 23, 454, 1979.
31. **Jensen, O. M.**, *Cancer Morbidity and Causes of Death among Danish Brewery Workers*, International Agency for Research on Cancer, Lyon, 1980.
32. **Robinette, C. D., Hrubec, Z., and Fraumeni, J. F., Jr.**, Chronic alcoholism and subsequent mortality in World War II veterans, *Am. J. Epidemiol.*, 109, 687, 1979.
33. **Klatsky, A. L., Friedman, G. D., and Siegelaub, A. B.**, Alcohol and mortality: a ten-year Kaiser-Permanente experience, *Ann. Intern. Med.*, 95, 139, 1981.
34. **Hirayama, T.**, Prospective studies on cancer epidemiology based on census population in Japan, in *Proceedings of the XIth International Cancer Congress*, Florence, 1974; *Cancer Epidemiology, Environmental Factors*, Vol. 3, Bucalossi, P., Veronesi, U., and Cascinelli, N., Eds., Excerpta Medica, Amsterdam, 1975, 26.

35. **Hirayama, T.,** Prospective studies on cancer epidemiology based on census population in Japan, in *Prevention and Detection of Cancer, Vol. 1, Etiology,* Nieburgs, H. E., Ed., Marcel Dekker, New York, 1978, 1139.

36. **Hirayama, T.,** A cohort study on cancer in Japan, in *Statistical Methods for Cancer Epidemiology,* Blot, W. J., Hirayama, T., and Hoel, D. G., Eds., Radiation Effects Research Foundation, Hiroshima, 1985, 73.

37. **Heuch, I., Kvale, G., Jacobsen, B. K., and Bjelke, E.,** Use of alcohol, tobacco and coffee, and risk of pancreatic cancer, *Br. J. Cancer,* 48, 637, 1983.

38. **IARC,** IARC monographs on the evaluation of carcinogenic risks to humans, *Alcohol Drinking,* Vol. 44, Lyon, 1988.

39. **Kono, S., Ikeda, M., Ogata, M., Tokudome, S., Nishizumi, M., and Kuratsune, M.** The relationship between alcohol and mortality among Japanese physicians, *Int. J. Epidemiol.,* 12, 437, 1983.

40. **Kono, S., Ikeda, M., Tokudome, S., Nishizumi, M., and Kuratsune, M.,** Alcohol and mortality: a cohort study of male Japanese physicians, *Int. J. Epidemiol.,* 15, 527, 1986.

41. **Nicholls, P., Edwards, G., and Kyle, E.,** Alcoholics admitted to four hospitals in England. II. General and cause-specific mortality, *Q. J. Stud. Alcohol,* 35, 841, 1974.

42. **Blackwelder, W. C., Yano, K., Rhoads, G. G., Kagan, A., Gordon, T., and Palesch, Y.,** Alcohol and mortality: the Honolulu Heart Study, *Am. J. Cancer,* 68, 164, 1980.

43. **Schmidt, W. and Popham, R. E.,** The role of drinking and smoking in mortality from cancer and other causes in male alcoholics, *Cancer,* 47, 1031, 1981.

44. **Hiatt, R. A., Klatsky, A. L., and Armstrong, M. A.,** Pancreatic cancer, blood glucose, and beverage consumption, *Int. J. Cancer,* 41, 794, 1988.

45. **Ishii, K., Nakamura, K., Ozaki, H., Yamada, N., and Takeuchi, T.,** Epidemiology of pancreatic cancer, *Jpn. J. Clin. Med.,* 26, 1839, 1968 (in Japanese).

46. **Ishii, K., Takeuchi, T., and Hirayama, T.,** Chronic calcifying pancreatitis and pancreatic carcinoma in Japan, *Digestion,* 9, 429, 1973.

47. **Raymond, L., Infante, F., Tuyns, A. J., Voirol, M., and Lowenfelds, A. B.,** Diet and pancreatic cancer, *Gastroenterol. Clin. Biol.,* 11, 488, 1987 (in French).

48. **Durbec, J. P., Chevillotte, G., Bidart, J. M., Berthezene, P., and Sarles, H.,** Diet, alcohol, tobacco, and risk of cancer of the pancreas: a case-control study, *Br. J. Cancer,* 47, 463, 1983.

49. **Olsen, G. W., Mandel, J. S., Gibson, R. W., Wattenberg, L. W., and Schuman, L. M.,** A case-control study of pancreatic cancer and cigarettes, alcohol, coffee and diet, *Am. J. Public Health,* 79, 1016, 1989.

50. **Cuzick, J. and Babiker, A. G.,** Pancreatic cancer, alcohol, diabetes mellitus and gallbladder disease, *Int. J. Cancer,* 43, 415, 1989.

51. **Wynder, E. L., Mabuchi, K., Maruchi, N., and Fortner, J. G.,** A case-control study of cancer of the pancreas, *Cancer,* 31, 641, 1973.

52. **Wynder, E. L., Hall, N. E. L., and Polansky, M.,** Epidemiology of coffee and pancreatic cancer, *Cancer Res.,* 43, 3900, 1983.

53. **Williams, R. R. and Horm, J. W.,** Association of cancer sites with tobacco and alcohol consumption and socioeconomic status of patients: interview study from the Third National Cancer Survey, *J. Natl. Cancer Inst.,* 58, 525, 1977.

54. **MacMahon, B., Yen, S., Trichopoulos, D., Warren, K., and Nardi, G.,** Coffee and cancer of the pancreas, *New Engl. J. Med.,* 304, 630, 1981.

55. **Manousos, O., Trichopoulos, D., Koutseliinis, A., Papadimitriou, C., Polychronopoulou, A., and Zavitsanos, X.,** Epidemiologic characteristics and trace elements in pancreatic cancer in Greece, *Cancer Det. Prev.,* 4, 439, 1981.

56. **Haines, A. P., Moss, A. R., Whittemore, A., and Quivey, J.,** A case-control study of pancreatic carcinoma, *J. Cancer Res. Clin. Oncol.,* 103, 93, 1982.

57. **Kodama, T. and Mori, W.,** Morphological behaviour of carcinoma of the pancreas. I. Histological classification and electron microscopical observation, *Acta Pathol. Jpn.,* 33, 467, 1983.

58. **Kodama, T., and Mori, W.,** Morphological lesions of the pancreatic ducts. Significance of pyloric gland metaplasia in carcinogenesis of exocrine and endocrine pancreas, *Acta Pathol. Jpn.,* 33, 645, 1983.

59. **Gold, E. B., Gordis, L., Diener, M. D., Seltser, R., Boitnott, J. K., Bynum, T. E., and Hutcheon, D. F.,** Diet and other risk factors for cancer of the pancreas, *Cancer,* 44, 460, 1985.

60. **Falk, R. T., Pickle, L. W., Fontham, E. T., Correa, P., and Fraumeni, J. F., Jr.,** Life-style risk factors for pancreatic cancer in Louisiana: a case-control study, *Am. J. Epidemiol.,* 128, 324, 1988.

61. **Clavel, F., Benhamou, E., Auquier, A., Tarayre, M., and Flamant, R.,** Coffee, alcohol, smoking and cancer of the pancreas: a case-control study, *Int. J. Cancer,* 43, 17, 1989.

62. **Bouchardy, C., Clavel, F., Vecchia, C., La, Raymond, L., and Boyle, P.,** Alcohol, beer and cancer of the pancreas, *Int. J. Cancer,* 45, 842, 1990.

63. **Farrow, D. C. and Davis, S.,** Risk of pancreatic cancer in relation to medical history and the use of tobacco, alcohol and coffee, *Int. J. Cancer,* 45, 816, 1990.

64. **Mack, T. M., Yu, M. C., Hanisch, R., and Henderson, B. E.,** Pancreas cancer and smoking, beverage consumption, and past medical history, *J. Natl. Cancer Inst.,* 76, 49, 1986.

65. **Norell, S. E., Ahlbom, A., Erwald, R., Jacobson, G., Linberg-Navier, I., Olin, R., Törnberg, B., and Wiechel, K.-L.,** Diet and pancreatic cancer: a case-control study, *Am. J. Epidemiol.,* 124, 894, 1986.

66. **Cubilla, A. L. and Fitzgerald, P. J.,** Classification of pancreatic cancer (nonendocrine), *Mayor Clin. Proc.,* 54, 449, 1979.

67. **Morohoshi, T., Held, G., and Kloppel, G.,** Exocrine pancreatic tumours and their histological classification; a study based on 167 autopsy and 97 surgical cases, *Histopathology,* 7, 645, 1983.

68. **Pour, P. M.,** Experimental pancreatic ductal (ductular) tumors, *Monogr. Pathol.,* 21, 111, 1980.

69. **Hosoda, S., Suzuki, H., and Suzuki, M.,** Spontaneous tumours and atypical proliferation of pancreatic acinar cells in Mastomys (praomys) natalensis, *J. Natl. Cancer Inst.,* 57, 1341, 1976.

70. **Rowlatt, U.,** Spontaneous epithelial tumours of the pancreas of mammals, *Br. J. Cancer,* 21, 82, 1967.

71. **Takahashi, M. and Pour, P. M.,** Spontaneous alterations in the pancreas of the aging Syrian golden Hamster, *J. Natl. Cancer Inst.,* 60, 355, 1978.

72. **Longnecker, D. S.,** Experimental models of exocrine pancreatic tumors, in *The Exocrine Pancreas: Biology, Pathobiology, and Diseases,* Go, V. L. W., Ed., Raven Press, New York, 1986, 443.

73. **Longnecker, D. S. and Crawford, B. G.,** Hyperplastic nodules and adenomas of exocrine pancreas in azaserine-treated rats, *J. Natl. Cancer Inst.,* 53, 573, 1974.

74. **Longnecker, D. S. and Curphey, T. J.,** Adenocarcinoma of the pancreas in azaserine-treated rats, *Cancer Res.,* 35, 2249, 1975.

75. **Longnecker, D. S., Roebuck, B. D., Yager, J. D., Lilja, H. S., and Siegmund, B.,** Pancreatic carcinoma in azaserine-treated rats: induction, classification and dietary modulation of incidence, *Cancer,* 47, 1562, 1981.

76. **Scherer, E., Bax, J., and Woutersen, R. A.,** Pathogenic interrelationship of focal lesions, nodules, adenomas and carcinomas in the multistage evolution of azaserine-induced rat pancreas carcinogenesis, in *Biologically-Based Methods for Cancer Risk Assessment,* Travis, C. C., Ed., Plenum Press, New York, 1989, 41.

77. **Pour, P. M. and Althoff, J.,** Short communication: induction of pancreatic neoplasms by 2,2′-dioxopropyl-N-propylnitrosamine, *Cancer Lett.,* 1, 3, 1975.

78. **Pour, P. M., Althoff, J., Gingell, R., and Kupper, R.,** A further pancreatic carcinogen in Syrian golden hamsters: *N*-nitroso-bis-(2-acetoxypropyl)-amine, *Cancer Lett.,* 1, 197, 1976.

79. **Pour, P. M., Althoff, J., Krüger, F. W., and Mohr, U.,** Improvement of the pancreatic cancer model by modified treatment with *N*-nitroso-bis(2-oxopropyl)amine, *Cancer Lett.,* 2, 233, 1977a.

80. **Pour, P. M., Althoff, J., Krüger, F. W., and Mohr, U.,** A potent pancreatic carcinogen in Syrian hamsters: *N*-nitroso-bis(2-oxopropyl)amine, *J. Natl. Cancer Inst.,* 58, 1449, 1977b.

81. **Pour, P. M., Salmasi, S. Z., and Runge, R. G.,** Selective induction of pancreatic ductular tumours by single doses of *N*-nitroso-bis(2-oxopropyl)amine in Syrian golden hamsters, *Cancer Lett.,* 4, 317, 1978.

82. **Pour, P. M., Runge, R. G., Birt, D., Gingell, R., Lawson, T., Nagel, D., Wallcave, L., and Salmasi, S. Z.,** Current knowledge of pancreatic carcinogenesis in the hamster and its relevance to the human disease, *Cancer,* 47, 1573, 1981.

83. **Takahashi, M., Pour, P. M., and Althoff, J.,** Sequential alteration of the pancreas during carcinogenesis in Syrian hamster by *N*-nitroso-bis(2-oxopropyl)amine, *Cancer Res.,* 37, 4602, 1977.

84. **Woutersen, R. A., van Garderen-Hoetmer, A., and Longnecker, D. S.,** Characterization of a four months protocol for the evaluation of BOP-induced preneoplastic lesions in hamsters and its application in studying the modulating effects of dietary fat, *Carcinogenesis,* 8, 833, 1987.

85. **Pour, P. M.,** Histogenesis of exocrine pancreatic cancer in the hamster model, *Environ. Health Perspect.,* 56, 229, 1984.

86. **Pour, P. M.,** Mechanism of pseudoductular (tubular) formation during pancreatic carcinogenesis in the hamster model. An electron-microscopic and immuno-histochemical study, *Am. J. Pathol.,* 130, 335, 1988.

87. **Meijers, M., Bruijntjes, J. P., Hendriksen, E. G. J., and Woutersen, R. A.,** Histogenesis of early preneoplastic lesions induced by *N*-nitrosobis(2-oxopropyl)amine in exocrine pancreas of hamsters, *Int. J. Pancreatol.,* 4, 127, 1989.

88. **Levitt, M. H., Harris, C. C., Squire, R., Springer, S., Wenk, M., Mollelo, C., Thomas, D., Kingsbury, E., and Newkirk, C.,** Experimental pancreatic carcinogenesis. I. Morphogenesis of pancreatic adenocarcinoma in the Syrian golden hamster induced by *N*-nitroso-bis(2-hydroxypropyl)amine, *Am. J. Pathol.,* 88, 5, 1977.

89. **Takahashi, M., Arai, H., Kokubo, T., Furukawa, F., Kurata, Y., and Ito, N.,** An ultrastructural study of precancerous and cancerous lesions of the pancreas in Syrian golden hamsters induced by *N*-nitroso-bis(2-oxopropyl)amine, *Gann,* 71, 816, 1980.

90. **Flaks, B. J., Moore, M. A., and Flaks, A.,** Ultrastructural analysis of pancreatic carcinogenesis. I. Morphological characterization of *N*-nitroso-bis(2-hydroxypropyl)-amine-induced neoplasms in Syrian hamster, *Carcinogenesis,* 1, 423, 1980.

91. **Flaks, B. J., Moore, M. A., and Flaks, A.,** Ultrastructural analysis of pancreatic carcinogenesis. IV. Pseudoductular transformation of acini in the hamster pancreas during *N*-nitroso-bis(2-hydroxypropyl)amine carcinogenesis, *Carcinogenesis,* 2, 1241, 1981.

92. **Flaks, B. J., Moore, M. A., and Flaks, A.,** Ultrastructural analysis of pancreatic carcinogenesis. VI. Early changes in hamster acinar cells induced by *N*-nitroso-bis(2-hydroxopropyl)amine, *Carcinogenesis,* 3, 1063, 1982.

93. **Flaks, B. J.,** Histogenesis of pancreatic carcinogenesis in the hamster, ultrastructural evidence, *Environ. Health Perspect.,* 56, 187, 1984.

94. **Carre-Llopis, A., Loridon-Rosa, B., and Escribano, M. J.,** Ultrastructural changes in acinar cells of hamster pancreas in chemically induced carcinogenesis, *Cell Biol. Int. Rep.,* 11, 665, 1987.

95. **Burns, W. A., Matthews, M. J., Hamosh, M., van de Weide, G., Blum, R., and Johnson, E. B.,** Lipase-secreting acinar cell carcinomas of the pancreas with polyarthropy: a light and electron microscopical histochemical study, *Cancer,* 33, 1002, 1974.

96. **Kakudo, K., Sakurai, M., Miyasi, T., Ikeda, Y., Satani, M., and Manabe, H.,** Pancreatic carcinoma in infancy: an E.M. study, *Acta. Pathol. Jpn.,* 26, 719, 1976.

97. **Longnecker, D. S., Shinozuka, H., and Dekker, A.,** Focal acinar cell dysplasia in human pancreas, *Cancer,* 45, 534, 1980.

98. **Woutersen, R. A., van Garderen-Hoetmer, A., Bax, J., Feringa, A. W., and Scherer, E.,** Modulation of putative preneoplastic foci in exocrine pancreas of rats and hamsters. I. Interaction of dietary fat and ethanol, *Carcinogenesis,* 7, 1587, 1986.

99. **Horie, A., Kohchi, S., and Kuratsune, M.,** Carcinogenesis in the esophagus. II. Experimental production of esophageal cancer by administration of ethanolic solution of carcinogens, *Gann,* 56, 429, 1965.

100. **Woutersen, R. A., van Garderen-Hoetmer, A., Bax, J., and Scherer, E.,** Modulation of dietary fat-promoted pancreatic carcinogenesis in rats and hamsters by chronic ethanol ingestion, *Carcinogenesis,* 10, 453, 1989.

101. **Pour, P. M., Reber, H. A., and Stepan, K.,** Modification of pancreatic carcinogenesis in the hamster model. XII. Dose-related effect of ethanol, *J. Natl. Cancer Inst.,* 71, 1085, 1983.

102. **Tweedie, J. H., Reber, H., Pour, P. M., and Ponder, D. M.,** Protective effect of ethanol on the development of pancreatic cancer, *Surg. Forum,* 32, 222, 1981.

103. **Johnson, J. R. and Zintel, H. A.,** Pancreatic calcification and cancer of the pancreas, *Surg. Gynecol. Obstet.,* 117, 585, 1979.

104. **Sarles, H. and Tiscornia, O.,** Ethanol and chronic calcifying pancreatitis, *Med. Clin. North Am.,* 58, 1333, 1974.

105. **Sarles, H., Figarella, C., Tiscornia, O., Colomb, E., Guy, O., Verine, H., De Caro, A., Multigner, L., and Lechene, P.,** Chronic calcifying pancreatitis (CCP). Mechanism of formation of the lesions. New data and critical study, in *The Pancreas,* Fitzgerald, P. J. and Morrison, A. B., Eds., Williams & Wilkins, Baltimore, 1980, 48.

106. **Singh, M.,** Ethanol and the pancreas, in *The Exocrine Pancreas: Biology, Pathobiology, and Disease,* Go, V. L. W., et al., Eds., Raven Press, New York, 1986, 423.

107. **Ammann, R. W., Muench, R., Otto, R., Buehler, H., Freiburghaus, A. U., and Siegenthaler, W.,** Evolution and regression of pancreatic calcification in chronic pancreatitis. A prospective long-term study of 107 patients, *Gasteroenterology,* 95, 1018, 1988.

108. **Singh, M. and Simsek, H.,** Ethanol and the pancreas: current status, *Gastroenterology,* 98, 1051, 1990.

109. **Sarles, H., Lebreuil, G., Tasso, F., Figarella, C., Clemente, F., Devaux, M. A., Fagonde, B., and Payan, H.,** A comparison of alcoholic pancreatitis in rat and man, *Gut,* 12, 377, 1971.

110. **Jalovaara, P., Rämö, J., and Apaja-Sarkkinen, M.,** Occurrence of pancreatic ductal cell dysplasia in rats fed with a high fat diet and ethanol, *Histol. Histopathol.,* 1, 377, 1986.

111. **Rämö, O. J.,** Antecedent long term ethanol consumption in combination with different diets alters the severity of experimental acute pancreatitis in rats, *Gut,* 28, 64, 1987.

112. **Mikal, S. and Campbell, A.,** Carcinoma of pancreas: diagnostic and operative criteria based on 100 consecutive autopsies, *Surgery,* 28, 961, 1950.

113. **Paulino-Netto, A., Dreiling, D. A., and Boronofsky, I. D.,** The relationship between pancreatic calcification and cancer of the pancreas, *Ann. Surg.,* 151, 530, 1960.

114. **Becker, V.,** Cancer of the pancreas and chronic pancreatitis, a possible relationship, *Acta Hepatogastroenterol.,* 25, 257, 1978.

115. **Rocca, G., Gaia, E., Iuliano, R., Caselle, M. T., Rocca, N., Calcamuggi, G., and Emanuelli, G.,** Increased incidence of cancer in chronic pancreatitis, *J. Clin. Gastroenterol.,* 9, 175, 1987.

116. **Haas, O., Guillard, G., Rat, P., Friedman, S., and Favre, J.-P.,** Pancreatic carcinoma developing in chronic pancreatitis: a report of four cases, *Hepato-gastroenterol.,* 37, 350, 1990.

117. **Feron, V. J. and Woutersen, R. A.**, Role of tissue damage in nasal carcinogenesis, in *Nasal Carcinogenesis in Rodents: Relevance to Human Health Risk*. Proc. TNO-CIVO/ NYU, Nose Symposium, Feron, V. J. and Bosland, M. C., Eds., Wageningen, Pudoc, 1989, 76.

118. **Laroye, G. J.**, How efficient is immunological surveillance against cancer and why does it fail?, *Lancet*, I, 1097, 1974.

119. **Berenblum, I.**, Irritation and carcinogenesis, *Arch. Pathol.*, 38, 233, 1944.

120. **Bennett, D. E., Sasser, W. F., and Ferguson, T. B.**, Adenocarcinoma of the lung in men, *Cancer*, 23, 431, 1969.

121. **Grasso, P.**, Persistent organ damage and cancer production in rats and mice, *Arch. Toxicol.*, Suppl. 11, 75, 1987.

122. **Woutersen, R. A., Appelman, L. M., Wilmer, J. W. G. M., Falke, H. E., and Feron, V. J.**, Inhalation toxicity of acetaldehyde in rats. III. Carcinogenicity study, *Toxicology*, 41, 213, 1986.

123. **Kerns, W. D., Pavkov, K. L., Donofrio, D. J., Gralla, E. J., and Swenberg, J. A.**, Carcinogenicity of formaldehyde in rats and mice after long-term inhalation exposure, *Cancer Res.*, 43, 4382, 1983.

124. **Spiegelhalder, B., Eisenbrand, G., and Preussmann, R.**, Occurrence of volatile nitrosamines in food: a survey of the West German market, in *N-Nitroso Compounds: Analysis, Formation, and Occurrence*, Walker, E. A., Griciute, L., Castegnaro, M., and Börzsönyi, M., Eds., IARC Publication, Lyon, 31, 467, 1980.

125. **Sen, H. P., Seaman, S., and McPherson, M.**, Further studies on the occurrence of volatile and nonvolatile nitrosamines in foods, in *N-Nitroso Compounds: Analysis, Formation, and Occurrence*, Walker, E. A., Griciute, L., Castegnaro, M., and Börzsönyi, M., Eds., IARC Publication, Lyon, 31, 457, 1980.

Chapter 14

ALCOHOL AND CANCER: BIOCHEMICAL AND IMMUNOLOGICAL MECHANISMS

Raz Yirmiya, Shamgar Ben-Eliyahu, and Anna N. Taylor

TABLE OF CONTENTS

257

I. INTRODUCTION

Considerable data suggest an association between alcohol consumption and increased cancer risk. The evidence for this association derives from epidemiological studies in humans and from experimental studies in both humans and animals. Several biochemical mechanisms by which alcohol might affect cancer, particularly the initiation and promotion of chemical carcinogen-induced cancers, have been proposed. Only few studies have focused on the effects of alcohol on tumor progression and the mechanisms mediating these effects. Although there have been suggestions that the effects of alcohol on cancer, particularly on tumor progression, may be mediated by its effects on the immune system, there is little experimental evidence to support this hypothesis.

In the following chapter we review the epidemiological and experimental studies that provide evidence for the existence of an association between alcohol and cancer. In addition, we review the proposed biochemical mechanisms that account for the effects of alcohol as a cocarcinogen and tumor promoter. Finally, we discuss the possible mediation of the effects of alcohol on tumor progression by the immune system, particularly our recent work on the mediation of alcohol's effects on tumor metastases in rats by natural killer (NK) cells.

II. ALCOHOL AND CANCER: EPIDEMIOLOGICAL STUDIES

Epidemiological studies show a correlation between alcohol consumption and several types of cancer, particularly cancers of the alimentary and respiratory systems, liver, large bowel, and to a lesser extent, cancers of the pancreas, stomach, bladder, breast, and lung (see Chapter 1 of this volume). In general, cancer rates are higher in persons with excessive alcohol consumption, in occupations with high-alcohol exposure (e.g., brewers), and in regions where alcohol consumption is particularly high.[1,2] In contrast, cancer rates are lower in populations with restricted alcohol consumption, such as in Mormons and Seventh Day Adventists.[3,4]

There is strong evidence for a relationship between alcohol consumption and cancer of the upper digestive and respiratory systems, including cancers of the tongue, oral cavity, nasopharynx, larynx, and esophagus (see Chapter 10 of this volume). A study conducted in France in 1910 was the first to show a correlation between high consumption of absinthe and cancer of the esophagus.[5] Since then, many epidemiological studies relating national or regional per capita alcohol consumption to cancer mortality, as well as case-control and prospective cohort studies, were conducted in other regions of the world. These studies confirmed and extended this first observation, showing that alcohol increases esophageal and other head and neck cancers in a dose-response relationship.[6-9] Alcohol and tobacco have synergistic effects on head and neck cancers. For example, in two similar studies, the risk for developing esophageal cancer was 5 to 7.4 times higher in smokers who do not drink, relative to nonsmoking-nondrinkers, but this relative risk increased to 38 to 100 times in smokers who also drink.[10,11] It is estimated that elimination of alcohol consumption could prevent more than 50% of all cancers of the upper alimentary and respiratory systems.[12]

Strong evidence also relates alcohol consumption and cancer of the liver (see Chapters 10 and 11 of this volume). Case-control studies conducted in the U.S. and Japan showed increasing risk for hepatocellular carcinoma with increasing consumption of alcohol.[13-15] Similar results were obtained in prospective cohort studies.[16] Overall, alcohol consumption increases the risk of primary liver cancer by two- to eightfold.[17] Alcohol is a major factor in development of cirrhosis, which in turn is strongly associated with development of hepatocellular carcinoma (see Chapter 11 of this volume). Hepatocellular carcinoma may also be related to hepatitis B infection, which can synergize with alcohol during hepatocellular carcinogenesis.[18,19] Overall, about 36% of liver cancers in the U.S. are attributable to alcohol consumption.[12]

Several reports suggest that alcohol may be involved in cancer of the rectum, and to a somewhat smaller extent, cancer of the colon (see Chapter 12 of this volume). Retrospective cohort studies showed increased morbidity and mortality from colorectal cancer.[20-22] Similar results were obtained in case-control studies, comparing alcohol consumption in patients with colorectal cancer and controls,[23] and in prospective studies.[24,25]

Studies on the effects of alcohol on pancreatic cancer are inconclusive (see Chapter 13 of this volume). Whereas some correlative,[26] case-control,[27] and prospective[28] studies report an increased risk for pancreatic cancer in alcoholics, other studies failed to find such an association.[29-31]

Other types of cancer which have been suggested to be associated with alcohol consumption are cancers of the stomach,[32] urinary tract,[33] and breast.[34,35] However, for each of these cancers there are negative reports, showing no association between alcohol and cancer incidence.

III. ALCOHOL AND CANCER INITIATION AND PROMOTION: MEDIATING MECHANISMS

Several mechanisms have been suggested as mediators of alcohol's effects on cancer (for review, see References 36 to 38). Some studies examined mechanisms related to the direct interaction between alcohol and established carcinogens. Other studies explored mechanisms by which alcohol indirectly affects carcinogenesis, particularly the role of carcinogens other than ethanol in alcoholic beverages and alcohol-associated malnutrition.

Experimental studies in animals found that alcohol is not a direct carcinogen,[39] and thus focused on the role of alcohol as a cocarcinogen, and the biochemical mechanisms involved. In most of these studies alcohol was chronically administered before and/or during and/or after administration of a particular carcinogen, or served as the solvent for the carcinogen, and the incidence of tumors was measured. Such studies revealed that alcohol consumption increased tumor incidence, and decreased the latency for developing experimental head and neck tumors caused by tobacco-associated carcinogens (e.g., nitrosamines).[40,41] Alcohol administration was also found to enhance hepatic carcinogenesis induced by nitrosamines or other carcinogens,[42-44] and increase the incidence of experimental rectal cancer initiated by acetoxymethylmethylnitrosamine,[45] pancreatic cancer initiated by azaserine,[46] gastric cancer initiated by *N*-methyl-*N'*-nitro-*N*-nitrosoguanidine,[47,48] and mammary adenocarcinoma initiated by dimethylbenzanthracene (DMBA).[49] It should be noted that the effects of alcohol on experimental carcinogenesis can be importantly altered by the timing of alcohol administration in relation to the carcinogen exposure, and by the method of administration. For example, in most studies, alcohol enhancement of hepatic carcinogenicity is found when alcohol is administered after carcinogen administration,[50,51] whereas administration of alcohol before or with carcinogen had either no effect or inhibited carcinogenesis.[52,53]

Several biochemical mechanisms have been proposed as the basis for alcohol's effect as a cocarcinogen and tumor promoter (Figure 1). Many carcinogens enter the body as procarcinogens and require metabolic activation by microsomal cytochrome-P-dependent enzymes. Chronic alcohol consumption in animals has been shown to induce such carcinogen-activating enzymes in several tissues in which alcohol has been suggested to be associated with cancer, including the liver, esophagus, and intestines (for review, see Reference 54). The effects on microsomal enzymes may be specific to a particular tissue, substance, gender, or species. For example, alcohol consumption enhanced the activation of the procarcinogen in tobacco pyrolyzate, but not tryptophan pyrolyzate, by lung microsomal enzymes. The opposite was true for the effect of alcohol on activation of these procarcinogens by intestinal microsomal enzymes.[55]

Alcohol has also been shown to increase the generation of reactive oxygen intermediates by microsomes.[56] These intermediates increase lipid peroxidation in the alcohol-treated animals,[57] which in turn can promote the carcinogenic process.[58] Another mechanism by which alcohol exacerbates the production of lipid peroxides and carcinogen-DNA adducts is by reducing the process of detoxification of these compounds. This effect is mainly produced by reducing the levels of glutathione (which is a major detoxifier of electrophiles and peroxides) in the liver of alcohol-treated animals.[59]

The promoting effects of alcohol on cancer may be related to the interference by alcohol and its major metabolite, acetaldehyde, with DNA metabolism. Alcohol was found to inhibit the ability of cells to repair DNA that was damaged by carcinogens. For example, the alkylation of DNA in the

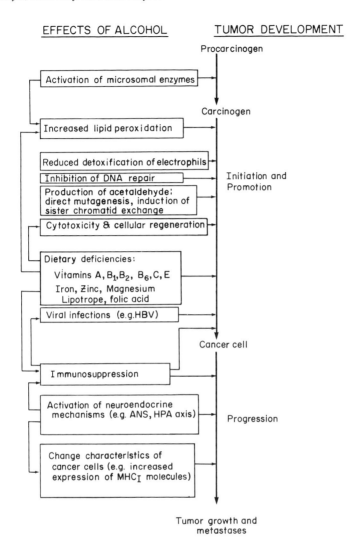

EFFECTS OF ALCOHOL   TUMOR DEVELOPMENT

FIGURE 1. Summary of the mechanisms that have been suggested to mediate the effects of alcohol on cancer. The direct effects of alcohol that contribute to tumorigenesis are presented in the boxes on the left side, with arrows pointing to the phase of tumor development in which this mechanism plays a role. Arrows between the boxes on the left side represent a secondary contribution of one effect of alcohol to another of its effects (see text for details).

liver by the carcinogen DMN persisted longer in alcohol-fed animals compared to control animals, due to alcohol-induced suppression of the activity of the enzyme that normally repairs this damage.[60] Acetaldehyde was also found to induce sister chromatid exchange in both experimental animals and human cells *in vitro*.[61,62] This process, along with other chromosomal aberrations that are elevated in alcoholic patients,[63] could increase the possibility that recessive mutations will be expressed[64] and lead to carcinogenesis.

Cellular injury followed by regeneration increases the risk of carcinogenicity, since replicating DNA is more reactive with chemical carcinogens (see, for example, Reference 65). Alcohol-induced cellular injury and mitogenesis were observed in the esophagus,[66] stomach,[67] liver,[36,68] and rectum,[69] and could account for the alcohol-induced increase in carcinogenesis observed in these tissues.

Several studies report an association between locally prepared alcoholic drinks which contain particular carcinogens and the incidence of cancer in these regions. Additionally, there seems to be a more global association between specific types of alcoholic beverages and specific types of cancers, e.g., an association between beer consumption and colon cancer.[24,26] However, other studies failed to report such specific relationships.[70]

Alcohol consumption in humans is often associated with malnutrition.[71] In fact, alcoholism is the major cause of malnutrition in countries with adequate food supply.[2] The nutritional deficiencies, particularly of certain vitamins and minerals, can in turn affect cancer via several pathways, which are described below. Alcohol administration in humans and experimental animals has been shown to be associated with reduced levels of several vitamins, including vitamin A,[72] B2 (riboflavin),[73] B6 (pyridoxin),[74] C,[73] and E.[75] These deficiencies have all been shown to be associated with increased cancer risk.[76-80] Furthermore, in experimental models, alcohol was found to have a synergistic effect with vitamin deficiency in increasing the risk of cancer.[81] Alcohol consumption has also been shown to alter the levels of minerals, such as iron[82] and zinc,[83] which are also associated with promotion of neoplasia.[84,85]

IV. ALCOHOL AND CANCER PROGRESSION: MEDIATION BY THE IMMUNE SYSTEM

The experimental studies described so far focused on the role of alcohol as a cocarcinogen, i.e., the interaction between chronic administration of alcohol and chemical carcinogens on the incidence and growth of experimental tumors in animals. However, almost no research focused on the effects of alcohol on animals that already have cancer, particularly not on the process of metastatic spread. One important mechanism that can mediate such enhancement of tumor progression, is alcohol-mediated immune suppression.

Recent studies indicate that both acute and chronic alcohol exposure impair both cellular and humoral immunity.[2,86] Alcohol consumption in humans and experimental animals decreases the number of T lymphocytes, and alters their function (see Chapters 1 and 2 of this volume). For example, chronic alcohol consumption in animals depresses mitogen-driven blastogenic transformation,[87,88] and suppresses the ability of blast cells to proliferate in response to exogenously added interleukin-2 (IL-2).[89,90] Alcohol administration affects macrophages by decreasing their number,[91] modulating their surface receptors,[92] impairing their phagocytic activity,[92-94] and inhibiting signal transduction in superoxide production by rat alveolar macrophages.[95,96] Exposure to alcohol can suppress NK cell activity (see Chapter 4 of this volume, and the discussion in Section IV.B of this chapter). Alcohol inhibits several neutrophil functions normally activated by inflammation and infection, such as delivery or migration to the site of inflammation, adherence of activated neutrophils to endothelial monolayers, and killing of bacteria.[97-99] Alcohol suppresses humoral immunity, as demonstrated by reduced antibody production to several antigens, e.g., sheep erythrocytes, in rats,[100] decreased immunization with hepatitis B vaccine in humans,[101] blunted mitogen-induced proliferation in the presence of alcohol,[102] and inhibition of antigen-induced B cell proliferation.[103] A recent study correlated alcohol-induced suppression of antibody production with an alcohol-induced decrease in resistance against the intestinal parasite *Trichinella spiralis*.[104] Finally, alcohol has profound effects on the release and function of many cytokines (see Chapter 5 of this volume). Of particular importance to resistance to tumors may be the effects of alcohol on tumor necrosis factor (TNF), which is a protein secreted by macrophages and which mediates the inflammatory cascade, stimulates phagocyte function, and may be involved in tumor necrosis (see Chapter 6 of this volume). Alcohol was found to suppress both serum and/or lung TNF secretion in response to endotoxin or lipopolysaccharide.[105,106] Interestingly, plasma TNF was found to predict decreased long-term survival in severe alcoholic hepatitis.[107]

The functional significance of the alcohol-induced alterations in immune function are still not fully understood. However, they are correlated with the greater susceptibility to diseases of both human alcoholics and experimental animals exposed to alcohol to diseases. For example, alcoholic patients are known to be prone to contract a number of infectious diseases,[108] including listeria,[109] tuberculosis,[110] bacterial pneumonia,[111] peritonitis,[112] endocarditis,[113] and viral disorders.[114] Experimental animals administered with alcohol are also more susceptible to infections,[115] and show a lower delayed cutaneous hypersensitivity-like response to PHA.[116]

The immunosuppressive effects of alcohol may also be related to decreased resistance to tumor progression. In the following sections, our work on alcohol and tumor progression and metastases is presented, and possible mechanisms mediating alcohol's effects on immunological resistance to cancer are described.

A. ALCOHOL AND TUMOR PROGRESSION IN RAT MODELS OF BREAST CANCER AND LEUKEMIA

The effects of alcohol on tumor progression have to be studied experimentally in animals with established cancer. This can be achieved by injecting tumor cells to animals and examining the effects of alcohol on the progression and metastases of the resulting tumors. This approach may be particularly important if some of alcohol's effects on cancer are mediated by the immune system, which is known to be involved in resistance to tumor progression and metastases.[117] Recent studies in our laboratory were designed to examine the influence of alcohol administration on tumor progression in rat models of breast cancer and leukemia.[118] In the first set of studies we used MADB106 mammary adenocarcinoma, syngeneic to Fischer 344 (F344) rats.

Subjects were F344 male rats, 10 to 12 weeks old. In chronic ethanol-exposure experiments, rats were housed individually and divided into three groups, receiving either a liquid diet containing ethanol (5% w/v, 35% ethanol-derived calories), pair-feeding of an isocaloric diet, or normal rat chow and water. After two weeks on these diets, animals were injected into the tail vein with 10^5 MADB106 cells. Animals were kept on their diets for three weeks when they were euthanized, lungs were removed, and visible surface metastases were counted. In acute ethanol exposure experiments, animals were divided into four groups and injected intraperitoneally (i.p.) with saline, or 1.5, 2.5, or 3.5 g/kg ethanol diluted in saline to 20% w/v. One hour later, animals were injected with MADB106 tumor cells. Animals were sacrificed three weeks after tumor inoculation, and surface lung metastases were enumerated.

Our data indicate that chronic ethanol consumption increases the number of breast cancer metastases in rats. In the chronic ethanol exposure experiment, mean ($\pm$ standard error of the mean [SEM]) number of metastases were 9.4 (± 1.0, normal chow), 20.1 (± 4.8, pair-fed), and 50.0 (± 8.2, ethanol). This result represented a significant increase in metastases by chronic ethanol exposure, compared to both pair-fed and normal groups. The difference between the latter groups was not significant. Body weight in the ethanol and pair-fed groups was similarly decreased during the first week of feeding, recovering thereafter. Experimental animals consumed 8.9 g/kg/day ethanol at the beginning of the experiment, increased their consumption in the first two weeks on the diet, and stabilized at about 12.0 g/kg/day. Mean ($\pm$ SEM) blood ethanol level, measured spectrophotometrically at the beginning of the dark period two weeks after initiation of the diet, was 1.63 (± 0.24) mg/ml.

Animals injected acutely with saline, 1.5, 2.5, or 3.5 g/kg ethanol had 43.1 (± 3.4), 84.6 (± 25.8), 144.7 (± 25.9), and 174.9 (± 33.2) lung metastases, respectively. Thus, rats administered with either 2.5 or 3.5 g/kg ethanol had significantly more MADB106 metastases than animals injected with saline or 1.5 g/kg ethanol. The increase following injection of 1.5 g/kg ethanol was not significant. Mean ($\pm$ SEM) blood ethanol concentration, measured in other rats one hour after injection of 1.5, 2.5, or 3.5 g/kg ethanol was 1.36 (± 0.61), 2.82 (± 0.60), and 3.41 (± 0.33) mg/ml, respectively.

In a second set of studies we used the CRNK-16 leukemia model. This leukemia occurs spontaneously, and is a major cause of death in aged F344 rats.[119] In chronic ethanol consumption experiments, rats were housed individually and divided into three groups, receiving either a liquid diet containing ethanol, pair-feeding of an isocaloric diet, or normal rat chow and water. After two weeks on this diet, animals were injected in the tail vein with 5×10^3 CRNK-16 cells. Animals remained on the diet, and survival was recorded. In acute ethanol experiments, animals were divided into four groups and injected i.p. with saline, 1.5, 2.5, or 3.5 g/kg ethanol. One hour later, animals were injected with CRNK-16 tumor cells. Animals were kept undisturbed in their cages, and survival was recorded.

The median survival times for animals in the chronic experiment were 21 (ethanol diet), 22 (pair-fed), and 22 (normal chow) days. The difference between the ethanol-treated and the other two control groups was not statistically significant. The median survival time for rats injected acutely with saline, 1.5, 2.5, or 3.5 g/kg of ethanol was 22, 21, 20, and 18.5 days, respectively. Statistical analysis showed that rats acutely injected with 1.5, 2.5, or 3.5 g/kg ethanol survived significantly less time than saline-injected rats. Additionally, survival was briefer in rats injected with 3.5 g/kg of ethanol than in rats injected with 1.5 g/kg ethanol.

B. MECHANISMS OF ALCOHOL'S EFFECTS ON METASTASES
1. Role of NK Cells
a. Previous Studies on the Effects of Alcohol on NK Activity

As discussed earlier, alcohol was found to suppress almost all of the immune functions that were measured after its administration. NK cells are one component of the immune system involved in resistance to tumor growth in general and metastases in particular.[117] Several lines of evidence indicate that exposure to alcohol modulates the cytotoxic activity of NK cells, although the relationships between alcohol administration and NK activity are complex, and many conflicting results have been reported (see Chapter 4 of this volume). Some of these inconsistencies may be explained by factors other than alcohol exposure, which also affect NK activity such as age, gender, and nutritional and emotional status.[117] For example, such inconsistent results were reported in studies of alcohol consumption *in vivo,* in which NK activity in alcoholic patients was reported to be decreased,[120] not affected,[121] or increased.[122] Some of this variability could be accounted for by considering such factors as liver damage, nutritional status, smoking, and depression. In alcoholic patients with liver damage, NK activity was suppressed, although there was no relationship between NK activity and the level of liver function.[123] In such patients, the percentage of blood NK cells was increased in comparison to patients who abstained from drinking for at least two weeks.[124] Both smoking[125] and depression[120] were found to lower NK activity in alcoholic patients. In the latter study, depressed patients with a history of alcohol abuse had lower NK activity than depressed patients without alcohol abuse, and alcoholic patients with secondary depression had lower NK activity than alcoholic patients without depression.[120]

Studies in rodents usually showed that chronic consumption of relatively low amounts of alcohol (i.e., lower than 19 g/kg body weight/day in mice) either had no effect on NK activity[126,127] or enhanced NK activity.[128] The enhancing effects were observed only after several weeks of consumption.[128] Consumption of higher levels of alcohol (i.e., above 22 g/kg body weight/day) significantly suppressed NK activity in mice.[127,129,130] This suppressive effect was observed as early as 7 days after initiation of alcohol consumption, and continued for the rest of the examined period (up to 70 days).

Studies conducted *in vitro* with human NK cells also report inconsistent results. Several studies show that addition of alcohol to the NK assay media reduces the cytotoxic activity of NK cells.[131,132] This inhibition was reported to occur even at low concentrations (e.g., 0.05% w/v) in one study,[132] or only at higher ethanol concentrations (above 0.2%) in another study.[133] In contrast, enhancement of NK activity has also been reported after addition of ethanol to the incubation medium.[93] In other studies, effector cells were incubated in ethanol-containing solutions, and then washed before the NK assay. These studies report that NK activity is either enhanced[134,135] or not affected by preincubation with low concentrations of ethanol, but decreased by incubation with higher concentrations of ethanol.[133] Studies of the effects of ethanol *in vitro* on rodent NK activity are more consistent, showing decreased NK activity when ethanol is present during the assay, which returns to baseline upon removal of ethanol.[136,137]

b. Mediation of Alcohol's Effects on Metastases by NK Cells

We have recently sought to provide more conclusive evidence for a causal relationship between the effects of alcohol on NK activity and tumor growth by using the MADB106 model described above. A direct role of NK cells in controlling metastases of the MADB106 tumor was previously reported.[138] For example, depletion of NK cells by treating rats with antibodies against NK cell surface markers, i.e., either with anti-asialo GM1 antiserum[138] or the more specific monoclonal antibody mAb 3.2.3.,[139] diminished the animal's ability to destroy circulating MADB106 cells, leading to a greatly increased number of lung metastases. Treatment with anti-asialo GM1 inhibited NK activity without affecting T cell-mediated immunity and macrophage cytotoxicity.[138] Finally, adoptive transfer of large granular lymphocytes with high NK activity, but not T cells, restored the ability of NK-depleted rats to inhibit the development of lung metastases.[138] We have recently used this same model to provide evidence for a causal relationship between the NK-suppressive and tumor-enhancing effects of swim-stress,[139] surgical-stress,[140] and opiates.[141]

For this reason, in addition to studying the effects of ethanol on MADB106 metastases *in vivo*, we also assessed the effects of ethanol on the cytotoxic activity of NK cells against this tumor *in vitro*. The application of this investigation to the CRNK-16 leukemia model is not clear, because a relationship between NK cells and CRNK-16 leukemia has not been fully established.

However, it should be mentioned that CRNK-16 tumor cells are sensitive to lymphokine-activated killer activity,[141] which is attributable to IL-2 stimulated NK cells.[143]

To assess NK activity *in vitro*, the same chronic and acute ethanol administration procedures described above were repeated, and the cytotoxic activity of spleen or blood NK cells against MADB106 or YAC-1 target cells was measured in a ^{51}Cr release assay. In chronic ethanol exposure experiments, rats were sacrificed after two weeks on their assigned diet, whereas in the acute studies, animals were sacrificed 1 to 2 h after administration of saline, 1.5, 2.5, or 3.5 g/kg ethanol.

Splenic NK activity was determined by dissociating spleen cells into single cell suspensions, washing them twice in phosphate buffered saline, filtering them through a nylon mesh, counting and adjusting their number, and then incubating them with a certain number of radiolabeled target cells for several hours, and measuring the amount of radioactivity released to the incubation media by killed target cells. Using this standard assay, we observed no effects of either chronic or acute ethanol administration on splenic NK activity against tumor target cells. Since blood NK cytotoxicity may be more relevant to the killing of tumor cells that are intravenously inoculated *in vivo*, we also assessed blood NK activity. In this experiment, rats were injected with either ethanol (2.5 g/kg body weight) or saline, two hours before 3 ml of heparinized cardiac blood were drawn. Half of the blood was washed (i.e., the serum was replaced by RPMI 1640 media), whereas the other half was not washed. Aliquots of the washed and unwashed blood were incubated with various concentrations of ^{51}Cr-labeled YAC-1 target cells, and cytotoxicity was determined in a 4-h release assay. In order to provide evidence that cytotoxicity in this assay is mediated by NK cells, several rats in this experiment were treated 24 h before the assay with the monoclonal antibody mAb 3.2.3, which is directed specifically at NK cells. We found that administration of 2.5 g/kg ethanol significantly suppressed NK cytotoxicity in both washed and unwashed blood. In the same assay, animals treated with mAb 3.2.3 had no detectable NK activity, suggesting that the cytotoxicity observed in the other rats was indeed mediated by NK cells.

The finding that ethanol suppressed blood NK activity in the whole blood assay, but had no effect on splenic NK activity, could have two explanations. One possibility is that NK cells in these two compartments are modulated differentially by ethanol, such that only blood NK activity is affected. The whole blood assay is sensitive, not only to the cytotoxic function of effector cells, but also to their number. Thus, another possibility is that ethanol reduces the number of NK cells in the blood (e.g., by directing them to other compartments, but not to spleen, where NK activity is unaffected by ethanol), and this decrease in number is reflected by the reduced NK activity. These possibilities are currently being investigated by assessing the activity of blood NK cells in a traditional NK assay, and by examining the effects of ethanol on the number and percentage of NK cells in different compartments.

In order to examine a possible direct effect of ethanol on NK activity *in vitro*, NK and target cells were cocultured in media containing ethanol in a range of concentrations approximating the actual blood levels seen, as reported above. Additionally, incubation of YAC-1 or MADB106 cells (without effector cells) in media containing ethanol at concentrations between 0 to 20.0 mg/ml was used to determine the effects of ethanol on spontaneous ^{51}Cr release. The results showed that incubation of spleen cells with MADB106 or YAC-1 target cells in media containing ethanol at concentrations 1.0 mg/ml and higher, or 5.0 mg/ml and higher, respectively, suppressed NK cell activity. There was no effect of any concentration of ethanol on spontaneous ^{51}Cr release by tumor cells.

The effects of ethanol on NK activity were also assessed *in vivo* by measuring the clearance of radiolabeled MADB106 cells from the lungs after intravenous (i.v.) inoculation. In this experiment, rats were injected with either saline or ethanol (2.5 g/kg body weight), and 2 h later were inoculated with 10^5 ^{51}Cr-labeled MADB106 cells. Rats were sacrificed either 2 or 24 h after the inoculation, and the amount of radioactivity retained in the lungs was measured. In saline-injected rats, the amount of radioactivity retained in the lungs was 11% after 2 h, and almost undetectable after 24 h. In contrast, ethanol-injected rats had more than 40% radioactivity retained in the lungs after 2 h, reducing to 5% after 24 h. These results indicate that ethanol exposure reduces the clearance of i.v. inoculated tumor cells, providing one possible mechanism for the increase in lung metastases observed three weeks after tumor inoculation. Animals that were injected with the monoclonal antibody 3.2.3, which abolishes NK activity, showed no clearance of the tumor cells at this period, indicating that the clearance was dependent on NK cells.

To evaluate further the hypothesis that NK cells are involved in the increase in MADB106 metastases produced by ethanol administration, we studied the effect of ethanol on metastases in rats whose NK activity was either abolished by administration of anti-asialo GM1 monoclonal antibody (anti-asGM1) or enhanced by administration of the interferon inducer, poly I:C. In the first study, rats were injected in the tail vein with either normal rabbit serum (NRS) or anti-asGM1, at a dilution of 1:5 (Wako Industries, Osaka, Japan). As mentioned earlier, this antibody has previously been shown to abolish NK activity against MADB106 cells *in vitro*, and increase lung metastases more than tenfold.[138,139] Two days later, rats within each group were further divided into two subgroups and injected i.p. either with saline or ethanol (2.5 g/kg). One hour later, two NRS-groups that received either saline or ethanol were injected i.v. with 10^5 MADB106 cells. The other two NRS-treated groups, and the two groups treated with anti-asGM1, were injected with 2×10^3 MADB106 cells at that time. Preliminary studies had indicated that injecting anti-asGM1-treated rats with the usual number of MADB106 cells (10^5) produced more than 300 metastases, making it im-

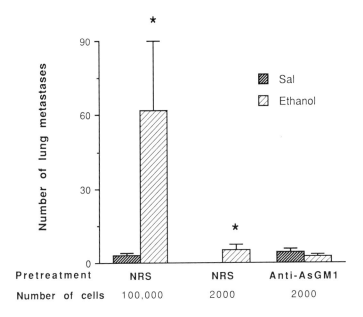

FIGURE 2. Mean ($\pm$ SEM) number of surface MADB106 metastases of both lungs in saline- and ethanol-injected rats. Rats were divided into two groups injected into the tail vein with either normal rabbit serum (NRS) or anti-asialo GM1 monoclonal antibody (anti-asGM1). Two days later, rats within each group were further divided into two subgroups and injected i.p. either with saline or ethanol (2.5 g/kg). One hour later, animals pretreated with NRS were injected with either 10^5 or 2×10^3 MADB106 cells, and anti-asGM1-treated rats were injected with 2×10^3 MADB106 cells. *Significantly different from saline-injected animals.

possible to observe any further increase with ethanol administration. Therefore, no groups treated with anti-asGM1 were injected with 10^5 MADB106 cells. We found that ethanol administration produced a significant increase in the number of lung metastases in animals treated with NRS and injected with 2×10^3 as well as 10^5 MADB106 cells, but had no effect in animals treated with anti-asGM1 (Figure 2). This finding was reflected by a significant treatment (NRS vs. anti-asGM1) by injection (saline vs. ethanol) interaction.

In the experiment with Poly I:C, rats were divided into two groups and injected with either saline or Poly I:C (1 mg/rat). One day later, animals within each group were further divided into two subgroups and injected with either saline or ethanol (2.5 g/kg in 20% w/v of saline). One hour after the second injection, all rats were inoculated with 2×10^5 MADB106 cells, and metastases were enumerated three weeks later. The results showed that Poly I:C treatment significantly reduced the number of MADB106 lung metastases (Figure 3). Ethanol increased the number of metastases in both saline and Poly I:C-treated animals; however, this increase was significant only in the latter group. These results are consistent with a role for NK cells in controlling metastases of the MADB106 tumor. Poly I:C is an interferon inducer, known

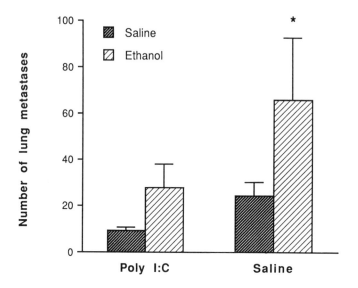

FIGURE 3.   Mean ($\pm$ SEM) number of surface MADB106 metastases of both lungs in saline- and ethanol-injected rats. Rats were divided into two groups injected with either Poly I:C or saline. One day later, rats within each group were further divided into two subgroups and injected i.p. either with saline or ethanol (2.5 g/kg). One hour after the second injection, all rats were inoculated with 2×10^5 MADB106 cells. *Significantly different from saline-injected animals.

to augment NK activity.[144] Thus, the finding that ethanol significantly enhanced metastases in the saline, but not Poly I:C-treated rats could provide support for a common mechanism (e.g., NK activity), which is enhanced by Poly I:C and suppressed by ethanol. However, since ethanol did enhance the number of metastases also in the Poly I:C-treated rats, such a conclusion should be taken cautiously until this experiment is repeated with similar findings.

The increase in metastases and tumor progression following acute administration of ethanol probably results from suppression of NK activity during a narrow time window (i.e., approximately 24 h, which is the time it takes F344 rats to completely eliminate ethanol from the body after an injection of 2.5 g/kg ethanol).[118] NK cells are known to be especially important in controlling the early stages of the metastatic process.[138] In fact, we have recently demonstrated that an increase in MADB106 metastases following exposure to acute swimming stress is also produced during a narrow time window (i.e., the stressor is effective when administered one hour before, but not one day before or after tumor inoculation).[139] These findings serve to explain how even a brief exposure to ethanol can influence tumor progression measured several weeks later.

A summary of the relationships between the effects of ethanol on NK activity against MADB106 tumor cells *in vitro* and metastases of this tumor

TABLE 1
Summary of the Relationship between the Effects of Ethanol on NK Activity against MADB106 Tumor Cells *In Vitro* and on MADB106 Metastases *In Vivo*

Ethanol exposure	Effect on NK activity	Effect on metastases
Acute	Splenic NK activity — no effect Blood NK activity — suppression	Increased number of metastases; Decreased clearance of tumor cells from the lungs
Chronic	Splenic NK activity — no effect Blood NK activity — not tested	Increased number of metastases
In vitro	Splenic NK activity — suppression	Incubation of MADB106 cells with ethanol decreased their proliferation
Acute (NK depleted rats)	No NK activity	Increased number of metastases in NK depleted rats, but no further increase by ethanol
Acute (Poly I:C treated rats)	Enhanced NK activity	Decreased number of metastases in Poly I:C treated rats; reversal of ethanol's effect by Poly I:C

in vivo is presented in Table 1. In conclusion, the findings that ethanol administration increases lung metastases in a tumor model in which NK cells are demonstrably important in controlling metastases, that blood NK activity against this same tumor is suppressed in ethanol-treated animals, that incubation with ethanol decreases NK activity *in vitro*, that ethanol administration reduces the clearance of these same tumor cells from the lungs, and that ethanol has no effect on metastases in animals in which NK activity has been abolished, strongly suggest a causal relationship between the effects of ethanol on NK activity and on metastases.

c. Effects of Alcohol on the Binding of NK to Tumor Cells

Alcohol has been found to inhibit binding of NK cells to YAC-1 target cells, and this inhibition correlates with alcohol's suppressive effect on NK activity.[136] We have recently tested the effects of ethanol *in vitro* on the binding of effector cells to MADB106 target cells. Spleens were removed and dissociated into single-cell suspensions, and splenic mononuclear cells were isolated by the Ficoll-Hypaque procedure. The target binding assay was a modification of one described by Roder.[145] MADB106 cells (10^6) and effector cells (10^6) were mixed in 200 μl of complete media, and then additional 50 μl of either media alone or media containing ethanol were added.

The final concentrations of ethanol in the solutions were 0, 1.6, 4, or 8 mg/ml. The mixtures of cells were centrifuged, placed on ice for 30 min, and then transferred to hemocytometers. The percentage of effector cells binding to MADB106 cells was then determined by direct microscopic observation of 200 to 250 MADB106 target cells. MADB106 cells are three to four times larger than lymphocytes, making it easy to distinguish between the two cell populations without specific labeling.

Ethanol significantly inhibited the binding of effector to MADB106 cells in a dose-related manner. Mean $\pm$ SEM percent binding of effector to target cells at the various ethanol solutions was 8.10 $\pm$ 1.49 (no ethanol), 5.30 $\pm$ 0.95 (1.6 mg/ml), 4.88 $\pm$ 1.37 (4 mg/ml), and 3.98 $\pm$ 0.75 (8 mg/ml). Statistical analysis showed that effector to target binding was reduced in each of the solutions containing ethanol, compared to the control solution.

One possible explanation of this decreased binding is ethanol's effect on the expression of MHC class I antigens by tumor cells. Acute ethanol intoxication increases expression of MHC class I antigens in humans.[146] In mice, increased expression of MHC class I antigens correlates with increased metastatic potential of several experimental tumors.[147] This increased metastatic potential is associated with a reduction in sensitivity to lysis by NK cells *in vitro,* and with reduced effectiveness of NK cells in controlling metastases *in vivo.*[148] Recently, strong evidence was provided that reduced MHC class I is a major mechanism by which NK cells recognize their targets.[149] Thus, an ethanol-induced increase in MHC class I antigens could account for impaired recognition and binding of tumor cells by NK cells.

2. Mediation by Neuroendocrine Factors

Several studies implicate hormones and the central nervous system (CNS) as modulators of the immune response to ethanol. Connections between the nervous and immune systems include activation of the hypothalamic-pituitary-adrenal (HPA) axis which causes release of glucocorticoids from the adrenal gland, activation of the autonomic nervous system which causes secretion of catecholamines and endorphins by sympathetic nerve terminals and the adrenal medulla, secretion of other pituitary and gonadal hormones, and secretion of cytokines by activated immune cells.[150,151] There is ample evidence that alcohol affects several of these neuroendocrine and neurotransmitter mechanisms by which the nervous and immune system interact, including glucocorticoids, catecholamines, and opioids. The possible relevance of these neuroendocrine effects of alcohol to alcohol's effects on tumor progression are discussed below.

Both acute and chronic alcohol exposure activate the sympathetic nervous system (SNS) and produce increases in norepinephrine and epinephrine levels in plasma and urine (for review, see Reference 152). Ethanol also stimulates corticotropin-releasing factor (CRF) release,[153] which has been shown to activate the SNS and reduce splenic NK cytotoxicity.[154] Association between alteration of the SNS and immune function by alcohol were found in a study in which young adult mice exposed to alcohol prenatally displayed immune impairment and altered noradrenergic synaptic transmission, including enhanced norepinephrine turnover, and reduced norepinephrine levels and β-adrenoceptor density in the thymus and spleen, but not the heart.[155] Activation of the SNS may affect the metastatic process in several ways. The hemodynamic and thermoregulatory changes associated with SNS activation may enhance the survival of the metastases in the circulation, e.g., by changing blood flow and turbulence, which are known to affect the incidence of metastases.[156] Additionally, the SNS has been shown to modulate immune function (for review, see Reference 157). For example, we have recently shown that the suppression of NK activity against MADB106 target cells, and the increase in number of MADB106 metastases produced by exposure to swim stress are mediated by adrenal epinephrine.[158] We are currently investigating whether the effects of alcohol on NK activity and metastases are similarly mediated.

Glucocorticoids have been shown to affect both immune function[159] and tumor growth[160] when administered exogenously, and to mediate at least some of the effects of stress on tumor growth.[161,162] The effects of glucocorticoids on tumor growth may be either direct[163] or mediated by suppression of immune function, including macrophages and NK cells (for review, see Reference 164). Evidence that glucocorticoids play a role in the immunosuppressive effects of alcohol has been provided. One study[165] showed that reduced mitogen-induced proliferation of T cells of rats withdrawn from alcohol treatment was abrogated by adrenalectomy. In another study[166] lymphocyte transformation was enhanced when thymocytes from intact rats were assayed in the presence of serum from castrated animals. Furthermore, serum from adrenalectomized rats also had an enhancing effect, additive to serum from castrate-adrenalectomized animals. To determine if the effects of alcohol on tumor growth might involve glucocorticoids, we measured corticosterone levels by radioimmunoassay. In an experiment with chronic alcohol consumption after two weeks of feeding (Figure 4), corticosterone levels were significantly higher in the pair-fed group than in either the ethanol or normal groups; the latter did not differ significantly from each other. Plasma corticosterone levels measured one hour after a single injection of either saline or ethanol are presented in Figure 5 (upper panel). The elevation in corticosterone levels in all ethanol-injected rats was significant. Similar results were seen in a measurement of plasma ACTH levels in these animals (Figure 5, lower panel). There were no significant differences among the ethanol-injected groups in either corticosterone or ACTH levels.

These results show that there is no relationship between the effects of alcohol on HPA hormones and on metastases. Rats that consumed ethanol chronically did not have higher blood corticosterone levels, but did have significantly more metastases than controls. Additionally, whereas acutely administered ethanol at all three doses caused a similar increase in ACTH

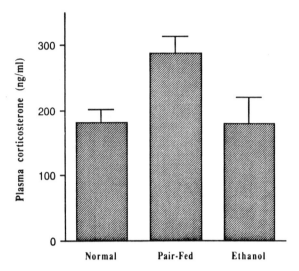

FIGURE 4.   Mean (± SEM) levels of corticosterone in the plasma of rats after two weeks of consumption of an ethanol-containing diet, pair-feeding of an isocaloric diet, or normal chow. Corticosterone levels were measured in the beginning of the dark phase of the light cycle.

and corticosterone levels, significant increases in lung metastases were seen only at the higher two doses. This lack of correlation with ACTH and corticosterone levels argues that activation of the HPA axis is not the mechanism underlying alcohol's effect on tumor progression.

Acute and chronic alcohol administration can affect several endogenous opioid systems. For example, acute alcohol treatment stimulates the release of β-endorphin from the pituitary,[167] and increases its levels in the hypothalamus.[168] Alcohol administration was also found to alter opiate receptor characteristics (see, for example, Reference 169). Endogenous opioid peptides can regulate tumor growth upon exogenous administration.[170,171] Additionally, the NK suppressive and tumor-enhancing effects of some stressful stimuli were shown to be blocked by naltrexone,[172,173] indicating that endogenous opioid peptides released by environmental stimuli may increase tumor development. We have recently demonstrated a causal relationship between the NK suppressive effects of opiate agonists (morphine and fentanyl) and their enhancement of the incidence of pulmonary MADB106 tumor metastases.[141,174]

We recently examined the role of opioids in mediating ethanol's effects on metastatic growth by examining interactions between ethanol and the opiate antagonist, naltrexone. Rats were divided into two groups, injected with either naltrexone (10 mg/kg) or saline. Each of these groups was further divided into two subgroups (n = 9 to 10), and injected 20 min later with either saline or 2.5 g/kg ethanol (20% w/v in saline). One hour after the second injection,

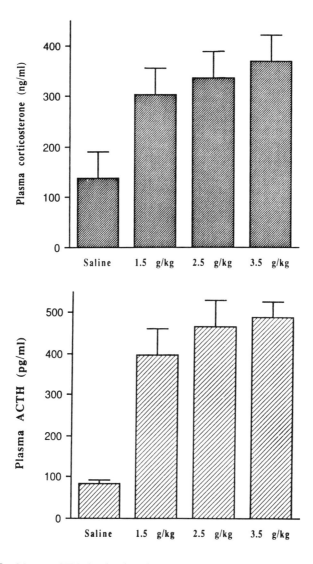

FIGURE 5. Mean (± SEM) levels of corticosterone in the plasma of rats one hour after administration of saline, 1.5, 2.5, or 3.5 g/kg body weight of ethanol (upper panel). Mean (± SEM) levels of adrenocorticotropin (ACTH) in the plasma of rats one hour after administration of saline, 1.5, 2.5, or 3.5 g/kg body weight of ethanol (lower panel).

all animals were inoculated with 10^5 MADB106 cells, and number of lung metastases was enumerated three weeks later. Ethanol administration significantly increased the number of metastases in both naltrexone- and saline-treated animals (Figure 6). However, naltrexone had no effect on this ethanol-induced increased number of metastases, suggesting that these effects are not mediated by an interaction between ethanol and endogenous opioids.

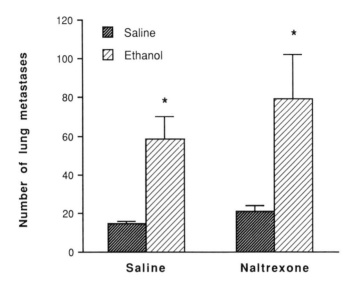

FIGURE 6.   Mean ($\pm$ SEM) number of surface MADB106 metastases of both lungs in saline- and ethanol-injected rats. Rats were divided into two groups injected with either naltrexone (10 mg/kg) or saline. Twenty minutes later, rats within each group were further divided into two subgroups and injected i.p. either with saline or ethanol (2.5 g/kg). One hour after the second injection, all rats were inoculated with 10^5 MADB106 cells. *Significantly different from saline-injected animals.

3. Direct Effects of Alcohol on Tumor Cells

In order to determine the direct effect of alcohol on tumor cells, MADB106 and CRNK-16 cells were incubated for five days in solution containing ethanol in a range of concentrations approximating blood levels observed following acute and chronic ethanol administration. CRNK-16 (3×10^5) or MADB106 (5×10^5) cells were incubated in tissue culture flasks containing either 0, 1.0, 2.0, 5.0, or 10.0 mg/ml ethanol in complete media. Number of tumor cells was counted five days later. Tests were performed in triplicates. The results showed that ethanol at concentrations of 2.0 or 5.0 mg/ml or higher significantly inhibited growth of MADB106 and CRNK tumor cells, respectively (Figure 7). Therefore, the increased metastatic effect observed *in vivo* cannot be explained by a direct effect of ethanol on tumor cells. Furthermore, it seems that ethanol has two opposing effects on tumor growth: one, a direct suppressive effect on tumor development seen in this *in vitro* assay, and the other, an indirect effect of enhanced tumor progression seen in the *in vivo* experiments reported above.

V. CONCLUSIONS

Mounting evidence indicates that alcohol consumption may be considered as a risk factor for the initiation, promotion, and progression of cancer.

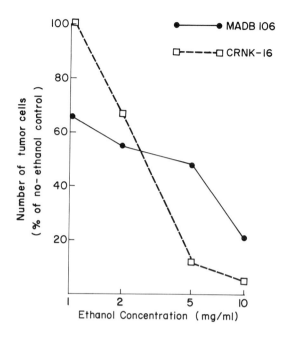

FIGURE 7. Mean numbers of tumor cells, five days after incubation of CRNK-16 (3×10^5) or MADB106 (5×10^5) cells in tissue culture flasks containing various concentrations of ethanol in complete media (expressed as percent of the number of cells incubated in media containing no ethanol). Ethanol at concentrations of 2.0 or 5.0 mg/ml or higher significantly inhibited growth of MADB106 and CRNK tumor cells, respectively.

Epidemiological studies provide strong evidence for a relationship between alcohol and several types of neoplasia, particularly cancers of the upper respiratory and alimentary systems, the liver and the rectum, and somewhat less strong evidence for an association with cancers of the pancreas, bladder, stomach, breast, and lung. Experiments in both humans and animals indicate that alcohol can serve as a cocarcinogen and tumor promoter. Several mechanisms by which alcohol produces its cocarcinogenic and tumor promoting effects have been described (see Figure 1).

Our data indicate that alcohol administration increases tumor progression and metastases in two different tumor models in rats. These effects were observed even with a single, intoxicating dose of alcohol. The MADB106 is a rat mammary adenocarcinoma and a possible model of breast cancer in humans.[175] Associations between alcohol and breast cancer were demonstrated in some epidemiological studies, where the incidence of breast cancer in alcohol drinkers (even with moderate alcohol consumption of one to two drinks per day) is 10 to 100% higher than in nondrinkers.[34] Since large numbers of women drink moderately,[176] and about 10% of women in the United States develop breast cancer, half of them already metastatic at diagnosis,[177] future research should examine whether alcohol consumption also increases breast cancer metastases. Moreover, with respect to cancer in general, in the United States alone more than one million new cases of cancer are diagnosed every year,[178] of which more than half are metastatic.[179] Our data show that even one acute administration of alcohol can dramatically increase the number of tumor metastases. It will need to be determined whether the results with acute alcohol exposure in rats are applicable to cancer in humans, epidemiological studies having investigated only the effects of long-term, averaged alcohol consumption on cancer risk. If one, or even several discrete episodes of alcohol intoxication can increase tumor progression, then the deleterious effects of alcohol on cancer in humans have been underestimated.

ACKNOWLEDGMENTS

This research has been supported by National Institute for Alcoholism and Alcohol Abuse Grant AA 06744, the Veterans Administration Medical Research Service, and Trent and Mary Wells (Anna N. Taylor); by National Institutes of Health Grant NS07628 (J. C. Liebeskind); by Grants from the National Institute for Psychobiology in Israel, the Israel Cancer Association, and the Israel Ministry of Science and Technology (Raz Yirmiya); and by the UCLA Psychoneuroimmunology Program (Raz Yirmiya and Shamgar Ben-Eliyahu).

REFERENCES

1. **Driver, H. E. and Swann, P. F.**, Alcohol and human cancer (review), *Anticancer Res.*, 7, 309, 1987.
2. **Watson, R. R.**, Ethanol, immunomodulation and cancer, *Prog. Food Nutrit. Sci.*, 12, 189, 1988.
3. **Lyon, J. L., Klauber, M. R., Gardner, J. W., and Smart, C. R.**, *New Engl. J. Med.*, 294, 129, 1976.
4. **Wynder, E. L., Lemon, F. R., and Bross, I. J.**, *Cancer*, 12, 1016, 1956.
5. **Lamy, L.**, Etude de statistique clinique de 134 cas de cancer de l'oesophage et du cardia, *Arch. Mal. Appar. Dis.*, 4, 451, 1910.
6. **Keller, A. Z.**, The epidemiology of oesophageal cancer in the west, *Prev. Med.*, 9, 607, 1980.
7. **Pottern, L. M.**, Oesophageal cancer among black men in Washington, D.C. I. Alcohol, tobacco, and other risk factors, *J. Natl. Cancer. Inst.*, 67, 777, 1981.
8. **Tuyns, A. J., Pequignot, G., and Abbatucci, J. S.**, Oesophageal cancer and alcohol consumption: importance of the type of beverage, *Int. J. Cancer*, 23, 443, 1979.
9. **Hinds, M. W., Kolonel, L. N., Lee, J., and Hirohata, T.**, Associations between cancer incidence and alcohol/cigarette consumption among five ethnic groups in Hawaii, *Br. J. Cancer*, 41, 929, 1980.
10. **Tuyns, A. J.**, Oesophageal cancer in nonsmoking drinkers and in nondrinking smokers, *Int. J. Cancer*, 32, 443, 1983.

11. **Blot, W. J., McLaughlin, J. K., Winn, D. M., Austin, D. F., Greenberg, R. S., et al.,** Smoking and drinking in relation to oral and pharyngeal cancer, *Cancer Res.,* 48, 3282, 1988.

12. **Rothman, K., Garfinkel, L., Keller, A. Z., Muir, C. S., and Schottenfeld, D.,** The proportion of cancer attributable to alcohol consumption, *Prev. Med.,* 9, 174, 1980.

13. **Yu, C. M., Mack, T., Hanisch, R., Peters, R. L., Henderson, B. E., and Pike, M. C.,** Hepatitis, alcohol consumption, cigarette smoking, and hepatocellular carcinoma in Los Angeles, *Cancer Res.,* 43, 6077, 1983.

14. **Austin, H., Delzell, E., Grufferman, S., Levine, R., Morrison, A. S., Stolley, P. D., and Cole, P. A.,** Case-control study of hepatocellular carcinoma and the hepatitis B virus, cigarette smoking and alcohol consumption, *Cancer Res.,* 46, 962, 1986.

15. **Oshima, T., Tsukuma, H., Hiyama, T., Fujimoto, I., Yamano, H., and Tanaka, M.,** Follow up study of HB_sAg-positive blood donors with special reference to effect of drinking and smoking on development of liver cancer, *Int. J. Cancer,* 34, 775, 1984.

16. **Kono, S., Ikeda, M., Tokudome, S., Nishizumi, M., and Kurastune, M.,** Cigarette smoking, alcohol, and cancer mortality: a cohort study of male Japanese physicians, *Gann,* 78, 1323, 1987.

17. **Yu, H., Harris, R. E., Kabat, G. C., and Wynder, E. L.,** Cigarette smoking, alcohol consumption and primary liver cancer: a case-control study in the U.S.A., *Int. J. Cancer,* 42, 325, 1988.

18. **Brechot, C., Nalpas, B., Courouce, A., Duhamel, G., Callard, P., et al.,** Evidence that hepatitis B virus has a role in liver cell carcinoma in alcoholic liver disease, *N. Engl. J. Med.,* 306, 1384, 1982.

19. **Ohnishi, K., Iida, S., Iwama, S., Goto, N., Nomura, F., et al.,** The effect of chronic habitual alcohol intake on the development of liver cirrhosis and hepatocellular carcinoma: relation to hepatitis B surface antigen carriers, *Cancer,* 49, 672, 1982.

20. **McMichael, A. J., Potter, J. D., and Hetzel, B. S.,** Time trends in colorectal cancer mortality in relation to food and alcohol consumption: U.S.A., U.K., Australia, and New Zealand, *Int. J. Epidemiol.,* 8, 295, 1979.

21. **Knox, E. G.,** Foods and diseases, *Br. J. Prevent. Soc. Med.,* 31, 71, 1977.

22. **Freudenheim, J. L., Graham, S., Marshall, J. R., Haughes, B. P., and Wilkinson, G.,** Lifetime alcohol intake and risk of rectal cancer in western New York, *Nutr. and Cancer,* 13, 101, 1990.

23. **Potter, J. D. and McMichael, A. J.,** Diet and cancer of the colon and rectum: a case-control study, *J. Natl. Cancer Inst.,* 76, 557, 1986.

24. **Pollack, E. A., Nomura, A. M. Y., Heilburn, L. K., Stemmermann, G. N., and Green, S. B.,** Prospective study of alcohol consumption and cancer, *N. Engl. J. Med.,* 310, 617, 1984.

25. **Wu, A. H., Paganini-Hill, A., Ross, R. K., and Henderson, B. E.,** Alcohol, physical activity, and other risk factors for colorectal cancer: a prospective study, *Br. J. Cancer,* 55, 687, 1987.

26. **Breslow, N. E. and Enstrom, J. E.,** Geographic correlates between cancer of the pancreas: a correlative hypothesis, *J. Natl. Cancer Inst.,* 53, 631, 1974.

27. **Olsen, G. W., Mandel, J. S., Gibson, R. W., Wattenberg, L. W., and Schuman, L. M.,** A case-control study of pancreatic cancer and cigarettes, alcohol, coffee and diet, *Am. J. Public Health,* 79, 1016, 1989.

28. **Klatsky, A. L., Friedman, G. D., and Siegelaub, A. B.,** Alcohol and mortality: a ten-year Kaiser-Permanente experience, *Ann. Intern. Med.,* 95, 139, 1981.

29. **Blot, W. J., Fraumeni, J. F., Jr., and Stone, B. J.,** Geographic correlates of pancreas cancer in the United States, *Cancer,* 42, 373, 1978.

30. **Haines, A. P., Moss, A. R., Whittemore, A., and Quivey, J.,** A case-control study of pancreatic carcinoma, *J. Cancer Res. Clin. Oncol.,* 103, 93, 1982.

31. **Hakulinen, T., Lehtimaki, L., Lehtonen, M., and Teppo, L.,** Cancer morbidity among two male cohorts with increased alcohol consumption in Finland, *J. Natl. Cancer Inst.,* 52, 1711, 1974.

32. **Gordon, T. and Kannel, W. B.,** Drinking and mortality: the Framingham study, *Am. J. Epidemiol.,* 120, 97, 1984.

33. **Kunze, E., Claude, J., and Frentzel-Beyme, R.,** Association of cancer of the lower urinary tract with consumption of alcoholic beverages. A case-control study, *Carcinogenesis,* 7, 163, 1986.

34. **Longnecker, M. P., Berlin, J. A., Orza, M. J., and Chalmers, T. C.,** A meta-analysis of alcohol consumption in relation to risk of breast cancer, *JAMA,* 260, 652, 1988.

35. **Lowenfels, A. B. and Zevola, S. A.,** Alcohol and breast cancer: an overview, *Alcohol.: Clin. Exp. Res.,* 13, 109, 1989.

36. **Lieber, C. S., Seitz, H. K., Garro, A. J., and Worner, T. M.** Alcohol-related diseases and carcinogenesis, *Cancer Res.,* 39, 2863, 1979.

37. **Seitz, H. K. and Simanowski, U. A.,** Alcohol and carcinogenesis, *Annu. Rev. Nutr.,* 8, 99, 1988.

38. **Garro, A. J. and Lieber, C. S.,** Alcohol and cancer, *Annu. Rev. Pharmacol. Toxicol.,* 30, 219, 1990.

39. **Ketcham, A. S., Wexler, H., and Mantel, N.,** Effect of alcohol on mouse neoplasia, *Cancer Res.,* 23, 667, 1963.

40. **Elzay, R. P.,** Effects of alcohol and cigarette smoke as promoting agents in hamster pouch carcinogenesis, *J. Dent. Res.,* 48, 1200, 1969.

41. **Konishi, N., Kitahori, Y., and Shimoyama, T.,** Effects of sodium chloride and alcohol on experimental esophageal carcinogenesis induced by *N*-nitrosopiperidine in rats, *Jpn. J. Cancer Res.,* 77, 446, 1986.

42. **Radike, M. J., Stemmer, K. L., Brown, P. B., Larson, E., and Bingham, E.,** Effect of ethanol and vinyl chloride on the induction of liver tumors, *Environ. Health Perspect.,* 21, 153, 1977.

43. **Tanaka, T., Nishikawa, A., and Iwata, H.,** Enhancing effect of ethanol on aflatoxin B1-induced hepatocarcinogenesis in male ACI/N rats, *Jpn. J. Cancer Res.,* 80, 526, 1989.

44. **Yanagi, S., Yamashita, M., and Hiasa, Y.,** Effect of ethanol on hepatocarcinogenesis initiated in rats with 3'-methyl-4-dimethylaminoazobenzene in the absence of liver injuries, *Int. J. Cancer,* 44, 681, 1989.

45. **Seitz, H. K., Simanowski, U. A., and Garzon, F. T.,** Possible role of acetaldehyde in ethanol-related rectal cocarcinogenesis in the rat, *Gastroenterology,* 98, 406, 1990.

46. **Woutersen, R. A., Van Garderen-Hoetmer, A., Bax, J., Feringa, A. W., and Scherer, E.,** Modulation of putative preneoplastic foci in exocrine pancreas of rats and hamsters. I. Interaction of dietary fat and ethanol, *Carcinogenesis,* 7, 1587, 1986.

47. **Takahashi, M., Hasegawa, R., and Furukawa, F.,** Effects of ethanol, potassium metabisulfite, formaldehyde and hydrogen peroxide on gastric carcinogenesis in rats after initiation with *N*-methyl-*N'*-*N*-nitrosoguanidine, *Jpn. J. Cancer Res.,* 77, 118, 1986.

48. **Iishi, H., Tatsuta, M., and Baba, M.,** Promotion by ethanol of gastric carcinogenesis induced by *N*-methyl-*N'*-nitro-*N*-nitrosoguanidine in Wistar rats, *Br. J. Cancer,* 59, 719, 1989.

49. **Grubbs, C. J., Juliana, M. M., and Whitaker. L. M.,** Effect of ethanol on initiation of methylnitrosourea (MNU) and dimethylbenzanthracene (DMBA)-induced mammary cancers, *Proc. Annu. Meet. Am. Assoc. Cancer Res.,* 29, A590, 1988.

50. **Driver, H. E. and McLean, A. E. M.,** Dose-response relationships for initiation of rat liver tumors by diethylnitrosamine and promotion by phenobarbitone or alcohol, *Food Chem. Toxicol.,* 24, 241, 1986.

51. **Takada, A., Nei, J., Takase, S., and Matsuda, Y.,** Effects of ethanol on experimental hepatocarcinogenesis, *Hepatology,* 6, 65, 1986.

52. **Habs, M. and Schmahl, D.,** Inhibition of the hepatocarcinogenic activity of diethyl-nitrosamine (DENA) by ethanol in rats, *Acta Gastroenterol.,* 28, 242, 1981.
53. **Teschke, R., Minzlaff, M., Oldiges, H., and Frenzel, H.,** Effect of chronic alcohol consumption on tumor incidence due to dimethylnitrosamine administration, *J. Cancer Res. Clin. Oncol.,* 106, 58, 1983.
54. **Lieber, C. S., Baraona, E., Leo, M. A., and Garro, A. J.,** Metabolism and metabolic effects of ethanol, including interaction with drugs, carcinogens and nutrition, *Mutat. Res.,* 186, 201, 1987.
55. **Seitz, H. K., Garro, A. J., and Lieber, C. S.,** Enhanced pulmonary and intestinal activation of procarcinogens and mutagens after chronic ethanol consumption in the rat, *Eur. J. Clin. Invest.,* 11, 33–38, 1981.
56. **Dicker, E. and Cederbaum, A. I.,** Hydroxyl radical generation by microsomes after chronic ethanol consumption, *Alcohol.: Clin. Exp. Res.,* 11, 309, 1987.
57. **Dianzani, M. U.,** Lipid peroxidation in ethanol poisoning: a clinical reconsideration, *Alcohol,* 20, 161, 1985.
58. **Perera, M. I. R., Katyal, S. L., and Shinozuka, H.,** Choline deficient diet enhances the initiating and promoting effects of methapyrilene hydrochloride in rat liver as assayed by the induction of gamma-glutamyltranspeptidase-positive hepatocyte foci, *Br. J. Cancer,* 56, 774, 1987.
59. **Guerri, C. and Grisolia, S.,** Changes in glutathione in acute and chronic alcohol intoxication, *Pharmacol. Biochem. Behav.,* 13, 53, 1980.
60. **Garro, A. J., Espina, N., Farinati, F., and Salvagnini, M.,** The effect of chronic ethanol consumption on carcinogen metabolism and on O^6-methyl-guanine transferase-mediated repair of alkylated DNA, *Alcohol.: Clin. Exp. Res.,* 10, 73s, 1986.
61. **Obe, G. and Back, B.,** Mutagenic activity of aldehydes, *Drug Alcohol Depend.,* 4, 91, 1979.
62. **Lambert, B. and He, S.-M.,** DNA and chromosomal damage induced by acetaldehyde in human lymphocytes *in vitro, Ann. N.Y. Acad. Sci.,* 534, 369, 1988.
63. **Obe, G. and Ristow, H.,** Mutagenic, carcinogenic and teratogenic effects of alcohol, *Mutat. Res.,* 65, 229, 1979.
64. **Kinsella, A. R. and Radman, M.,** Tumor promoter induces sister chromatid exchanges: relevance to mechanisms of carcinogenesis, *Proc. Natl. Acad. Sci. U.S.A.,* 75, 6149, 1978.
65. **Craddock, V. M.,** Cell proliferation and induction of liver cancer, in *Primary Liver Tumors,* Bolt, H., Bannaschi, P., and Popper, H., Eds., MTP Press, Lancaster, England, 377, 1978.
66. **Winship, D. H., Carlton, R. C., Zaboralskie, F. F., and Hagan, W. J.,** Deterioration of esophageal peristalsis in patients with alcoholic neuropathy, *Gastroenterology,* 55, 173, 1968.
67. **Dinoso, V. P., Chey, W. Y., Braverman, S. P., Rosen, A. P., and Ottenberg, D.,** Gastric secretion and gastric mucosal morphology in chronic alcoholics, *Arch. Intern. Med.,* 130, 715, 1972.
68. **Tuyns, A. J.,** Alcohol and cancer, *Alcohol. Health Res. World,* 2, 20, 1978.
69. **Simanowski, U. A., Seitz, H. K., Baier, B., Kommerell, B., and Schmidt-Gayk, H.,** Chronic ethanol consumption selectively stimulates rectal cell proliferation in the rat, *Gut,* 27, 278, 1986.
70. **Williams, R. R. and Horn, J. W.,** Association of cancer sites with tobacco and alcohol consumption and socioeconomic studies of patients: interview study from Third National Cancer Survey, *J. Natl. Cancer Inst.,* 58, 525, 1977.
71. **Windham, C. T., Wyse, B. W., and Hansen, R. G.,** Alcohol consumption and nutrient density of diets in the nationwide food consumption survey, *J. Am. Diet Assoc.,* 82, 364, 1983.

72. **Sato, M. and Lieber, C. S.,** Hepatic vitamin A depletion after chronic ethanol consumption in baboons and rats, *J. Nutr.,* 111, 2015, 1981.
73. **Baines, M.,** Detection and incidence of B and C vitamin deficiency in alcohol-related illness, *Ann. Clin. Biochem.,* 15, 307, 1978.
74. **Lumeng, L. and Li, T.,** Vitamin B6 metabolism in chronic alcohol abuse, *J. Clin. Invest.,* 53, 693, 1974.
75. **Losowsky, M. S. and Leonard, P. J.,** Evidence of vitamin E deficiency in patients with malabsorption or alcoholism and the effects of therapy, *Gut,* 8, 539, 1967.
76. **Ziegler, R. G.,** A review of epidemiologic evidence that carotenoids reduce the risk of cancer, *J. Nutr.,* 119, 116, 1989.
77. **Wynder, E. L. and Chan, P. C.,** The possible role of riboflavin deficiency in epithelial neoplasia. II. Effect on skin tumor development, *Cancer,* 26, 1221, 1970.
78. **Wynder, E. L.,** Nutrition and cancer, *Fed. Proc.,* 35, 1309, 1976.
79. **McKeown-Eyssen, G. E. and Bright-See, E.,** Dietary factors in colon cancer, *Nutr. Cancer,* 6, 160, 1984.
80. **Wald, N. J., Boreham, J., Hayward, J. L., and Bulbrook, R. D.,** Plasma retinol, carotene and vitamin E levels in relation to the future risk of breast cancer, *Br. J. Cancer,* 49, 321, 1984.
81. **Mak, K. M., Leo, M. A., and Lieber, C. S.,** Potentiation by ethanol consumption of tracheal squamous metaplasia caused by vitamin A deficiency in rats, *J. Natl. Cancer Inst.,* 79, 1001, 1987.
82. **Burton, W. N. and Gladstone, L.,** Laboratory clues to the diagnosis of alcoholism, *Ill. Med. J.,* 161, 265, 1982.
83. **Sullivan, J. F. and Lankford, H. G.,** Urinary excretion of zinc in alcoholism and postalcoholic cirrhosis, *Am. J. Clin. Nutr.,* 10, 153, 1962.
84. **Vitale, J. J. and Gottlieb, L. S.,** Alcohol and alcohol-related deficiencies as carcinogens, *Cancer Res.,* 35, 3336, 1975.
85. **Gabrial, G. N., Schrager, T. F., and Newberne, P. M.,** Zinc deficiency, alcohol, and a retinoid: association with esophageal cancer in rats, *J. Natl. Cancer Inst.,* 68, 785, 1982.
86. **MacGregor, R. R.,** Alcohol and immune defense, *JAMA,* 256, 1474, 1986.
87. **Jerrells, T. R., Marietta, C. A., Eckardt, M. J., Majchrowicz, E., and Weight, F. F.,** Effects of ethanol administration on parameters of immunocompetency in rats, *J. Leukocyte Biol.,* 39, 499, 1986.
88. **Roselle, G. A. and Mendenhall, C. L.,** Ethanol-induced alterations in lymphocyte function in the guinea pig, *Alcohol: Clin. Exp. Res.,* 8, 62, 1984.
89. **Kaplan, D. R.,** A novel mechanism of immunosuppression mediated by ethanol, *Cellular Immunol.,* 102, 1, 1986.
90. **Jerrells, T. R., Perritt, D., Eckardt, M. J., and Marietta, C.,** Alterations in interleukin-2 utilization by T cells from rats treated with an ethanol-containing diet, *Alcohol.: Clin. Exp. Res.,* 14, 245, 1990.
91. **Watson, R. R., Prabhala, R. H., Abril, E., et al.,** Changes in lymphocyte subsets and macrophage functions from high, short term dietary ethanol in C57/BL6 mice, *Life Sci.,* 43, 865, 1988.
92. **Bagasra, O., Howeedy, A., and Kajdacsy-Ball, A.,** Macrophage function in chronic experimental alcoholism. I. Modulation of surface receptors and phagocytosis, *Immunology,* 65, 405, 1988.
93. **Mufti, S. J., Prabhala, R., Moriguchi, S., Glenn Sipes, I., and Watson, R. R.,** Functional and numerical alterations induced by ethanol in the cellular immune system, *Immunopharmacology,* 15, 85, 1988.
94. **Rimland, D.,** Mechanisms of ethanol-induced defects of alveolar macrophage function, *Alcohol.: Clin. Exp. Res.,* 8, 73, 1983.

95. **Dorio, R. J. and Forman, H. J.,** Ethanol inhibition of signal transduction in superoxide production by rat alveolar macrophages, *Annal. Clin. Lab. Sci.,* 18, 190, 1988.

96. **Dorio, R. J., Hoek, J. B., Rubin, E., and Forman, H. J.,** Ethanol modulation of rat alveolar macrophage superoxide production, *Biochem. Pharmacol.,* 37, 3528, 1988.

97. **Arstry, C. L., Warr, G. A., and Jakab, G. J.,** Impairment of polymorphonuclear leukocyte immigration as a mechanism of alcohol-induced suppression of pulmonary antibacterial defences, *Am. Rev. Respir. Dis.,* 128, 113, 1983.

98. **McGregor, B. R., Safford, M., and Shalit, M.,** Effect of ethanol on functions required for the delivery of neutrophils to sites of inflammation, *J. Infec. Dis.,* 157, 682, 1988.

99. **Brayton, R. G., Stokes, P. E., Schwartz, M. S., and Louria, D. B.,** Effect of alcohol and various diseases on leukocyte mobilization, phagocytosis, and intracellular bacterial killing, *N. Engl. J. Med.,* 282, 123, 1970.

100. **Bagasra, O., Howeedy, A., Dorio, R., and Kajdacsy-Balla, A.,** Functional analysis of T cell subsets in chronic experimental alcoholism, *Immunology,* 61, 63, 1987.

101. **Mendenhall, C., Roselle, G. A., Lybecker, L., et al.,** Hepatitis B vaccination, response of alcoholic with and without liver injury, *Dig. Dis. Sci.,* 33, 263, 1988.

102. **Glassman, A. B., Bennet, C. E., and Randall, C. L.,** Effects of ethyl alcohol on human peripheral lymphocytes, *Arch. Pathol. Lab. Med.,* 109, 540, 1985.

103. **Aldo-Benson, M.,** Mechanisms of alcohol-induced suppression of B cell response, *Alcohol.: Clin. Exp. Res.,* 13, 469, 1989.

104. **Steven, W. M., Kumar, S. N., Stewart, C. L., and Seelig, L. L.,** The effects of ethanol consumption on the expression of immunity to *trichinella spiralis* in rats, *Alcohol.: Clin. Exp. Res.,* 14, 87, 1990.

105. **Nelson, S., Bagby, G., and Summer, W. R.,** Alcohol suppresses lipopolysaccharide-induced tumor necrosis factor activity in serum and lung, *Life Sci.,* 44, 673, 1989.

106. **D'Souza, N. B., Bagby, G. J., Nelson, S., Lang, C. H., and Spitzer, J. J.,** Acute alcohol infusion suppresses endotoxin-induced serum tumor necrosis factor, *Alcohol.: Clin. Exp. Res.,* 13, 295, 1989.

107. **Flever, M. E., Mezey, E., McGuire, M., Mitchell, M. C., Herlong, F., Veech, G. A., and Veech, R. L.,** Plasma tumor necrosis factor alpha predicts decreased long-term survival in severe alcoholic hepatitis, *Alcohol.: Clin. Exp. Res.,* 14, 255, 1990.

108. **Straus, B. and Berenyi, M. R.,** Infection and immunity in alcoholic cirrhosis, *Mt. Sinai J. Med.,* 40, 631, 1973.

109. **Cherubin, C. E., Marr, J. S., Sierra, M. F., and Becker, S.,** Listeria and gram-negative bacillary meningitis in New York City (1972–1979), *Am. J. Med.,* 71, 199, 1981.

110. **Fingold, A. D.,** Association of alcoholism and tuberculosis, *South. Med.,* 69, 1336, 1976.

111. **Heineman, H. O.,** Alcohol and the lung, *Am. J. Med.,* 63, 81, 1977.

112. **Correia, J. F. and Conn, H. O.,** Spontaneous bacterial peritonitis in cirrhosis: endemic or epidemic? Symposium on disease of the liver, *Med. Clin. N. Am.,* 59, 963, 1975.

113. **Yoshikawa, T. T. and Schwabe, A. D.,** Bacterial endocarditis and cirrhosis of the liver, *Am. J. Dig. Dis.,* 13, 664, 1968.

114. **Cotte, J., Forestier, F., Quero, A. M., Bourrinet, P., and German, A.,** The effect of alcohol ingestion on the susceptibility of mice to viral infections, *Alcohol.: Clin. Exp. Res.,* 6, 239, 1982.

115. **Louria, D. B.,** Susceptibility to infection during experimental alcohol intoxication, *Trans. Assoc. Am. Physicians,* 76, 102, 1963.

116. **Dehne, N. E., Mendenhall, C. L., Roselle, G. A., and Grossman, C. J.,** Cell-mediated immune responses associated with short term alcohol intake: time course and dose dependency, *Alcohol.: Clin. Exp. Res.,* 13, 201, 1989.

117. **Whiteside, T. L. and Herberman, R. B.,** The role of natural killer cells in human disease, *Clin. Immunol. Immunopathol.,* 53, 1, 1989.

118. **Yirmiya, R., Ben-Eliyahu, S., Gale, R. P., Shavit, Y., Liebeskind, J. C., and Taylor, A. N.,** Ethanol increases tumor progression in rats: possible involvement of natural killer cells, *Brain Behav. Immun.,* 6, 74, 1992

119. **Ward, J. M. and Reynolds, C. W.,** Large granular lymphocyte leukemia, *Am. J. Pathol.,* 111, 1, 1983.

120. **Irwin, M., Caldwell, C., Smith, T. L., Brown, S., Schuckit, M. A., and Gillin, J. C.,** Major depressive disorder, alcoholism, and reduced natural killer cell cytotoxicity, *Arch. Gen. Psychiatr.,* 47, 713, 1990.

121. **Ericsson, C. D., Kohl, S., Pickering, L. K., Davis, J., Glass, G. S., and Faillace, L. A.,** Mechanisms of host defense in well-nourished patients with chronic alcoholism, *Alcohol.: Clin. Exp. Res.,* 4, 261, 1980.

122. **Saxena, Q. B., Mezey, E., and Adler, W. H.,** Regulation of natural killer activity *in vivo.* II. The effect of alcohol consumption on human peripheral blood natural killer activity, *Int. J. Cancer,* 23, 413, 1980.

123. **Charpentier, B., Franco, D., Paci, L., Charra, M., Martin, B., Vuitton, D., and Fries, D.,** Deficient natural killer cell activity in alcoholic cirrhosis, *Clin. Exp. Immunol.,* 58, 107, 1984.

124. **Jovanovic, R., Worner, T., Lieber, C. S., and Paronetto, F.,** Lymphocyte subpopulations in patients with alcoholic liver disease, *Dig. Dis. Sci.,* 31, 125, 1986.

125. **Chadha, K. C., Whitney, R. B., Cummings, M. K., Norman, M., Windle, M., and Stadler, I.,** Evaluation of interferon system among chronic alcoholics, in *Alcohol, Immunomodulation, and AIDS,* Seminara, D., Watson, R. R., and Pawlowski, A., Eds., Alan R. Liss, New York, 1990, 123.

126. **Abdallah, R. M., Starkey, J. R., and Meadows, G. G.,** Alcohol and related dietary effects on mouse natural killer cell activity, *Immunology,* 50, 131, 1983.

127. **Abdallah, R. M., Starkey, J. R., and Meadows, G. G.,** Toxicity of chronic high alcohol intake on mouse natural killer cell activity, *Res. Commun. Chem. Path. Pharm.,* 59, 245, 1988.

128. **Saxena, Q. B., Saxena, R. K., and Adler, W. H.,** Regulation of natural killer activity *in vivo.* IV. High natural killer activity in alcohol drinking mice, *Indian J. Exp. Biol.,* 19, 1001, 1981.

129. **Meadows, G. G., Blank, S. E., and Duncan, D. D.,** Influence of ethanol consumption on natural killer cell activity in mice, *Alcohol.: Clin. Exp. Res.,* 13, 476, 1989.

130. **Blank, S. E., Duncan, D. A., and Meadows, G. G.,** Suppression of natural killer cell activity by ethanol consumption and food restriction, *Alcohol.: Clin. Exp. Res.,* 15, 16, 1991.

131. **Suthanthiran, M., Solomon, S. D., Williams, P. S., Rubin, A. L., Novogrodsky, A., and Stenzel, K. H.,** Hydroxy radical scavengers inhibit human natural killer cell activity, *Nature (London),* 307, 276, 1984.

132. **Stacy, N. H.,** Inhibition of antibody-dependent cell-mediated cytotoxicity by ethanol, *Immunopharmacology,* 8, 155, 1984.

133. **Nair, M. P. N., Kronfol, Z. A., and Schwartz, S. A.,** Effects of alcohol and nicotine on cytotoxic functions of human lymphocytes, *Clin. Immunol. Immunopathol.,* 54, 395, 1990.

134. **Rice, C., Hudig, D., Lad, P., and Mendelsohn, J.,** Ethanol activation of human natural cytotoxicity, *Immunopharmacology,* 6, 303, 1983.

135. **Kendall, R. A. and Targan, S.,** The dual effect of prostaglandin (PGE2) and ethanol on the natural killer cytolytic process: effector activation and NK-cell-target cell conjugate lytic inhibition, *J. Immunol.,* 125, 2770, 1980.

136. **Ristow, S. S., Starkey, J. R., and Haas, G. M.,** Inhibition of natural killer cell activity *in vitro* by alcohols, *Biochem. Biophys. Res. Commun.,* 105, 1315, 1982.

137. **Walia, A. S., Pruitt, K. M., Rodgers, J. D., and Lemon, E. W.,** *In vitro* effect of ethanol on cell-mediated cytotoxicity by murine spleen cells, *Immunopharmacology,* 13, 11, 1987.

138. **Barlozzari, T., Leonhardt, J., Wiltrout, R. H., Herberman, R. B., and Reynolds, C. W.,** Direct evidence for the role of LGL in the inhibition of experimental tumor metastases, *J. Immunol.,* 134, 2783, 1985.

139. **Ben-Eliyahu, S., Yirmiya, R., Liebeskind, J. C., Taylor, A. N., and Gale, R. P.,** Stress increases metastatic spread of a mammary tumor in rats: evidence for mediation by the immune system, *Brain Behav. Immun.,* 5, 193, 1991.

140. **Page, G., Ben-Eliyahu, S., Yirmiya, R., and Liebeskind, J. C.,** Surgical stress promotes metastatic growth and suppresses natural killer cell function in rats, *J. Pain Symptom Manag.,* 6, 180, 1991.

141. **Yirmiya, R., Ben-Eliyahu, S., Shavit, Y., Gale, R. P., Page, G., Talor, A. N., and Liebeskind, J. C.,** Opiates increase tumor progression in rats: evidence for mediation by natural killer cells, *Brain Behav. Immun.,* in press.

142. **Long, G. S., Hiserodt, J. C., Harnaha, J. B., and Cramer, D. V.,** Lymphokine-activated killer cell purging of leukemia cells from bone marrow prior to syngeneic transplantation, *Transplantation,* 46, 433, 1988.

143. **Herberman, R. B., Balch, R., Bolhius, S., Golub, J., Hiserodt, J., Lanier, L., Latzova, E., Phillips, J., and Vujanovic, N.,** Most lymphokine-activated killer (LAK) activity mediated by blood and splenic lymphocytes is attributable to stimulation of natural killer (NK) cells by interleukin-2 (IL-2), *Immunol. Today,* 8, 178, 1987.

144. **Djeu, J. Y., Heinbaugh, J. A., Holden, H. T., and Herberman, R. B.,** Augmentation of mouse natural killer cell activity by interferon and interferon inducers, *J. Immunol.,* 143, 175, 1978.

145. **Roder, J. C., Kiessling, R., Biderfeld, P., and Andersson, B.,** Target-effector interaction in the natural killer (NK) cell system. II. The isolation of NK cells and studies on the mechanisms of killing, *J. Immunol.,* 6, 2509, 1978.

146. **Singer, D. S., Parent, L. J., and Kobler, M. A.,** Ethanol: an enhancer of transplantation antigen expression. *Alcohol.: Clin. Exp. Res.,* 13, 480, 1989.

147. **Katzav, S., DeBaetselier, P., Tartakovsky, B., Feldman, M., and Segal, S.,** Alteration in MHC phenotypes of clonal T10 sarcoma cells are associated with shifts from non-metastatic to metastatic cells, *J. Natl. Cancer Inst.,* 71, 317, 1983.

148. **Karre, K., Ljunggren, H. G., Piontek, G., and Kiessling, R.,** Selective rejection of H-2 deficient lymphoma variants suggests alternative immune defense strategy, *Nature (London),* 319, 675, 1986.

149. **Liao, N., Bix, M., Zijlstra, M., Jaenisch, R., and Raulet, D.,** MHC class I deficiency: susceptibility to natural killer (NK) cels and impaired NK activity, *Science,* 253, 199, 1991.

150. **Ader, R., Felten, D., and Cohen, N., Eds.,** *Psychoneuroimmunology,* 2nd ed., Academic Press, New York, 1991.

151. **Bateman, A., Singh, A., Krai, T., and Solomon, S.,** The immune-hypothalamic-pituitary adrenal axis, *Endocrine Rev.,* 10, 92, 1989.

152. **Patel, V. A. and Pohorecky, L. A.,** Interaction of stress and ethanol: effect of b-endorphin and catecholamines, *Alcohol.: Clin. Exp. Res.,* 12, 785, 1988.

153. **Redei, E., Branch, B. J., Gholami, S., Lin, E. Y. R., and Taylor, A. N.,** Effect of ethanol on CRF release *in vitro, Endocrinology,* 123, 2736, 1988.

154. **Irwin, M., Hauger, R. L., Brown, M. and Britton, K. T.,** CRF activates autonomic nervous system and reduces natural killer cytotoxicity, *Am. J. Physiol.,* 255, R744, 1988.

155. **Gottesfeld, Z., Christie, R., Felten, D. L., and LeGrue, S. J.,** Prenatal ethanol exposure alters immune capacity and noradrenergic synaptic transmission in lymphoid organs of the adult mouse, *Neuroscience,* 29, 715, 1990.

156. **Sugarbaker, E. V.,** Cancer metastasis: a product of tumor-host interactions, *Current Probs. Cancer,* 3, 1, 1979.

157. **Madden, K. S. and Livnat, S.,** Catecholamine action and immunologic reactivity, in *Psychoneuroimmunology,* 2nd ed., Ader, R., Felten, D., and Cohen, N., Eds., Academic Press, New York, 283, 1991.

158. **Ben-Eliyahu, S., Yirmiya, R., Page, G., Weiner, H., Tan, A., Taylor, A. N., and Liebeskind, J. C.**, Stress-induced sympathetic activation suppresses blood natural killer cytotoxicity and increases metastatic spread in rats: mediation by adrenal epinephrine, *Soc. Neurosci. Abst.*, 17, 829, 1991.

159. **Munck, A. and Guyre, P. M.**, Glucocorticoids and immune function, in *Psychoneuroimmunology*, 2nd ed., Ader, R., Felten, D., and Cohen, N., Eds., Academic Press, New York, 447, 1991.

160. **Peters, L. J. and Kelley, H.**, The influence of stress and stress hormones on the transplantability of a nonimmunogenic syngeneic murine tumor, *Cancer*, 39, 1482, 1977.

161. **Riley, V.**, Psychoneuroendocrine influences on immunocompetence and neoplasia, *Science*, 214, 1104, 1981.

162. **Sapolsky, R. M. and Donnelly, T. M.**, Vulnerability to stress-induced tumor growth increases with age in rats: role of glucocorticoids, *Endocrinology*, 117, 662, 1985.

163. **Laue, L., Peacock, J., Brandon, D. D., Gallucci, W. T., Cutler, G. B., Jr., Loriaux, D. L., Chrousos, G. P., and Norton, J. A.**, Glucocorticoid receptor-mediated effects on rat fibrosarcoma growth, *Cancer Res.*, 48, 2703, 1988.

164. **Fitzmaurice, M. A.**, Physiological relationships among stress, viruses, and cancer in experimental animals, *Intern. J. Neurosci.*, 39, 307, 1988.

165. **Jerrells, T. R., Perritt, D., Marietta, C., and Eckardt, M. J.**, Mechanisms of suppression of cellular immunity induced by ethanol, *Alcohol.: Clin. Exp. Res.*, 13, 490, 1989.

166. **Roselle, G. A., Mendenhall, C. L., and Grossman, C. J.**, Ethanol and soluble mediators of host response, *Alcohol.: Clin. Exp. Res.*, 13(4), 494, 1989.

167. **Gianoulakis, C. and Barcomb, A.**, Effects of acute ethanol *in vivo* and *in vitro* on the β-endorphin system in the rat, *Life Sci.*, 40, 19, 1987.

168. **Schulz, R., Wuster, M., Duka, T., and Herz, A.**, Acute and chronic ethanol treatment changes endorphin levels in brain and pituitary, *Psychopharmacology*, 68, 221, 1980.

169. **Charness, M. E., Gordon, A. S., and Diamond, I.**, Ethanol modulation of opiate receptors in cultured neural cells, *Science*, 222, 1246, 1983.

170. **Zagon, I. S. and McLaughlin, P. J.**, Endogenous opioids and the growth regulation of a neural tumor, *Life Sci.*, 43, 131, 1988.

171. **Simon, R. H., Arbo, T. E., and Lundi, J.**, β-endorphin injected into the nucleus of the raphe magnus facilitates metastatic tumor growth, *Brain Res. Bull.*, 12, 487, 1984.

172. **Lewis, J. W., Shavit, Y., Terman, G. W., Nelson, L. R., Gale, R. P., and Liebeskind, J. C.**, Apparent involvement of opioid peptides in stress-induced enhancement of tumor growth, *Peptides*, 4, 635, 1983.

173. **Shavit, Y., Lewis, J. W., Terman, G. W., Gale, R. P., and Liebeskind, J. C.**, Opioid peptides mediate the suppressive effects of stress on natural killer cell cytotoxicity, *Science*, 223, 188, 1984.

174. **Yirmiya, R., Shavit, Y., Ben-Eliyahu, S., Gale, R. P., Liebeskind, J. C., Taylor, A. N., and Weiner, H.**, Modulation of immunity and neoplasia by neuropeptides released by stressors, in *Stress, Neuropeptides, and Systemic Disease*, McCubbin, J. A., Kaufmann, P. G., and Nemeroff, C. B., Eds. Academic Press, San Diego, 261, 1991.

175. **Van Zwieten, M. J.**, *The Rat as Animal Model in Breast Cancer Research*, Martinus Nijhoff, Boston, 1984.

176. **Schoenborn, C. A. and Cohen, B. H.**, Trends in smoking, alcohol consumption and other health practices among U.S. adults, 1977 and 1983. *National Center for Health Statistics*, Advance Data from Vital and Health Statistics, No. 118. DHHS Publ. No. (PHS) 86-1250, Hyattsville, MD, Public Health Service, 1983.

177. **DeVita, V. T., Jr., Young, R. C., and Canellos, G. P.**, Combination versus single agent chemotherapy: a review of the basis for selection of drug treatment of cancer, *Cancer*, 35, 98, 1975.

178. **Boring, C. C., Squires, T. S., and Tong, T.**, Cancer Statistics, 1991, *CA*, 41, 19, 1991.

179. **Henderson, I. C. and Canellos, G. P.**, Cancer of the breast, *N. Engl. J. Med.*, 302, 17, 1980.

Index

INDEX